The Latest Exploration of Cerebrovascular Diseases: From Preclinical Research to Treatment

The Latest Exploration of Cerebrovascular Diseases: From Preclinical Research to Treatment

Guest Editors

Basil Grüter
Martina Sebök

MDPI

Basel • Beijing • Wuhan • Barcelona • Belgrade • Novi Sad • Cluj • Manchester

Guest Editors
Basil Grüter
Department of Neurosurgery
and Institute of
Neuroradiology
Aarau Cantonal Hospital
Aarau
Switzerland

Martina Sebök
Department of Neurosurgery
University Hospital Zurich
Zurich
Switzerland

Editorial Office
MDPI AG
Grosspeteranlage 5
4052 Basel, Switzerland

This is a reprint of the Special Issue, published open access by the journal *Brain Sciences* (ISSN 2076-3425), freely accessible at: https://www.mdpi.com/journal/brainsci/special_issues/SL8VLT5BOP.

For citation purposes, cite each article independently as indicated on the article page online and as indicated below:

Lastname, A.A.; Lastname, B.B. Article Title. *Journal Name* **Year**, *Volume Number*, Page Range.

ISBN 978-3-7258-7488-0 (Hbk)
ISBN 978-3-7258-7489-7 (PDF)
https://doi.org/10.3390/books978-3-7258-7489-7

Contents

About the Editors

Basil Grüter

Basil Grüter is a board-certified neurosurgeon with additional specialization in diagnostic and interventional neuroradiology. He serves as a group leader and co-chair of the Cerebrovascular Research Group at the Department for BioMedical Research (DBMR), University of Bern. His research focuses on the biological and biomechanical mechanisms involved in the formation, growth, rupture, and healing of intracranial aneurysms in a preclinical environment, with the overarching goal of improving clinical outcomes for patients with cerebrovascular disease. In parallel, he is actively engaged in the development as well as the preclinical and clinical evaluation of novel endovascular devices, contributing to advances in minimally invasive cerebrovascular therapies with enhanced safety and efficacy.

Martina Sebök

Martina Sebök is a consultant vascular neurosurgeon at the Department of Neurosurgery, University Hospital Zurich, and serves as a junior group leader in the BOLD-CVR research group. She completed a Clinical Fellowship in Cerebrovascular Neurosurgery at Toronto Western Hospital in Ontario, Canada. As a Clinical Scientist, Dr. Sebök is at the forefront of cerebrovascular research, advancing the understanding of cerebrovascular diseases and neurosurgery through the innovative application of advanced MRI techniques, specifically BOLD cerebrovascular reactivity.

brain sciences

Editorial

The Latest Exploration of Cerebrovascular Diseases: From Preclinical Research to Treatment

Basil Erwin Grüter [1,*] and Martina Sebök [2]

1 Department of Neurosurgery and Neuroradiology, HOCH Health Ostschweiz, 9000 St. Gallen, Switzerland
2 Department of Neurosurgery, Clinical Neuroscience Center, University Hospital Zurich, University of Zurich, 8091 Zurich, Switzerland; martina.seboek@usz.ch
* Correspondence: basil.grueter@h-och.ch

1. Introduction

Cerebrovascular diseases represent one of the most significant challenges in modern clinical neuroscience, encompassing a spectrum of disorders in which disturbances of cerebral blood flow, vascular integrity, and hemodynamic regulation culminate in devastating neurological sequelae [1,2]. Recognizing the complex interplay of these mechanisms, this *Special Issue* was conceived to capture cutting-edge research spanning mechanistic and preclinical investigations through to translational and clinical treatment studies. Particularly noteworthy are the rapid advances in imaging technologies, biomarker discovery, endovascular and microsurgical techniques, regenerative and neuroprotective strategies, and, more recently, the integration of artificial intelligence into cerebrovascular diagnostics and therapeutic planning.

In this Editorial, we provide an overview of the works published within this Special Issue, delineate persisting gaps in our understanding, and propose future research directions to guide the field toward more individualized and effective cerebrovascular care.

2. Overview of Published Works

The Special Issue brings together twenty articles that collectively map the broad continuum of cerebrovascular research—from computational modeling of aneurysm formation to clinical studies on complex vascular malformations, and from the refinement of imaging biomarkers to the development of novel drug delivery technologies. The publications can be grouped into four overarching research domains:

1. Mechanistic simulations and modeling studies;
2. Imaging and diagnostic biomarker investigations;
3. Interventional and therapeutic innovations;
4. Artificial Intelligence and decision-support systems.

Mechanistic studies have provided crucial insights into the pathophysiological processes underlying cerebrovascular disease, laying the foundation for improved clinical comprehension [3]. Advances in imaging and the development of vessel-wall biomarkers have expanded the diagnostic repertoire, improving both detection and risk stratification [4]. Large surgical and endovascular cohorts have offered valuable real-world data on treatment outcomes and procedural strategies, supporting the refinement of evidence-based decision-making.

At the therapeutic frontier, innovative delivery systems—such as ultrasound-mediated nimodipine release—have illustrated promising alternatives beyond conventional care paradigms. Meanwhile, the first explorations into the role of artificial intelligence and large

 https://doi.org/10.3390/brainsci15121281

language models in clinical decision analysis have signaled a future in which computational tools may augment, rather than replace, clinician judgment.

However, significant challenges persist. Mechanistic models, though increasingly sophisticated, remain distant from clinical integration. Imaging biomarkers require prospective validation in large, heterogeneous populations. Many treatment strategies continue to rely on expert consensus rather than robust randomized evidence, particularly for rare vascular malformations. Artificial intelligence applications remain preliminary, often limited to retrospective analysis without demonstrated impact on patient outcomes. Similarly, drug delivery systems and nanocarriers, while conceptually elegant, have yet to advance beyond preclinical evaluation [5].

3. Focus on Future Research Directions

Building on the collective contributions of this Special Issue, several key avenues for future research can be delineated:

1. Bridging mechanistic modeling and individualized risk prediction

Fluid–structure interaction studies of aneurysm initiation and modeling approaches in leukoaraiosis underscore the value of mechanistic insight. The next step lies in translating these models into patient-specific risk assessment tools—integrating hemodynamic, geometric, and histopathological parameters to form individualized treatment strategies [6].

2. Translating novel delivery and regenerative technologies

The development of nimodipine nanocarriers exemplifies the potential for controlled, on-demand pharmacologic interventions targeting subarachnoid hemorrhage, vasospasm, or focal ischemia [7]. To move toward clinical application, forthcoming studies should prioritize in vivo validation, toxicological safety profiling, and early-phase clinical trials, ideally within multidisciplinary translational frameworks.

3. Addressing venous and microvascular pathophysiology

While arterial mechanisms have dominated research, venous outflow resistance and microvascular dysfunction—implicated in entities such as leukoaraiosis—remain underexplored. Systematic investigations into the venous compartment, microcirculatory flow, and neurovascular unit integrity will be crucial to comprehensively understanding cerebrovascular disease [8].

4. Prospective validation of imaging biomarkers

Imaging markers, such as vessel-wall contrast enhancement in Moyamoya disease and intracranial aneurysms, have demonstrated potential as predictive tools. Prospective multicenter validation and integration into structured clinical algorithms are essential. Analogous biomarker development should extend to other pathologies, including AVMs and perforator aneurysms, to enable earlier and more stratified interventions [9].

5. Responsible integration of artificial intelligence

Initial evidence indicates that AI models can approximate multidisciplinary board decisions for unruptured intracranial aneurysms. Future research must evaluate real-world deployment, focusing on safety, interpretability, clinician acceptance, and measurable impact on outcomes [10]. Ethical oversight and medico-legal governance must evolve concurrently to ensure responsible adoption.

6. Advancing precision medicine and molecular targeting

The movement toward precision medicine will increasingly rely on genetic, hemodynamic, and anatomical phenotyping. In AVMs, for instance, emerging data on somatic KRAS and BRAF mutations suggest the feasibility of targeted molecular interventions [11]. Broader incorporation of molecular diagnostics into cerebrovascular management is likely to define the next decade of translational research.

7. Strengthening evidence through multicenter clinical trials

While large retrospective cohorts remain informative, randomized and multicenter prospective studies are urgently needed to refine decision-making, particularly for rare lesions such as AVMs, combined aneurysm–stenosis cases and surgical treatment of (acute) stroke [12,13]. Such studies will form the backbone of evidence-based cerebrovascular therapy.

4. Conclusions

The Special Issue "*The Latest Exploration of Cerebrovascular Diseases: From Preclinical Research to Treatment*" encapsulates the dynamic evolution of the field—from hemodynamic modeling to advanced imaging, from clinical cohorts to interventional innovation, and from artificial intelligence to precision nanomedicine. Yet, the translation of mechanistic insights into clinical applicability, the validation of biomarkers, the conduction of high-quality interventional trials, and the ethical integration of AI remain critical frontiers.

We invite the readership—clinicians, scientists, bioengineers, and data specialists alike—to engage with the comprehensive body of work presented herein, to build upon its foundations, and to contribute toward the next generation of cerebrovascular research. The convergence of mechanistic, imaging, therapeutic, and computational advances heralds a transformative era in cerebrovascular medicine—one defined by precision, personalization, and improved patient outcomes.

In this spirit, we already look forward to the second volume of the Special Issue, which will continue this trajectory toward bridging experimental insight and clinical translation in the management of cerebrovascular disease.

Conflicts of Interest: The authors report no conflict of interest.

References

1. Xie, X.; Atkins, E.; Lv, J.; Bennett, A.; Neal, B.; Ninomiya, T.; Woodward, M.; MacMahon, S.; Turnbull, F.; Hillis, G.S.; et al. Effects of intensive blood pressure lowering on cardiovascular and renal outcomes: Updated systematic review and meta-analysis. *Lancet* **2016**, *387*, 435–443. [CrossRef] [PubMed]
2. Hu, X.; De Silva, T.M.; Chen, J.; Faraci, F.M. Cerebral Vascular Disease and Neurovascular Injury in Ischemic Stroke. *Circ. Res.* **2017**, *120*, 449–471. [CrossRef] [PubMed]
3. Guo, Y.; Li, P.; Boltze, J. Recent advances in mechanistic, therapeutic, and diagnostic research of cerebrovascular diseases: Updates from brain & BrainPET 2022. *J. Cereb. Blood Flow Metab.* **2023**, *43* (Suppl. S2), 4–7. [CrossRef] [PubMed]
4. Mazzacane, F.; Mazzoleni, V.; Scola, E.; Mancini, S.; Lombardo, I.; Busto, G.; Rognone, E.; Pichiecchio, A.; Padovani, A.; Morotti, A.; et al. Vessel Wall Magnetic Resonance Imaging in Cerebrovascular Diseases. *Diagnostics* **2022**, *12*, 258. [CrossRef] [PubMed]
5. Akay, E.M.Z.; Hilbert, A.; Carlisle, B.G.; Madai, V.I.; Mutke, M.A.; Frey, D. Artificial Intelligence for Clinical Decision Support in Acute Ischemic Stroke: A Systematic Review. *Stroke* **2023**, *54*, 1505–1516. [CrossRef] [PubMed]
6. Bandhauer, B.; Gruber, P.; Andereggen, L.; Berberat, J.; Wanderer, S.; Cattaneo, M.; Schubert, G.A.; Remonda, L.; Marbacher, S.; Grüter, B.E. From conservative to interventional management in unruptured intracranial aneurysms. *J. Neurosurg.* **2024**, *142*, 619–625. [CrossRef] [PubMed]
7. Macdonald, R.L.; Hänggi, D.; Strange, P.; Steiger, H.J.; Mocco, J.; Miller, M.; Mayer, S.A.; Hoh, B.L.; Faleck, H.J.; Etminan, N.; et al. Nimodipine pharmacokinetics after intraventricular injection of sustained-release nimodipine for subarachnoid hemorrhage. *J. Neurosurg.* **2021**, *134*, 95–101. [CrossRef] [PubMed]
8. Stamenkovic, S.; Schmid, F.; Gurler, G.; Abolmaali, F.; Weitermann, N.A.; Takasaki, K.T.; Bonney, S.K.; Sosa, M.J.; Bennett, H.C.; Kim, Y.; et al. Impaired capillary-venous drainage contributes to gliosis and demyelination in mouse white matter during aging. *Nat. Neurosci.* **2025**, *28*, 1868–1882. [CrossRef] [PubMed]
9. Sebök, M.; Germans, M.R.; van Niftrik, C.H.B.; Kulcsár, Z.; Regli, L.; Fierstra, J. More pronounced hemodynamic alterations in patients with brain arteriovenous malformation-associated epilepsy. *Neurosurg. Focus.* **2022**, *53*, E4. [CrossRef] [PubMed]
10. Akhtar, M.; Farooqi, H.A.; Nabi, R.; Hasan, H. Advancing aneurysm management: The potential of AI and machine learning in enhancing safety and predictive accuracy. *Neurosurg. Rev.* **2024**, *47*, 432. [CrossRef] [PubMed]
11. Bameri, O.; Salarzaei, M.; Parooie, F. KRAS/BRAF mutations in brain arteriovenous malformations: A systematic review and meta-analysis. *Interv. Neuroradiol.* **2021**, *27*, 539–546. [CrossRef] [PubMed]

12. Molyneux, A.; Kerr, R.; Stratton, I.; Sandercock, P.; Clarke, M.; Shrimpton, J.; Yu, L.M.; Sneade, S.M.; Yarnold, J.A.; International Subarachnoid Aneurysm Trial (ISAT) Collaborative Group. International Subarachnoid Aneurysm Trial (ISAT) of neurosurgical clipping versus endovascular coiling in 2143 patients with ruptured intracranial aneurysms: A randomised trial. *Lancet* **2002**, *360*, 1267–1274. [CrossRef] [PubMed]
13. Magro, E.; Gentric, J.-C.; Darsaut, T.E.; Ziegler, D.; Bojanowski, M.W.; Raymond, J. Responses to ARUBA: A systematic review and critical analysis for the design of future arteriovenous malformation trials. *J. Neurosurg.* **2017**, *126*, 486–494. [CrossRef] [PubMed]

brain sciences

MDPI

Article

A Lumped Parameter Modelling Study of Leukoaraiosis Suggests Its Vascular Pathophysiology May Be Similar to Normal-Pressure Hydrocephalus

Grant A. Bateman [1,2,*] and Alexander R. Bateman [3]

1 Department of Medical Imaging, John Hunter Hospital, Newcastle, NSW 2310, Australia
2 College of Health, Medicine and Wellbeing, Newcastle University School of Medicine and Public Health, Callaghan Campus, Newcastle, NSW 2308, Australia
3 College of Engineering, Science and Environment, Newcastle University School of Engineering, Callaghan Campus, Newcastle, NSW 2308, Australia; alex.bateman@newcastle.edu.au
* Correspondence: grant.bateman@health.nsw.gov.au

Abstract

Introduction: Leukoaraiosis (LA) or white matter disease is a significant component of vascular dementia. There is a large overlap noted between normal-pressure hydrocephalus (NPH) and LA. A previously reported lumped parameter modelling study of NPH led to novel findings in this disease. Given the overlap between LA and NPH, the purpose of the current study is to perform a lumped parameter study into LA to see if the vascular pathophysiology is similar to NPH. Methods: A lumped parameter model originally developed to study normal-pressure hydrocephalus was extended to investigate LA. The model was constrained by the known cerebral blood flow and cerebral blood volumes found in LA, as derived from the literature. Results: Similar to NPH, in LA, the model predicted a balanced increase in arterial and venous outflow resistance, with the resulting ischemia affecting the white matter rather than the grey matter. However, unlike NPH, in LA, the findings are irreversible, most likely due to structural venous wall changes. Conclusions: The model suggests that the vascular physiology of LA maybe similar to NPH. A common pathophysiology is discussed based on a pulsation-induced increase in the venous outflow resistance.

Keywords: cerebral blood flow; cerebral blood volume; leukoaraiosis; normal-pressure hydrocephalus; pulsation; vascular dementia

1. Introduction

Neuroimaging often shows areas of low density on CT and a high T2 signal intensity on MRI within the white matter of the brain. This change is denoted as white matter disease or leukoaraiosis (LA) [1]. The term leukoaraiosis comes from the Greek language, leuko meaning white and araiosis meaning rarefaction [2]. Pathological studies have found demyelination and reactive gliosis [3] to be the cause of the imaging findings. The most significant correlation of leukoaraiosis is with aging [4]. There is also a strong vascular component to the aetiology of LA, with risk factors of hypertension, diabetes mellitis, and cardiac disease also being prominent [5]. Indeed, leukoaraiosis is a major determinant of vascular dementia [6], which is, by definition, known to be of vascular origin. There is also an interesting overlap between normal-pressure hydrocephalus (NPH) and LA [7]. Up to 73% of patients with NPH have significant degrees of leukoaraiosis within the deep white matter [8]. This suggests a possible degree of common causation between these two disorders.

In a previous study performed by the current authors, a lumped parameter vascular model was developed to study the vascular pathophysiology of NPH [9]. This model suggested that there was a balanced increase in the vascular resistance in the arterial inflow and the venous outflow in this disease. There was a significant difference between the findings in the grey matter and white matter, with significant ischemia within the white matter in NPH [10]. Given the model's previous findings in NPH, and the overlap between NPH and LA, the purpose of the current study is to extend the NPH lumped parameter modelling study [9], utilizing the parameters gleaned from the literature to study the vascular pathophysiology of leukoaraiosis.

2. Materials and Methods

2.1. Equations

The equations used in this study were extensively discussed previously [9] and can be reviewed in this study. However, the relevant equations will be reproduced here for convenience. Firstly, Ohm's law for hydraulic circuits is required:

$$\Delta P = Q \times R \tag{1}$$

ΔP is the pressure drop across the vascular segment, Q is the flow rate, and R is the resistance. Resistances in series are additive, therefore.

$$R_{art} + R_{cap} + R_{ven} + R_{cuf} = R_{tot} \tag{2}$$

R_{art}, R_{cap}, R_{ven}, R_{cuf}, and R_{tot} are the resistances of the artery, capillary, venous cuff, and the total system, respectively. Poiseuille's equation calculates the pressure drop across each of these segments:

$$\Delta P = \frac{8\mu LQ}{\pi r^4} \tag{3}$$

ΔP is the pressure drop across the vascular segment, μ the viscosity, L the vessel length, Q the fluid flow rate, π the circle proportionality constant, and r the radius. Given that the viscosity and vessel lengths are constants in this study, it can be shown that there is a direct relationship between a change in a segment's resistance and a change in its volume.

$$\Delta R = \Delta V^{-2} \tag{4}$$

where ΔR is the change in resistance, and ΔV the change in volume. It was previously shown that the venous outflow varies with the transmural pressure, as demomstrated using the following equation [9]:

$$\Delta TMP_{ven} = -0.033\Delta V_{ven}{}^{2} + 7.49 \times \Delta V_{ven} - 3.44 \tag{5}$$

ΔTMP_{ven} is the normalized increase in venous transmural pressure, and ΔV_{ven} is the change in venous volume.

2.2. Model Input Parameters

The input parameters used in this modelling are also unchanged from the previous study [9] and are summarized in Table 1. The details can be obtained from the original study. Of note, the normal sagittal sinus pressure is derived by subtracting the CSF-venous sinus pressure gradient from the ICP. The pre-outflow cuff pressure is obtained by adding the venous TMP to the ICP. The total CBV is obtained by taking the percentages of the brain made up of the grey and white matter and multiplying each by the brain weight and then the CBV for each of these components. The venous volume is obtained by subtracting the arterial and capillary volume from the total.

Table 1. Summary of the normal input parameters.

Parameter	Value	Reference
Brain size	1500 g	Bell et al. [11]
Cerebral blood flow	50 mL/100 g/min	Lassen et al. [12]
Arterial inflow volume	750 mL/min	Buijs et al. [13]
Mean arterial pressure	100 mmHg	Ursino [14]
Pre-capillary bed pressure	32 mmHg	Salmon et al. [15]
End-capillary bed pressure	15 mmHg	Cirovic et al. [16]
CSF pressure	11.5 mmHg	Fleishmann et al. [17]
Pressure gradient CSF-SSS	4 mmHg	Benabid et al. [18] Pollay et al. [19]
Sagittal sinus pressure	7.5 mmHg	Bateman et al. [9]
Cortical vein TMP	2.5 mmHg	Johnston et al. [20]
Pre-outflow cuff pressure	14 mmHg	Bateman et al. [9]
Grey matter CBV	4.6 mL/100 g	Helenius et al. [21]
White matter CBV	1.3 mL/100 g	Helenius et al. [21]
Brain grey matter percentage	65%	Good et al. [22]
Brain white matter percentage	35%	Good et al. [22]
Total CBV	51 mL	Bateman et al. [9]
Arterial volume	12.8 mL	Hua et al. [23]
Capillary volume	20.3 mL	Menéndez González [24]
Venous volume	17.9 mL	Bateman et al. [9]

Note: CBV, cerebral blood volume; SSS, superior sagittal sinus; TMP, transmural pressure.

2.3. Vessel Responses to Transmural Pressure Variations

It is assumed that the changes in arterial resistance and volume in this model depend entirely on active arterial constriction or dilatation and not the vessel transmural pressure.

The capillary and venous beds are assumed to be without active constriction or dilatation [25] but vary depending on their transmural pressures. It is further assumed that a moderate reduction in capillary TMP below normal does not change the capillary size, but a maximal increase in TMP will increase their volume. The previous study indicated that an increase in capillary TMP from 12 to 37.9 mmHg would increase the capillary volume by 44%. or a 1.7% increase in volume for each 1 mmHg pressure rise. Below a TMP of 12 mmHg, the volume is unchanged at 20.3 mL, and above a TMP of 37.9, the elastic limit is reached and the volume is set to 29.2 mL [9]. The veins are assumed to alter their size purely depending on their transmural pressures. In a previous modelling study [9], the function for outflow vein dilatation was found to be summarized by Equation (5).

The outflow cuff is the segment joining the cortical veins to the sinus wall. The collapse of this segment occurs due to the transmural pressure between the ICP and the sinus pressure, which is usually negative [26]. The segment is short, and it is mostly under a state of collapse secondary to physiological ICPs. The change in volume from this segment will be ignored in this model. However, its resistance will be taken into consideration.

3. Results

3.1. Whole-Brain Findings

The whole-brain modelling findings are summarized in Figure 1. The five vascular segments modelled are shown in Figure 1a, with the arterial in red, the capillaries in orange, the veins in yellow, the outflow cuff in green, and the sinus in blue. The pressures from

Table 1 have been appended to each vascular segment within the vessels in Figure 1a. The resistance of each segment can be calculated using Equation (1) and is appended below the vessels in Figure 1. The normal cerebral blood volume (CBV) values are shown below the resistances. The blue numbers represent the transmural pressure gradients for each vessel segment, which are obtained by subtracting the ICP from the segment pressure. The red figure is the average capillary TMP obtained by averaging the values from before and after the capillaries. Figure 1b represents the findings in leukoaraiosis. Figure 1c was obtained from the previous modelling study into NPH [9] and is appended for comparison. In these later two figures, the red segments represent the areas of increased resistance compared to the normal findings, and the green represent reduced resistance.

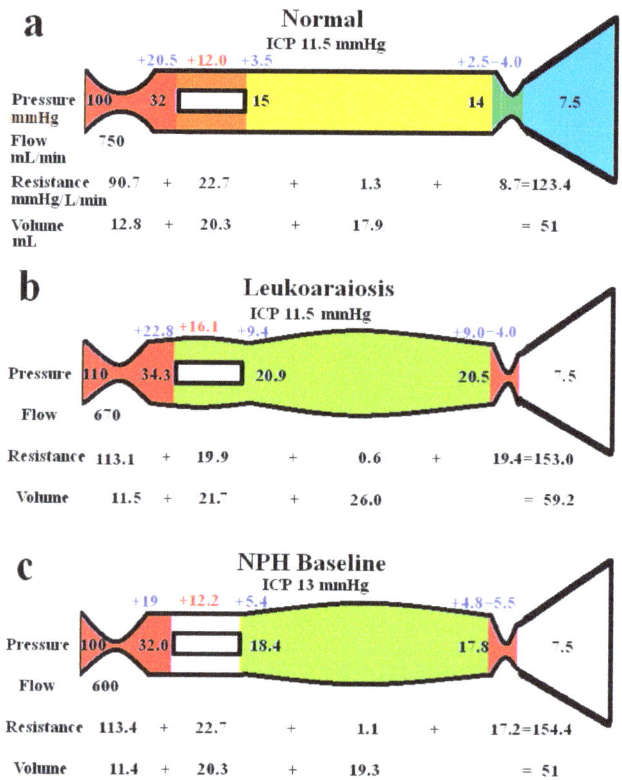

Figure 1. Results of modelling. (**a**) The normal findings. The segments are red for arterial, orange for the capillary, yellow for the veins, green for the outflow cuff, and blue for the venous sinus. The vascular pressures are shown within the vessels. The blue numbers are the transmural pressures at each site. The red number is the average capillary transmural pressure. The resistances and volumes for each segment are shown below the vessel. (**b**) The findings in leukoaraiosis. The red area indicates an increase in resistance in the arteries and outflow cuff, and the green decreased resistance in the capillaries and veins compared to normal. Both the capillary and venous TMP are increased, giving vascular dilatation. (**c**) The findings in NPH from a previous study. The overall findings are similar except the capillary TMP is lower and the pressure gradient across the sinus wall higher than in leukoaraiosis. Note: ICP, intracranial pressure; min, minute; and mmHg, millimetres of mercury. (**a**,**c**) are reproduced from [9] under a CC BY 4.0 commons licence.

In Figure 1b, the whole-brain findings in leukoaraiosis are modelled. The arterial inflow and venous outflow pressures, the ICP, the mean blood flow rate, and target CBV were obtained from the literature. The sinus pressure was assumed to be unchanged due to the normal ICP.

The pressure drop from the arteries to the sinus plus the blood flow through them allows the calculation of the total vascular resistance using Equation (1), i.e., it is increased to 153.0 mmHg/L/min compared to 123.4 mmHg/L/min in the normal model. The increase in resistance needed to be apportioned within the model. By necessity, a change in resistance changes the volume of the segment it affects. The TMP across the outflow cuff (obtained by subtracting the ICP from the sinus pressure) is normal. Therefore, the cuff outflow resistance was initially assumed to be normal. Knowing the cuff resistance and blood flow will allow for setting the blood pressure at the end of the veins by using Equation (1), which was therefore also normal. The normal TMP across the vein walls meant their volume using Equation (5) was normal. Similarly, the capillary resistance and volume were normal. In order for the total resistance to be balanced, the arterial inflow resistance needed to be set very high, but this reduced the arterial blood volume using Equation (4). The overall CBV at this stage undershot the target value of 59.2 mL by a large margin. Alternatively, placing all of the increased resistance on the venous side meant the CBV overshot the target by a large amount. Similar to the modelling we previously performed in NPH [9], a total resistance of 153.0 mmHg/L/min and a CBV of 59.2 mL constrained the model to a single solution, which was likely somewhere between an isolated increase in the arterial or venous outflow resistance. Using an iterative approach from both extremes, it was found the venous outflow resistance of 19.4 mmHg/L/min was the correct one. From this, the post-venous pressure could be calculated using Equation (1). Using this pressure, the venous CBV was calculated using Equation (4), and the resistance of this segment calculated using Equation (1). This gave the post-capillary pressure. Using the capillary tube law, the volume and resistance of this segment were calculated. The resultant volume of the capillaries was 21.7 mL. Knowing the total resistance and the other resistances, the arterial inflow resistance could be calculated using Equation (2). Figure 1b is the only valid solution to the constraints of the model, with all of the equations being satisfied. Note, there is an increase in both the arterial and the outflow cuff resistance, with a reduction in resistance of the other segments due to the increased pressures and volumes compared to normal. There is an increase in the mean capillary transmural pressure.

In Figure 1c, the findings in NPH from the previous study are appended for comparison [9]. Note, the arterial and venous outflow resistances are almost identical to Figure 1b, i.e., they are both increased over baseline, suggesting a balanced increase in the arterial and venous resistances. The overall blood flow is less in NPH, and the capillary transmural pressure is lower than in Figure 1b, being closer to the normal figure.

3.2. Differences Between the Grey and White Matter

Figure 2 shows extended modelling to gauge the differences between the grey and white matter. The red segments represent the areas of increased resistance compared to the normal findings, and the green represent reduced resistance. In Figure 2a, the brain is modelled as if all of it was being affected in a way similar to the grey matter in LA. In the study by Markus et al. [27], the grey matter CBF was normal, and the CBV was increased by 28% in LA. We elected to leave the outflow resistance as unchanged from the previous global model (Figure 1b) and reduced the arterial resistance until the CBF increased back to normal at 750 mL/min. The result was a further dilatation of the capillary and venous beds, with an increase in the capillary and venous transmural pressures. The CBV was increased to 63.5 mL, which was only 2.8% less than the target of value of 65.3 mL, as suggested by Markus et al. [27]. Figure 2b indicates the findings when the blood flow was increased to normal in NPH, similarly to Figure 2a. The findings are very similar, except there is a slight increase in arterial resistance in LA. This is required to balance the increased inflow pressure. Figure 2c shows the findings for the white matter, with increased resistance throughout the vascular system, excluding the capillaries. Some venous wall thickening and stenosis was required, or the low CBV could not be attained. The wall thickening reduced the venous CBV to a level where the total CBV could be reached. Figure 2d is the findings in the white matter in NPH, which are similar overall. Note, no venous wall thickening was required to match the target CBV.

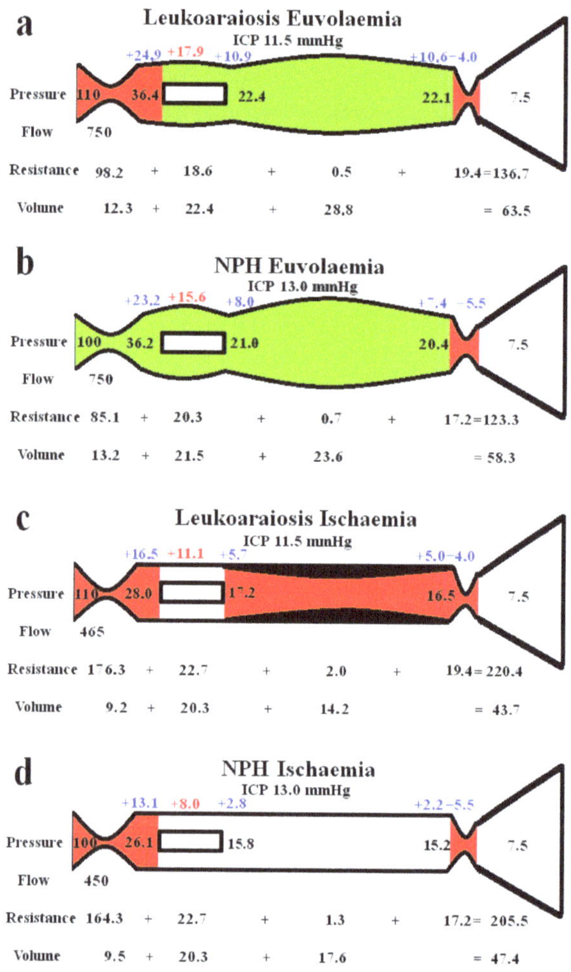

Figure 2. Modelling of grey and white matter. (**a**) Findings in leukoaraiosis following an increase in CBF back towards normal. There is an increase in arterial, capillary, and venous volumes, giving an overall CBV close to the target value. (**b**) Findings in NPH once the arterial inflow had been returned to normal from a previous study [10]. Note, the arterial resistance is less than in LA, but the remainder of the findings are very similar. The arterial resistance is slightly higher than normal in leukoaraiosis because of the higher inflow pressure. (**c**) Findings in leukoaraiosis once the CBF was reduced by 38%. The target CBV could not be attained unless the venous wall was thickened, giving an overall 50% reduction in venous volume compared to (**a**). (**d**) Findings in NPH from a previous study where the CBF was reduced. The overall findings are similar to (**c**), except the requirement for venous wall thickening as seen in (**c**) is not required in (**d**). (**b**,**d**) reproduced from [10] under a CC BY 4.0 commons licence.

4. Discussion

In this study, we have applied a lumped parameter model, previously developed to investigate NPH, to leukoaraiosis. The overall findings suggest that the vascular pathophysiology of LA may be similar to NPH. We have made many assumptions in this lumped parameter modelling study. We have tested the modelling we have performed by comparing the outcomes predicted by the model with the available literature. Previously, the model successfully predicted the cerebral blood volume changes found in the literature at the limits of autoregulation, in both human and animal studies [9]. The model also correctly predicted the cerebral blood volume changes in Alzheimer's disease [28] and in idiopathic intracranial hypertension [29].

4.1. Global Brain Changes in Leukoaraiosis

The global findings within the brain are summarised in Figure 1b. In a study by Markus et al., when using an MRI contrast first-pass technique, the cerebral blood flow (CBF) in the grey matter was normal, but in the white matter, the CBF was reduced by 38% [27]. Similarly, another study showed a normal CBF in the grey matter of leukoaraiosis patients without dementia [30]. Given that the grey matter averages 65% of the brain volume and the white matter 35% [22], we can calculate the global reduction in CBF in LA to be just over 10%. This figure is comparable to a study by Henry-Feugeas et al., where the global reduction in CBF in leukoaraiosis was found to be 6% by using an MRI phase-contrast flow quantification technique [31]. Thus, in the model, a CBF of 670 mL/min was used for the blood flow rate. The mean arterial pressure in patients with significant leukoaraiosis is 10% higher compared to those with minimal disease [32], so we have increased the arterial inflow pressure to 110 mmHg in the model. The ICP in NPH patients without LA (those patients had a normal ICP) was not significantly different compared to those with mild, moderate, or severe LA [33], so we have left the ICP unchanged in the model. Given that the ICP is normal in isolated LA, the venous sinuses are unlikely to be compressed, so the venous sinus pressure was left unchanged from normal. The cerebral blood volumes (CBVs) in LA found in the study by Markus et al. showed an increase of 28% in the grey matter but a reduction of 14% in the white matter [27]. The latter result failed to reach significance, but this was most likely due to this part of the study being under-powered and unable to confirm this finding. However, a study using positron emission tomography CT showed similar results to those of Markus et al., with a reduced white matter CBV of 15% [34]. Given that the CBV of the normal grey matter is 4.6 mL/100 g, and in the white matter, it is 1.3 mL/100 g [21], and given the percentage of the brain volume that each of these two components makes up (as already discussed), the global CBV would be increased by 16.1% in LA, so we used this as our target value. The CBF and CBF values constrained the model, meaning the findings in Figure 1b were the only ones that allowed all of the equations to be satisfied. Note, there is an increase in perfusion pressure due to the increased arterial inflow pressure. The model predicts that the arterial resistance in LA is increased by 24.7% above normal. Normally, an increase in the perfusion pressure from an increase in arterial pressure constricts the arterioles (as found in the model) and therefore also reduces the global CBV [35]. However, the global CBV is elevated in LA. Therefore, we required an increase in the venous outflow resistance to dilate the veins and capillaries in order to resolve the equations successfully. This outflow resistance increase appears to correlate with the literature. An increased diameter of the basal veins of Rosenthal and internal cerebral veins is associated with the white matter hyperintensity volume in LA [36]. In another study, the internal cerebral veins were enlarged, which was related to both aging and increased white matter hyperintensity independently [37]. Using an MRI susceptibility sequence, the number of pixels within the deep white matter (assumed to be within the larger deep medullary veins) was increased by 40% in leukoaraiosis, compared to controls and correlated with white matter disease volumes [32]. Given that the dilatation within the veins of the brain also extends into the subarachnoid space component, the venous outflow stenosis producing the dilatation must be between the distal ends of the veins and the sinuses.

It can be seen from Figure 1 that there are similarities between LA and NPH. There is an overall reduction in CBF compared to normal, which is slightly more pronounced in NPH than in LA. There is a 25% increase in arterial resistance compared to normal in both diseases and a 123% increase in venous outflow resistance in LA, which is more pronounced than the 98% increase in venous outflow resistance in NPH. The differences between the diseases are that NPH appears to be associated with a CSF outflow resistance increase, manifest as an increased pressure gradient across the arachnoid granulations within the sinus wall as compared to no change in LA. The capillary transmural pressure is higher in LA than NPH, which may bring about an increase in the overall CSF formation rate compared to NPH if the blood–brain barrier were to be disrupted in the former [9]. Patients with leukoaraiosis showed a 34% increase in the CSF-to-serum albumin ratio, signifying a breakdown in the blood–brain barrier [38]. This finding was independent of the degree of dementia, atrophy, or presence of cerebral infarction. Similarly, an MRI contrast technique indicated there was significant BBB breakdown in LA [39]. The lack of a significant increase in ICP in LA despite the BBB's expected increase in interstitial fluid leakage would suggest that the CSF outflow absorption is not deficient, unlike in NPH.

4.2. *Differences Between the Cortex and White Matter*

Figure 2 highlights the expected differences in physiology between the cortical grey matter and the deeper white matter. Figure 2a models the effect of increasing the blood flow back to normal, as per the findings within the LA literature in the grey matter, as already discussed. The outflow cuff resistance was unaltered from the previous model, and the effect was to dilate the arteries, capillaries, and veins, with an increase in total CBV from 59.2 mL in the original LA model to 63.5 mL. Thus, the euvolaemia model predicts the CBV to be only 2.8% less than the target value of 65.3 mL, as suggested by Markus et al. [27]. This tends to indicate that the modelling may be accurate enough for the current purposes. Figure 2b gives the results from previous modelling where the CBF was returned to normal in NPH [10]. The overall findings are very similar to Figure 2a, with the only significant difference being the 8.3% increase in arterial resistance in LA compared to normal. This mostly comes about due to the increased perfusion pressure from the increased arterial inflow pressure. It can be seen that LA is likely not predominately a disease of the cortex, despite the increased venous and capillary pressures, but is probably a disease of the white matter. Illustrating this, Brown et al., using Xenon CT before and after acetazolamide vasodilatation, found that the cortical blood flow increased normally in leukoaraiosis patients, but there was no significant increase in the white matter blood flow, indicating an exhaustion of autoregulation in the deeper regions and its preservation superficially [40]. However, the 61% increase in the cortical venous volume in LA as compared to normal may be expected to narrow the venous perivascular spaces [41] and thus impede the glymphatic outflow, as occurs in NPH [42]. Glymphatic disruption is noted to be a feature of LA [43], like NPH. The glymphatic flow is thought to pass from the arterial perivascular spaces, through the interstitium, and out via the venous perivascular spaces [44]. Most of the evidence suggests that the dilated perivascular spaces are around arteries and not the veins [44]. This would indicate that either there is a significant increase in glymphatic fluid inflow into the arterial perivascular spaces, which the outflow cannot handle (unlikely as the total glymphatic flow is not increased), or that the outflow passageway is obstructed, backing up the fluid further upstream. Dilatation of the veins within their perivascular spaces could provide this downstream obstruction.

Figure 2c illustrates the effect of reducing the CBF to match the reduction in blood flow found in the white matter in leukoaraiosis. The modelling was unable to reach the target CBV unless there was also wall thickening and stenosis added to the venous segment. Moody et al. studied the deep medullary veins of the brain from 20 to 800 μm diameter and found significant wall thickening in LA [45]. This thickening was termed venous collagenosis and was due to a large amount of collagen deposited within the walls. They found that 65% of subjects older than 60 years had at least a 50% stenosis of their periventricular veins [45]. They suggested that severe stenosis or occlusion of the deep cerebral veins may promote the development of leukoaraiosis [45]. In another study, collagenosis of small and medium-calibre veins was significantly worse in patients with larger volumes of LA [46]. In fact, the strongest predictor of LA score was stenosis of the large-calibre veins [46]. Venous collagenosis is a major difference between LA and pure NPH, with the NPH ischaemia model in Figure 2d not requiring wall thickening or stenosis. In those with mixed disease (LA and NPH), the LA is associated with more severe symptoms but may not affect the CSF shunting outcome [33].

In both NPH and LA, there was a large increase in arterial inflow resistance required in the white matter, despite the venous resistance increase. In LA, of the 97 mmHg/L/min increase in the white matter vascular resistance, 88.2% came from the arterioles, 11% from the venous outflow cuff, and only 0.7% from the venous bed, with the capillaries being unchanged in resistance. A major difference between NPH and LA is the reversibility of the reduced blood flow and presumably the reversibility of the large increase in arterial resistance. In NPH, there was a 53% increase in CBF in those who improved with shunting, indicating retained autoregulation [47]. This suggested to us that the brain was electing to limit the CBF in NPH, perhaps to minimize the ICP by reducing the CSF formation rate increase inherent when there is an opening of the blood–brain barrier [9,10]. There is no apparent residual autoregulation within the white matter in LA [40]. This would suggest that there may be some irreversible arterial disease as well as venous collagenosis in the deep white matter in LA. Some authors suggest that arteriolosclerosis is almost always detected within areas of LA [48], but not all studies show such a strong correlation. Both arteriolosclerosis and venular collagenosis are more prevalent with age. However, arterial sclerosis was associated with lacunar infarction and haemosiderin deposition but not leukoaraiosis severity in one study [49]. Conversely, venular collagenosis was not associated with lacunes or haemosiderin but was associated with leukoaraiosis in the same study [49]. In another study, arterial wall collagen deposition was not a predictor of white matter disease, but venous collagen deposition was such a predictor [50]. Brown et al. indicated that the increase in resistance may be due to arteriolar tortuosity rather than sclerosis of the wall [51]. The results of a meta-analysis suggest that although there is lower blood flow in LA, the findings did not strongly support causation. The results suggested that the reduced flow may reflect a reduction in supply required by the tissue secondary to decreased neuronal activity or atrophy [52]. The findings indicate that there may be a functional arterial cause rather than a structural cause for the lack of irreversibility of the reduced white matter blood flow in LA.

4.3. Pulsatility as a Cause of Leukoaraiosis

It is apparent that there is a reduction in blood flow to the white matter in LA, but as discussed, this may not be the causative factor. Previously, one of the current authors developed a theory suggesting that there was a common pathophysiology between Alzheimer's disease, vascular dementia, and NPH based on intracranial pulsation energy dissipation [53]. It was suggested that there was a spectrum of pulsation differences between these diseases, with the process termed pulse wave encephalopathy. The literature appears to support this hypothesis, as the percentage of the brains volume affected by LA increases in accordance with arterial pulse pressure quartiles in male subjects [2]. The severity of LA correlates with the middle cerebral artery pulsatility and the pulse wave velocity (a measure of aortic arterial stiffness) in multivariate analysis [54]. The authors concluded that increased arterial stiffening causes increased transmission of enhanced aortic pulsatility to the cerebral circulation, causing LA due to either decreased perfusion in diastole, increased endothelial shear stress, or impaired autoregulation [54]. However, the increased pulsation is not just limited to the arterial tree. Patients with dementia and moderate leukoaraiosis showed a 69%, 48%, and 34% increase in pulsatility in the blood flow of the arteries, sagittal sinus, and superficial cortical veins compared to dementia patients without leukoaraiosis [55]. In vascular dementia patients, the absolute pulsation volume of the straight sinus (which drains the deep white matter) is increased by 57% compared to normal elderly controls [56]. These venous findings correlate with NPH, where there was a 56% increase in the pulsatility index of the arteries and a 70% increase in this metric within the sagittal sinus compared to dementia patients without leukoaraiosis [55]. In NPH, the CSF pulse pressure increases by 6–8 times what is normal [57]. The CSF pulse pressure has not been measured in LA, but given the arterial, cortical vein, and sinus pulsation findings, it is likely to be increased similar to NPH. Interestingly, when veins are used as arterial bypass grafts and experience pulsatile flow, they become thickened similar to the collagenosis already discussed. In a porcine venous graft model, after the first week, wall thickening occurs largely due to extracellular matrix deposition (fibrosis) and neointimal smooth muscle cell proliferation [58]. Could pulsation energy deposited within the walls of the veins be behind the venous collagenosis noted in white matter disease as well?

The modelling highlights an apparent paradox. The previous NPH modelling suggested that a 37% increase in the pressure gradient across the outflow cuff led to a 98% increase in outflow resistance of this segment (see Figure 1c) [9]. In the current modelling, a normal pressure gradient across the outflow cuff in LA still resulted in a 123% increase in resistance of this segment (see Figure 1b). Where does this increase in resistance come from? We have previously suggested that this may be due to the effect of the CSF pulsation pressure inducing a phenomenon in the veins known as impedance pumping [59]. However, there may be a simpler explanation for this finding. The cortical veins are a series of collapsible tubes in which the pressure external to the tubes (ICP) exceeds the sinus pressure. This arrangement represents a Starling resistor. The collapse of the distal end of a Starling resistor maintains the pressure across the tube wall upstream to the collapse. This upstream transmural pressure (TMP) it is only very slightly positive in classical Starling resistors [60]. Thus, if the ICP were to increase, the venous TMP would be expected to remain nearly constant and the venous pressure to be minimally above the ICP [60]. It is apparent from the modelling that cortical veins do not act as traditional Starling resistors in this regard. The normal vein TMP is 2.5 mmHg (not close to zero as an ideal Starling resistor model would predict) and increases to 4.8 mmHg in our NPH model (see Figure 1c). It further increases to 9 mmHg in LA in our model. If the veins were ideal Starling resistors, then the upstream venous pressure would normally be just above the ICP, i.e., 11.5 mmHg. This would give a normal venous cuff resistance of 5.3 mmHg/L/min, but we estimate this resistance to be 8.7 mmHg/L/min in the normal model. The CSF pulse originates from the intracranial arterial pulse. It is dissipated by shifting CSF backwards and forwards through the foramen magnum and by compressing the cortical veins, making the venous outflow in the sagittal sinus pulsatile [55]. This sinus pulsation occurs due to compression of the outflow cuff. In MRV studies of humans with elevated ICP, 80% showed a narrow segment of the cortical vein, approximately 5 mm long at the level of the cuff. This appeared in only 10% of the control subjects [61]. The diameter of the cortical veins increased by 30% upstream from the cuff in those patients with raised ICP compared to controls, suggesting an increase in venous outflow resistance over and above that required to keep the veins open [61]. Increasing the ICP increases the CSF pulse pressure due to the intracranial compliance being reduced [62], suggesting that there may be a correlation between the ICP pulse pressure and venous outflow resistance. The peak flow in the cortical veins lags behind the peak flow in the sinus by 100 mS [55] despite the sinus being distal to the veins that drain into it. This suggests that cuff pulsation delays cortical vein emptying by generating a pressure wave going back towards the capillaries [55]. It may be envisaged that a rhythmic contraction of the vein cuff, which reduces its volume by 50% below its mean value and then increases its volume by 50% above the mean, would increase and decrease the resistance of the outflow by the same amount, and therefore they would cancel each other out. However, this may not be the case. The volume of a cylinder changes as the square of the radius, but Poiseuille's Equation (3) indicates that the outflow resistance varies with the inverse fourth power of the radius. Therefore, a systolic reduction in venous cuff volume of 50% would increase its outflow resistance by 4 times, but an increase in volume by 50% in diastole would decrease its resistance by only 0.44 times. Given that systole lasts for 40% of the cardiac cycle and diastole for 60% on average [63], the time-averaged cuff resistance over the entire cardiac cycle would be increased by 1.9 times normal with such a pulsation. Reducing the average cuff volume by 2/3 in systole and increasing it by 2/3 in diastole with a larger pulse pressure would increase the average outflow resistance by 4.9 times, suggesting that increasing the pulsation pressure may increase the venous outflow resistance. Thus, we suggest that an increase in the CSF pulse pressure in both NPH and LA would increase the outflow resistance and pressure and send a pressure wave back toward the capillaries. In LA, we suggest that this pulsation energy induces vein wall thickening, making the walls less compliant and propagating the pressure waves further towards the capillaries with a greater amplitude [55].

4.4. Clinical Utility

If we are correct and the CSF pulsations generate both an increase in the venous outflow pressure and a pulse pressure wave travelling back towards the capillaries, then this could explain the blood–brain barrier disruption in both diseases. A mouse model indicates that an increase in venous pressure will disrupt the blood–brain barrier without any other requirement [64]. Therefore, in order to limit the effects of this pulsation energy and the progression of LA, strategies aimed at reducing the pulsation amplitude in both the arterial inflow and the subarachnoid space could have therapeutic value. It has been suggested that syringomyelia of the cord (the development of a cystic cavity) secondary to a Chiari I malformation (foramen magnum being blocked by the cerebellum) is analogous to NPH [65]. There is a reduction in the spinal canal subarachnoid space compliance, increased CSF pulse pressures, and disruption of the blood spinal cord barrier in syringomyelia similar to NPH [65]. A dog model of syringomyelia showed dilatation of the venous outflow of the cord, similar to our findings in both NPH and LA [66]. A posterior fossa decompression increases the compliance of the spinal canal, reduces the CSF pulse pressure, and collapses the syrinx [65]. Interestingly, increasing the cranial compliance by posterior fossa decompression also improves Chiari I-associated hydrocephalus in 90% of cases without further treatment [67]. Similarly, subtemporal craniectomy is noted to significantly reduce the ventricle size in patients with shunt-dependant hydrocephalus [68]. Increasing the intracranial compliance by craniectomy would reduce the ICP pulse pressure. Could the same procedure halt the progression of LA?

4.5. Limitations

Poiseuille's equation requires that a Newtonian fluid should pass through a thin, rigid, circular tube, without turbulence, to be valid. If these assumptions hold, the findings would be accurate. However, despite the equation's limitations, it is commonly used in modelling the vasculature within the medical literature.

We have assumed the mean arterial inflow pressure to be increased in LA to 110 mmHg. We performed a sensitivity analysis to gauge any error induced by this assumption, by increasing the arterial inflow pressure to less than the cut-off for autoregulation failure at 150 mmHg [25]. We found the capillary pressure to be unchanged, because the arterial resistance must increase to keep the blood flow from increasing [29].

We assumed the ICP in leukoaraiosis to be unchanged from normal at 11.5 mmHg, but this was derived from a single reference [33]. We performed a sensitivity analysis by increasing the ICP by 9% to 12.5 mmHg to gauge the effect this would have on the model. The result was that the venous outflow cuff resistance needed to increase by 8% and the arterial resistance reduce by 0.9% for the target CBV increase of 16.1% to be reached. This does not materially change the findings of the model, which indicate that venous outflow resistance must be increased in leukoaraiosis.

We assumed that the sinus pressure was normal at 7.5 mmHg in our model. Given that the blood flow through the sinuses was 10% lower than normal, one could argue that the sinus pressure could be less than normal if the resistance to blood flow through the venous sinuses and neck was unchanged. A sensitivity analysis was performed by reducing the sinus pressure by 13% to 6.5 mmHg. This increased the required total resistance in the system by 1% to 154.5 mmHg/L/min. In order for the target CBV increase of 16.1% to be reached, the outflow cuff resistance needed to be increased by 15% and the arterial resistance reduced by 0.9%. Again, this does not materially change the finding that the outflow cuff resistance must be increased in leukoaraiosis for the CBV to be increased.

The model that assumes the capillary volume is unchanged as the capillary TMP is reduced below normal. This assumption was made because the critical buckling pressure for such a small tube as a capillary is very high and is never approached in this model. The critical transmural pressure at which buckling of a collapsible tube begins depends on several variables, such as the stiffness of the wall (Young's elastic modulus), Poisson's ratio (how the wall deforms under a tensile load), the wall thickness, the internal diameter of the vessel, and the vessel length [69]. The most important of these is the ratio of the wall thickness to the internal diameter, because the critical buckling pressure is proportional to the cube of this ratio. The buckling pressure is linearly related to the other variables [69]. The average internal diameter of a human cerebral capillary is 8 μm, and the wall thickness is 1 μm [70], giving a wall thickness-to-internal diameter ratio of 0.13. The average human cortical vein adjacent to the sagittal sinus has an internal diameter of 3.3 mm and a wall thickness of 0.044 mm [59], giving a ratio of 0.013 (tenfold less). The cube of the ratio of thickness divided by diameter for the capillaries compared to the veins is therefore 1000. The elastic modulus for the capillaries is 0.68 MPa [70], and for cortical veins, it is 0.16 MPa [59], indicating that the capillary walls are stiffer than the veins. Poisson's ratio for the tensile deformation in most materials varies between 0 and 0.5, with the value for blood vessels being 0.4 [70]. The capillaries are shorter than the cortical veins, making them harder to collapse from this viewpoint. Given that the critical buckling pressure is proportional to the cube of the thickness-to-diameter ratio, and the capillaries are stiffer and shorter than veins, then the capillaries and smallest veins will have a critical buckling pressure that is at least 1000 times greater than the distal cortical veins. The buckling pressure is probably very low in cortical veins, standing at approximately 0.1 mmHg in a dog model using the inferior vena cava [71]. The figure for capillaries will therefore be much larger, approximating 100 mmHg.

Some of the data we required is not available from human studies, and so animal studies were utilised. The data linking dilatation of the capillaries to the changes in TMP was taken from rodent studies, and the normal venous TMP was obtained from a primate study. We have no way of knowing if the animal data closely approximates human findings, so this is a limitation.

The modelling does not attempt to stratify the changes in the parameters that may occur due to differing burdens of white matter disease. This is because there is no published data to give the required CBV for the differing levels of LA. Interestingly, the reduction in CBF does not appear to be directly related to the degree to LA, with one study finding that there was no relationship between LA severity and measures of arterial inflow [72] and another indicating no clear change in CBF with the Fazekas score [55].

5. Conclusions

Our modelling suggests that the vascular physiology of LA may be similar to NPH. The model required thickening of the venous walls in LA, which was not required in NPH. The increase in venous outflow resistance can be explained by pulsation-derived compression and dilatation of the outflow cuff.

Author Contributions: Conceptualisation G.A.B., A.R.B.; Methodology G.A.B., A.R.B.; Validation A.R.B.; Writing—Original Draft Preparation G.A.B.; Writing—Review and Editing G.A.B., A.R.B. All authors have read and agreed to the published version of the manuscript.

Funding: This research received no external funding.

Institutional Review Board Statement: Not applicable.

Informed Consent Statement: Not applicable.

Data Availability Statement: The original contributions presented in this study are included in the article. Further inquiries can be directed to the corresponding author.

Conflicts of Interest: The authors declare no conflicts of interest.

References

1. Liu, C.K.; Miller, B.L.; Cummings, J.L.; Mehringer, C.M.; Goldberg, M.A.; Howng, S.L.; Benson, D.F. A quantitative MRI study of vascular dementia. *Neurology* **1992**, *42*, 138–143. [CrossRef] [PubMed]
2. Kim, S.H.; Shim, J.Y.; Lee, H.R.; Na, H.Y.; Lee, Y.J. The relationship between pulse pressure and leukoaraiosis in the elderly. *Arch. Gerontol. Geriatr.* **2012**, *54*, 206–209. [CrossRef]
3. van Gijn, J. Leukoaraiosis and vascular dementia. *Neurology* **1998**, *51*, S3–S8. [CrossRef] [PubMed]
4. Pantoni, L.; Garcia, J.H. The significance of cerebral white matter abnormalities 100 years after Binswanger's report. A review. *Stroke* **1995**, *26*, 1293–1301. [CrossRef]
5. Lindgren, A.; Roijer, A.; Rudling, O.; Norrving, B.; Larsson, E.M.; Eskilsson, J.; Wallin, L.; Olsson, B.; Johansson, B.B. Cerebral lesions on magnetic resonance imaging, heart disease, and vascular risk factors in subjects without stroke. A population-based study. *Stroke* **1994**, *25*, 929–934. [CrossRef]
6. Inzitari, D.; Diaz, F.; Fox, A.; Hachinski, V.C.; Steingart, A.; Lau, C.; Donald, A.; Wade, J.; Mulic, H.; Merskey, H. Vascular risk factors and leuko-araiosis. *Arch. Neurol.* **1987**, *44*, 42–47. [CrossRef] [PubMed]
7. Ades-Aron, B.; Yeager, S.; Miskin, N.; Fieremans, E.; George, A.; Golomb, J. Diffusional Kurtosis along the Corticospinal Tract in Adult Normal Pressure Hydrocephalus. *AJNR Am. J. Neuroradiol.* **2018**, *39*, 2218–2223. [CrossRef]
8. Tullberg, M.; Jensen, C.; Ekholm, S.; Wikkelso, C. Normal pressure hydrocephalus: Vascular white matter changes on MR images must not exclude patients from shunt surgery. *AJNR Am. J. Neuroradiol.* **2001**, *22*, 1665–1673.

9. Bateman, G.A.; Bateman, A.R. A lumped parameter modelling study of cerebral autoregulation in normal pressure hydrocephalus suggests the brain chooses to be ischemic. *Sci. Rep.* **2024**, *14*, 24373. [CrossRef]
10. Bateman, G.A.; Bateman, A.R. A Lumped Parameter Model Suggests That Infusion Studies Overestimate the Cerebrospinal Fluid Outflow Resistance in Normal Pressure Hydrocephalus. *Brain Sci.* **2024**, *14*, 1242. [CrossRef] [PubMed]
11. Bell, M.D.; Long, T.; Roden, A.C.; Cooper, F.I.; Sanchez, H.; Trower, C.; Martinez, C.; Hooper, J.E.; Autopsy Committee of the College of American, P. Updating Normal Organ Weights Using a Large Current Sample Database. *Arch. Pathol. Lab. Med.* **2022**, *146*, 1486–1495. [CrossRef]
12. Lassen, N.A. Normal Average Value of Cerebral Blood Flow in Younger Adults is 50 mL/100 g/min. *J. Cereb. Blood Flow Metab.* **1985**, *5*, 347–349. [CrossRef] [PubMed]
13. Buijs, P.C.; Krabbe-Hartkamp, M.J.; Bakker, C.J.; de Lange, E.E.; Ramos, L.M.; Breteler, M.M.; Mali, W.P. Effect of age on cerebral blood flow: Measurement with ungated two-dimensional phase-contrast MR angiography in 250 adults. *Radiology* **1998**, *209*, 667–674. [CrossRef] [PubMed]
14. Ursino, M. A mathematical study of human intracranial hydrodynamics. Part 1—The cerebrospinal fluid pulse pressure. *Ann. Biomed. Eng.* **1988**, *16*, 379–401. [CrossRef]
15. Salmon, J.H.; Timperman, A.L. Effect of intracranial hypotension on cerebral blood flow. *J. Neurol. Neurosurg. Psychiatry* **1971**, *34*, 687–692. [CrossRef]
16. Cirovic, S.; Walsh, C.; Fraser, W.D. Mathematical study of the role of non-linear venous compliance in the cranial volume-pressure test. *Med. Biol. Eng. Comput.* **2003**, *41*, 579–588. [CrossRef] [PubMed]
17. Fleischman, D.; Berdahl, J.P.; Zaydlarova, J.; Stinnett, S.; Fautsch, M.P.; Allingham, R.R. Cerebrospinal fluid pressure decreases with older age. *PLoS ONE* **2012**, *7*, e52664. [CrossRef]
18. Benabid, A.L.; De Rougemont, J.; Barge, M. Cerebral venous pressure, sinus pressure and intracranial pressure. *Neurochirurgie* **1974**, *20*, 623–632.
19. Pollay, M. The function and structure of the cerebrospinal fluid outflow system. *Cerebrospinal Fluid. Res.* **2010**, *7*, 9. [CrossRef]
20. Johnston, I.H.; Rowan, J.O. Raised intracranial pressure and cerebral blood flow. 3. Venous outflow tract pressures and vascular resistances in experimental intracranial hypertension. *J. Neurol. Neurosurg. Psychiatry* **1974**, *37*, 392–402. [CrossRef]
21. Helenius, J.; Perkio, J.; Soinne, L.; Ostergaard, L.; Carano, R.A.; Salonen, O.; Savolainen, S.; Kaste, M.; Aronen, H.J.; Tatlisumak, T. Cerebral hemodynamics in a healthy population measured by dynamic susceptibility contrast MR imaging. *Acta Radiol.* **2003**, *44*, 538–546. [CrossRef] [PubMed]
22. Good, C.D.; Johnsrude, I.; Ashburner, J.; Henson, R.N.; Friston, K.J.; Frackowiak, R.S. Cerebral asymmetry and the effects of sex and handedness on brain structure: A voxel-based morphometric analysis of 465 normal adult human brains. *Neuroimage* **2001**, *14*, 685–700. [CrossRef]
23. Hua, J.; Liu, P.; Kim, T.; Donahue, M.; Rane, S.; Chen, J.J.; Qin, Q.; Kim, S.G. MRI techniques to measure arterial and venous cerebral blood volume. *Neuroimage* **2019**, *187*, 17–31. [CrossRef]
24. Menéndez González, M. (Ed.) CNS Compartments: The Anatomy and Physiology of the Cerebrospinal Fluid. In *Liquorpheresis: Cerebrospinal Fluid Filtration to Treat CNS Conditions*; Springer Nature Switzerland: Cham, Switzerland, 2023; pp. 1–19.
25. Claassen, J.; Thijssen, D.H.J.; Panerai, R.B.; Faraci, F.M. Regulation of cerebral blood flow in humans: Physiology and clinical implications of autoregulation. *Physiol. Rev.* **2021**, *101*, 1487–1559. [CrossRef] [PubMed]
26. De Simone, R.; Ranieri, A.; Bonavita, V. Starling resistors, autoregulation of cerebral perfusion and the pathogenesis of idiopathic intracranial hypertension. *Panminerva Medica* **2017**, *59*, 76–89. [CrossRef] [PubMed]
27. Markus, H.S.; Lythgoe, D.J.; Ostegaard, L.; O'Sullivan, M.; Williams, S.C. Reduced cerebral blood flow in white matter in ischaemic leukoaraiosis demonstrated using quantitative exogenous contrast based perfusion MRI. *J. Neurol. Neurosurg. Psychiatry* **2000**, *69*, 48–53. [CrossRef]
28. Bateman, G.A.; Bateman, A.R. Brain Ischemia in Alzheimer's Disease May Partly Counteract the Disruption of the Blood–Brain Barrier. *Brain Sci.* **2025**, *15*, 269. [CrossRef]
29. Bateman, G.A.; Bateman, A.R. A Lumped Parameter Modelling Study of Idiopathic Intracranial Hypertension Suggests the CSF Formation Rate Varies with the Capillary Transmural Pressure. *Brain Sci.* **2025**, *15*, 527. [CrossRef]
30. Yao, H.; Sadoshima, S.; Ibayashi, S.; Kuwabara, Y.; Ichiya, Y.; Fujishima, M. Leukoaraiosis and dementia in hypertensive patients. *Stroke* **1992**, *23*, 1673–1677. [CrossRef]
31. Henry-Feugeas, M.C.; Roy, C.; Baron, G.; Schouman-Claeys, E. Leukoaraiosis and pulse-wave encephalopathy: Observations with phase-contrast MRI in mild cognitive impairment. *J. Neuroradiol.* **2009**, *36*, 212–218. [CrossRef]
32. Yan, S.; Wan, J.; Zhang, X.; Tong, L.; Zhao, S.; Sun, J.; Lin, Y.; Shen, C.; Lou, M. Increased visibility of deep medullary veins in leukoaraiosis: A 3-T MRI study. *Front. Aging Neurosci.* **2014**, *6*, 144. [CrossRef]
33. Cai, H.; Huang, K.; Yang, F.; He, J.; Hu, N.; Gao, H.; Feng, S.; Qin, L.; Wang, R.; Yang, X.; et al. The contribution of cerebral small vessel disease in idiopathic normal pressure hydrocephalus: Insights from a prospective cohort study. *Alzheimers Dement.* **2025**, *21*, e14395. [CrossRef] [PubMed]

34. Hatazawa, J.; Shimosegawa, E.; Satoh, T.; Toyoshima, H.; Okudera, T. Subcortical hypoperfusion associated with asymptomatic white matter lesions on magnetic resonance imaging. *Stroke* **1997**, *28*, 1944–1947. [CrossRef]
35. Gwinnutt, C.L.; Saha, B. Cerebral blood flow and intracranial pressure. *Anaesth. Intensive Care Med.* **2005**, *6*, 153–156. [CrossRef]
36. Houck, A.L.; Gutierrez, J.; Gao, F.; Igwe, K.C.; Colon, J.M.; Black, S.E.; Brickman, A.M. Increased Diameters of the Internal Cerebral Veins and the Basal Veins of Rosenthal Are Associated with White Matter Hyperintensity Volume. *AJNR Am. J. Neuroradiol.* **2019**, *40*, 1712–1718. [CrossRef]
37. Huang, Z.; Tu, X.; Lin, Q.; Zhan, Z.; Tang, L.; Liu, J. Increased internal cerebral vein diameter is associated with age. *Clin. Imaging* **2021**, *78*, 187–193. [CrossRef]
38. Pantoni, L.; Inzitari, D.; Pracucci, G.; Lolli, F.; Giordano, G.; Bracco, L.; Amaducci, L. Cerebrospinal fluid proteins in patients with leucoaraiosis: Possible abnormalities in blood-brain barrier function. *J. Neurol. Sci.* **1993**, *115*, 125–131. [CrossRef]
39. Uh, J.; Yezhuvath, U.; Cheng, Y.; Lu, H. In vivo vascular hallmarks of diffuse leukoaraiosis. *J. Magn. Reson. Imaging* **2010**, *32*, 184–190. [CrossRef]
40. Brown, M.M.; Pelz, D.M.; Hachinski, V. Proceedings of the Association of British Neurologists and the Society of British Neurological Surgeons, Bristol, 4–6 April 1990. *J. Neurol. Neurosurg. Psychiatry* **1990**, *53*, 808–817. [CrossRef]
41. Bateman, G.A.; Bateman, A.R. Syringomyelia Is Associated with a Reduction in Spinal Canal Compliance, Venous Outflow Dilatation and Glymphatic Fluid Obstruction. *J. Clin. Med.* **2023**, *12*, 6646. [CrossRef] [PubMed]
42. Kikuta, J.; Kamagata, K.; Taoka, T.; Takabayashi, K.; Uchida, W.; Saito, Y.; Andica, C.; Wada, A.; Kawamura, K.; Akiba, C.; et al. Water Diffusivity Changes Along the Perivascular Space After Lumboperitoneal Shunt Surgery in Idiopathic Normal Pressure Hydrocephalus. *Front. Neurol.* **2022**, *13*, 843883. [CrossRef]
43. Sabayan, B.; Westendorp, R.G.J. Neurovascular-glymphatic dysfunction and white matter lesions. *Geroscience* **2021**, *43*, 1635–1642. [CrossRef]
44. Yu, L.; Hu, X.; Li, H.; Zhao, Y. Perivascular Spaces, Glymphatic System and MR. *Front. Neurol.* **2022**, *13*, 844938. [CrossRef]
45. Moody, D.M.; Brown, W.R.; Challa, V.R.; Anderson, R.L. Periventricular venous collagenosis: Association with leukoaraiosis. *Radiology* **1995**, *194*, 469–476. [CrossRef]
46. Keith, J.; Gao, F.Q.; Noor, R.; Kiss, A.; Balasubramaniam, G.; Au, K.; Rogaeva, E.; Masellis, M.; Black, S.E. Collagenosis of the Deep Medullary Veins: An Underrecognized Pathologic Correlate of White Matter Hyperintensities and Periventricular Infarction? *J. Neuropathol. Exp. Neurol.* **2017**, *76*, 299–312. [CrossRef]
47. Tanaka, A.; Kimura, M.; Nakayama, Y.; Yoshinaga, S.; Tomonaga, M. Cerebral blood flow and autoregulation in normal pressure hydrocephalus. *Neurosurgery* **1997**, *40*, 1161–1165; discussion 1165–1167. [CrossRef]
48. Fazekas, F.; Kleinert, R.; Offenbacher, H.; Schmidt, R.; Kleinert, G.; Payer, F.; Radner, H.; Lechner, H. Pathologic correlates of incidental MRI white matter signal hyperintensities. *Neurology* **1993**, *43*, 1683–1689. [CrossRef]
49. Cao, Y.; Huang, M.Y.; Mao, C.H.; Wang, X.; Xu, Y.Y.; Qian, X.J.; Ma, C.; Qiu, W.Y.; Zhu, Y.C. Arteriolosclerosis differs from venular collagenosis in relation to cerebrovascular parenchymal damages: An autopsy-based study. *Stroke Vasc. Neurol.* **2023**, *8*, 267–275. [CrossRef]
50. Lahna, D.; Schwartz, D.L.; Woltjer, R.; Black, S.E.; Roese, N.; Dodge, H.; Boespflug, E.L.; Keith, J.; Gao, F.; Ramirez, J.; et al. Venous Collagenosis as Pathogenesis of White Matter Hyperintensity. *Ann. Neurol.* **2022**, *92*, 992–1000. [CrossRef]
51. Brown, W.R.; Moody, D.M.; Challa, V.R.; Thore, C.R.; Anstrom, J.A. Venous collagenosis and arteriolar tortuosity in leukoaraiosis. *J. Neurol. Sci.* **2002**, *203–204*, 159–163. [CrossRef]
52. Shi, Y.; Thrippleton, M.J.; Makin, S.D.; Marshall, I.; Geerlings, M.I.; de Craen, A.J.M.; van Buchem, M.A.; Wardlaw, J.M. Cerebral blood flow in small vessel disease: A systematic review and meta-analysis. *J. Cereb. Blood Flow Metab.* **2016**, *36*, 1653–1667. [CrossRef]
53. Bateman, G.A. Pulse wave encephalopathy: A spectrum hypothesis incorporating Alzheimer's disease, vascular dementia and normal pressure hydrocephalus. *Med. Hypotheses* **2004**, *62*, 182–187. [CrossRef]
54. Webb, A.J.; Simoni, M.; Mazzucco, S.; Kuker, W.; Schulz, U.; Rothwell, P.M. Increased cerebral arterial pulsatility in patients with leukoaraiosis: Arterial stiffness enhances transmission of aortic pulsatility. *Stroke* **2012**, *43*, 2631–2636. [CrossRef]
55. Bateman, G.A. Pulse-wave encephalopathy: A comparative study of the hydrodynamics of leukoaraiosis and normal-pressure hydrocephalus. *Neuroradiology* **2002**, *44*, 740–748. [CrossRef]
56. Bateman, G.A.; Levi, C.R.; Schofield, P.; Wang, Y.; Lovett, E.C. The venous manifestations of pulse wave encephalopathy: Windkessel dysfunction in normal aging and senile dementia. *Neuroradiology* **2008**, *50*, 491–497. [CrossRef]
57. Stephensen, H.; Tisell, M.; Wikkelso, C. There is no transmantle pressure gradient in communicating or noncommunicating hydrocephalus. *Neurosurgery* **2002**, *50*, 763–771; discussion 771–773. [CrossRef]
58. Shi, Y.; Pieniek, M.; Fard, A.; O'Brien, J.; Mannion, J.D.; Zalewski, A. Adventitial remodeling after coronary arterial injury. *Circulation* **1996**, *93*, 340–348. [CrossRef]
59. Bateman, G.A.; Bateman, A.R.; Subramanian, G.M. Dilatation of the bridging cerebral cortical veins in childhood hydrocephalus suggests a malfunction of venous impedance pumping. *Sci. Rep.* **2022**, *12*, 13045. [CrossRef]

60. Portnoy, H.D.; Chopp, M.; Branch, C.; Shannon, M.B. Cerebrospinal fluid pulse waveform as an indicator of cerebral autoregulation. *J. Neurosurg.* **1982**, *56*, 666–678. [CrossRef]
61. Si, Z.; Luan, L.; Kong, D.; Zhao, G.; Wang, H.; Zhang, K.; Yu, T.; Pang, Q. MRI-based investigation on outflow segment of cerebral venous system under increased ICP condition. *Eur. J. Med. Res.* **2008**, *13*, 121–126.
62. Nornes, H.; Aaslid, R.; Lindegaard, K.F. Intracranial pulse pressure dynamics in patients with intracranial hypertension. *Acta Neurochir.* **1977**, *38*, 177–186. [CrossRef]
63. Bachani, N.; Vijay, S.; Vyas, A.; Jadwani, J.; Panicker, G.; Lokhandwala, Y. The diastolic duration as a percentage of the cardiac cycle in healthy adults: A pilot study. *Indian Heart J.* **2025**, *77*, 73–77. [CrossRef]
64. Fulop, G.A.; Ahire, C.; Csipo, T.; Tarantini, S.; Kiss, T.; Balasubramanian, P.; Yabluchanskiy, A.; Farkas, E.; Toth, A.; Nyul-Toth, A.; et al. Cerebral venous congestion promotes blood-brain barrier disruption and neuroinflammation, impairing cognitive function in mice. *Geroscience* **2019**, *41*, 575–589. [CrossRef]
65. Bateman, G.A. Pulse wave myelopathy: An update of an hypothesis highlighting the similarities between syringomyelia and normal pressure hydrocephalus. *Med. Hypotheses* **2015**, *85*, 958–961. [CrossRef]
66. Yamada, H.; Yokota, A.; Haratake, J.; Horie, A. Morphological study of experimental syringomyelia with kaolin-induced hydrocephalus in a canine model. *J. Neurosurg.* **1996**, *84*, 999–1005. [CrossRef]
67. Koueik, J.; DeSanti, R.L.; Iskandar, B.J. Posterior fossa decompression for children with Chiari I malformation and hydrocephalus. *Childs Nerv. Syst.* **2022**, *38*, 153–161. [CrossRef]
68. Linder, M.; Diehl, J.; Sklar, F.H. Subtemporal decompressions for shunt-dependent ventricles: Mechanism of action. *Surg. Neurol.* **1983**, *19*, 520–523. [CrossRef]
69. Laudato, M.; Mosca, R.; Mihaescu, M. Buckling critical pressures in collapsible tubes relevant for biomedical flows. *Sci. Rep.* **2023**, *13*, 9298. [CrossRef]
70. Fung, Y.C.; Zweifach, B.W.; Intaglietta, M. Elastic environment of the capillary bed. *Circ. Res.* **1966**, *19*, 441–461. [CrossRef]
71. Moreno, A.H.; Katz, A.I.; Gold, L.D.; Reddy, R.V. Mechanics of distension of dog veins and other very thin-walled tubular structures. *Circ. Res.* **1970**, *27*, 1069–1080. [CrossRef]
72. Jolly, T.A.; Bateman, G.A.; Levi, C.R.; Parsons, M.W.; Michie, P.T.; Karayanidis, F. Early detection of microstructural white matter changes associated with arterial pulsatility. *Front. Hum. Neurosci.* **2013**, *7*, 782. [CrossRef] [PubMed]

brain sciences

MDPI

Article

Fluid–Structure Interaction Simulations of the Initiation Process of Cerebral Aneurysms

Jozsef Nagy [1], Wolfgang Fenz [2], Veronika M. Miron [3], Stefan Thumfart [2], Julia Maier [3], Zoltan Major [3], Harald Stefanits [4,5], Johannes Oberndorfer [4], Nico Stroh [4,5], Vanessa Mazanec [4,5], Philip-Rudolf Rauch [4,5], Andreas Gruber [4,5,6,*] and Matthias Gmeiner [4,5]

1 eulerian-solutions e.U., Leonfeldnerstraße 245, 4040 Linz, Austria; jozsef.nagy@eulerian-solutions.com
2 Unit Medical Informatics, RISC Software GmbH, Softwarepark 32a, 4232 Hagenberg, Austria; wolfgang.fenz@risc-software.at (W.F.); stefan.thumfart@risc-software.at (S.T.)
3 Institute of Polymer Product Engineering, Johannes Kepler University Linz, Altenberger Strasse 69, 4040 Linz, Austria; veronika.miron@biz-up.at (V.M.M.); julia.maier@jku.at (J.M.); zoltan.major@jku.at (Z.M.)
4 Medical Faculty, Johannes Kepler University Linz, Altenberger Strasse 69, 4020 Linz, Austria; harald.stefanits@kepleruniklinikum.at (H.S.); johannes.oberndorfer@kepleruniklinikum.at (J.O.); nico.stroh@kepleruniklinikum.at (N.S.); vanessa.mazanec@kepleruniklinikum.at (V.M.); philip-rudolf.rauch@kepleruniklinikum.at (P.-R.R.); matthias.gmeiner@kepleruniklinikum.at (M.G.)
5 Department of Neurosurgery, Kepler University Hospital, Wagner-Jauregg-Weg 15, 4020 Linz, Austria
6 Clinical Research Institute for Neuroscience, Johannes Kepler University Linz, 4020 Linz, Austria
* Correspondence: andreas.gruber_1@kepleruniklinikum.at

Abstract: Background: Hemodynamics during the growth process of cerebral aneurysms are incompletely understood. We developed a novel fluid–structure interaction analysis method for the identification of relevant scenarios of aneurysm onset. **Method:** This method integrates both fluid dynamics and structural mechanics, as well as their mutual interaction, for a comprehensive analysis. Patients with a single unruptured cerebral aneurysm were included. **Results:** Overall, three scenarios were identified. In scenario A, wall shear stress (WSS) was low, and the oscillatory shear index (OSI) was high in large areas within the region of aneurysm onset (RAO). In scenario B, the quantities indicated a reversed behavior, where WSS was high and OSI was low. In the last scenario C, a behavior in-between was found, with scenarios A and B coexisting simultaneously in the RAO. Structural mechanics demonstrated a similar but independent trend. Further, we analyzed the change in hemodynamics between the onset and a fully developed aneurysm. While scenarios A and C remained unchanged during aneurysm growth, 17% of aneurysms in scenario B changed into scenario A and 20% into scenario C. **Conclusions:** In conclusion, these findings suggest that WSS and the OSI are reciprocally regulated, and both low and high WSS/OSI conditions can lead to aneurysm onset.

Keywords: cerebral aneurysm; fluid–structure interaction simulation; hemodynamics; structural mechanics; initiation

1. Introduction

Cerebral aneurysms affect 2–5% of the general population [1]. An aneurysm rupture may cause a severe subarachnoid hemorrhage (SAH) with high mortality and morbidity rates [2]. Several studies have demonstrated various clinical, genetic, morphological, or hemodynamic factors contributing to the initiation, growth, and rupture of cerebral aneurysms [3].

Recent computational fluid dynamics (CFD) investigations revealed significantly different hemodynamics in ruptured versus unruptured aneurysms [4,5]. Hemodynamic phenomena can provide mechanical triggers, which are transduced into biological signals, leading to possible aneurysm growth and rupture [6].

Numerous attempts have been made to study the influence of the wall shear stress (WSS), one of the best-characterized fluid-dynamic parameters, on these processes [5–8]. Meng et al. described a novel view of aneurysm development, proposing that WSS plays a key mechanistic role, as suggested by their high-versus-low WSS theory [9]. In other studies, similar investigations were carried out, with conflicting results [10].

If the exact mechanisms of aneurysm formation could be determined, aneurysm rupture might be predicted and prevented [7]. Additionally, aneurysm growth may occur in up to 18% of affected patients and may be associated with aneurysm destabilization and rupture [2]. Similarly, other studies found a 12-fold increase in rupture risk in growing aneurysms [11].

Currently, several studies have analyzed hemodynamics in aneurysm initiation [7,8,12]. Although many detailed fluid dynamics simulation analyses, including complex flow patterns, were conducted [13–22], only a few studies have focused on structural dynamics calculations [23–26]. Most of these studies focused on abdominal aneurysms [24–26]. However, a comprehensive evaluation of individual hemodynamics should include the analysis of fluid as well as structural aspects using fluid–structure interaction (FSI) analysis. Therefore, basic research remains important for accurately characterizing and understanding mechanisms of cerebrovascular diseases to enable patient-specific treatment strategy optimization.

The aim of this study is to develop a novel FSI analysis method and investigate the impacts of both hemodynamics and structural mechanics on the initiation and growth of cerebral aneurysms in order to better understand the controversial dynamics of the initiation and growth process of cerebral aneurysms.

2. Methods

2.1. Patient Data

Patients with a single unruptured cerebral aneurysm treated at the Department of Neurosurgery, Kepler University Hospital Linz in 2020 were included for the identification of characteristic scenarios regarding the initiation and growth of cerebral aneurysms. Data were collected retrospectively, and fusiform and dissecting aneurysms were excluded. Additionally, we excluded large aneurysms with a size > 10 mm (n = 4) to minimize the effect of aneurysm size on the FSI analysis, as previously reported [7,27]. Overall, 44 patients were included (26 females, mean age 54 years; ranging from 34–76 years). Microsurgical or endovascular treatments were performed in 19 and 25 patients, respectively. The aneurysms were located at the internal carotid artery (n = 13), middle cerebral artery (MCA; n = 16), anterior communicating artery (n = 9), and posterior circulation (n = 6). This study was approved by the local ethics committee (Ethikkommission der medizinischen Fakultät der Johannes Kepler Universität; EK Nr: 1129/2022), and the requirement for the acquisition of informed consent from patients was waived, owing to the retrospective nature of the research.

2.2. Patient Image Data

We extracted the aneurysm geometries from medical image data obtained via digital subtraction angiography (DSA). Since these images showed only the cerebral blood vessels with high contrast and no other anatomical structures, segmentation was relatively straightforward and could be performed with intensity thresholding and minor editing of the voxel volume. A hydrodynamic entrance length of 5–10 times the inlet and outlet diameters was utilized for the inflow and outflow vessels, respectively, in order to define the cutoff positions during the reconstruction of the vascular geometry [28,29]. In case the quality of the DSA images did not allow such a length, the maximum possible length was taken. The segmentation was then converted into a surface mesh (STL format), the centerlines of the mesh were calculated, and inlet as well as outlet planes were placed perpendicular to these lines.

There are multiple alternatives to investigating the aneurysms onset. Possibly the most ideal approach is the investigation of de novo aneurysms, as shown with 10 aneurysms in [7]. Often, it is difficult to obtain patient data of a large number of de novo aneurysms; thus, in literature, a retrospective approach is used alternatively, where aneurysms are manually removed from the parent vessel. While this approach may have some limitations compared to the first approach, it is still mostly utilized in literature [8,27,30–34].

In this work, the retrospective approach was utilized, due to the available patient images. The CAD models in the form of the generated STL files of the aneurysms (see Figure 1 left) were modified in a subsequent step by removing the aneurysm sac with the help of a Laplacian smoother algorithm [35–38] in order to obtain the geometry of the parent vessel without the aneurysm sac (see Figure 1 center).

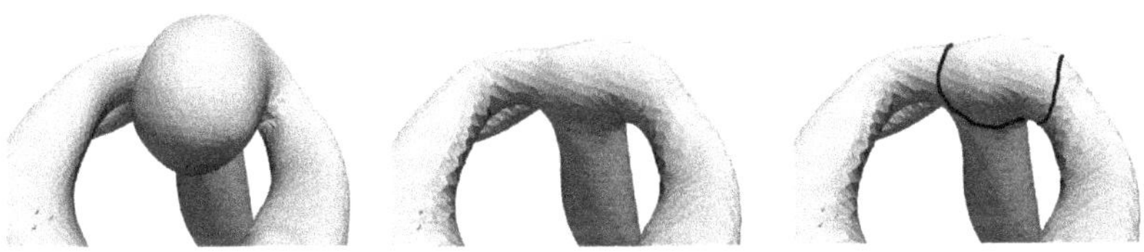

Figure 1. Typical CAD geometry of a cerebral artery, with aneurysm sac (**left**), aneurysm sac removed (**center**), and indicator line of the region of aneurysm onset (RAO, **right**).

In Figure 1, an estimated black line is shown, which indicates the approximate region of aneurysm onset (RAO). This region is important for understanding the initiation process of aneurysm growth.

The generated STL files (both with and without the aneurysm sac) were used to generate the volumetric calculation grid for the FSI simulations. In the first step, the fluid domain was established, and in the second subsequent step, the wall domain was created, with a constant wall thickness of 0.3 mm [22], by extruding and creating a separate vessel wall domain with the given thickness.

2.3. Hemodynamic and Structural Mechanical Modeling

A finite volume solver [39], based on the computational fluid dynamics framework OpenFOAM v2012 [40,41], alongside the fluid–structure interaction library solids4Foam [42], was utilized to numerically solve the unsteady equations of hemodynamics in the simulation process. The models applied the principles of mass and momentum conservation through both the continuity equation and the Navier–Stokes equations. For structural mechanics, Newton's second law was employed. These equations were solved in a sequential manner and were coupled with a fluid–structure interaction (FSI) boundary condition. The details, as well as the experimental validation of the simulation methods, were described in [39].

The fluid dynamic boundary conditions at the inflow were defined by a pulsatile flow profile, characterized by a temporal velocity curve derived from published data [43]. The outflow conditions were set to a time-dependent value defined by experimental pressure measurements [44]. Boundary conditions along the interior vessel walls assumed a no-slip condition. Blood was represented in the model as a Newtonian fluid, with viscosity set at 0.04 poise and a constant density of 1.06 g/cm^3. The simulation lasted for a single cardiac cycle of 1 s, corresponding to a heart rate of 60 beats per minute, discretized into 100 temporal increments ($\Delta t = 0.01$ s).

The vessel walls at the in- and outflow faces were fixed on the solid mechanical side. The vessel wall was assumed to be linear elastic, with a Young's modulus value E of 2490 kPa [45] and a Poisson's ratio ν of 0.49, which assumed an almost incompressible material, as described in [25,46]. Results for this Young's modulus are shown in Figures 2–4. We changed the Young's modulus from the defined value of 2490 kPa from [45] to 5700 and 500 kPa [23], respectively, to assess the influence of vessel wall stiffness.

The investigated parameter of the oscillatory shear index OSI was defined as:

$$OSI = 0.5\left(1 - \frac{\left|\int_0^T \boldsymbol{\tau} dt\right|}{\int_0^T |\boldsymbol{\tau}| dt}\right), \quad (1)$$

where $\boldsymbol{\tau}$ is the wall shear stress.

Investigated cohorts did not show normal distribution; thus, standard deviation was not given, and the significance of the difference between the means was determined with a Mann–Whitney U test (p-values < 0.05).

2.4. Convergence Analysis

In order to guarantee the accuracy of the simulations while maintaining a reasonable simulation runtime, the results of a convergence analysis are presented with the exemplary aneurysm in Figure 1. For this, the following numeric parameters were analyzed:

- Time step independence;
- Calculation mesh convergence;
- Newtonian vs. non-Newtonian fluid;
- One cardiac cycle vs. five cardiac cycles.

Table 1 shows the convergence results, including the required runtime for a simulation. A good time step convergence can be found, and a time step size of 0.01 s was utilized in all simulations, guaranteeing accuracy and also a reasonable simulation runtime.

Table 1. Convergence analysis of time step size and mesh size independence, as well as the influence of the non-Newtonian viscosity model and multiple cardiac cycles. (Base simulation settings consisted of Δt = 0.01 s, Δx = 0.2 mm, 3 solid cells, Newtonian model, and one single cardiac cycle).

	Parameter	WSS [Pa]	OSI [-]	ES [-]	MISES [kPa]	Runtime [s]
Time independence	Δt = 0.1 s	0.083	0.148	0.033	73.54	347
	Δt = 0.01 s	0.085	0.150	0.034	75.41	715
	Δt = 0.001 s	0.086	0.151	0.035	75.43	1872
Fluid mesh convergence	Δx = 0.3 mm	0.080	0.139	0.031	69.84	262
	Δx = 0.25 mm	0.083	0.145	0.033	72.14	426
	Δx = 0.2 mm	0.086	0.150	0.034	75.41	715
	Δx = 0.15 mm	0.088	0.152	0.035	76.11	1592
Solid mesh convergence	2 cells	0.086	0.150	0.032	73.94	578
	3 cells	0.086	0.150	0.034	75.41	715
	4 cells	0.086	0.151	0.034	75.42	1643
Viscosity model	Newtonian	0.085	0.150	0.034	75.41	715
	Non-Newtonian	0.086	0.151	0.034	75.41	727
Number of cardiac cycles	1	0.085	0.150	0.034	75.41	715
	5	0.085	0.150	0.034	75.41	3512

The change in the fluid volume element edge length delivered a good convergence at 0.2 mm. The given values were target values for the meshing algorithm, and due to the irregularity of the geometry, small local deviations were possible.

The change in the solid volume element size was defined by the utilized number of cells over the thickness of the vessel wall; as in all simulations, a constant thickness of 0.3 mm [22] was utilized. Three cells over the thickness offered the best compromise between accuracy and simulation runtime.

The influence of a non-Newtonian viscosity model was also compared to the constant-viscosity approach by utilizing the Carreau–Yasuda model, as presented in [47]. Since the investigated aneurysms were located in arteries, the arterial blood flow with the assumed volume flux from [43] seemed to be dominated by high shear rates, thus resulting in a negligible change in fluid parameters, due to non-Newtonian effects, and no considerable change in structural mechanical parameters.

Since neither fluid nor solid mechanical properties were assumed to be viscoelastic, no time delay was introduced into the simulations. Due to the almost incompressibility of both the fluid as well as the vessel wall material [25,46], no significant differences can be seen when comparing one single cycle to five cycles.

Thus, all simulations were run with the base simulation settings of Δt = 0.01 s, Δx = 0.2 mm, 3 solid cells, constant viscosity, and one single cardiac cycle.

3. Results

3.1. Hemodynamic Scenarios in the Parent Artery and Cerebral Aneurysm

Three different scenarios can be identified (see first and third columns in Figure 2 for behavior without the aneurysm sac).

- In **Scenario A**, a large area with low WSS (<~0.1 Pa) and an increased OSI (>~0.1) was clearly visible.
- In **Scenario B**, high WSS values (i.e., large area with WSS > ~0.5 Pa) were observed, while OSI values remained low (<~0.05).
- In **Scenario C**, an intermediate behavior was observed, where certain parts of the region of aneurysm growth clearly showed low WSS, while other regions displayed high WSS values.

We did not find low WSS/low OSI or high WSS/high OSI scenarios in this study.

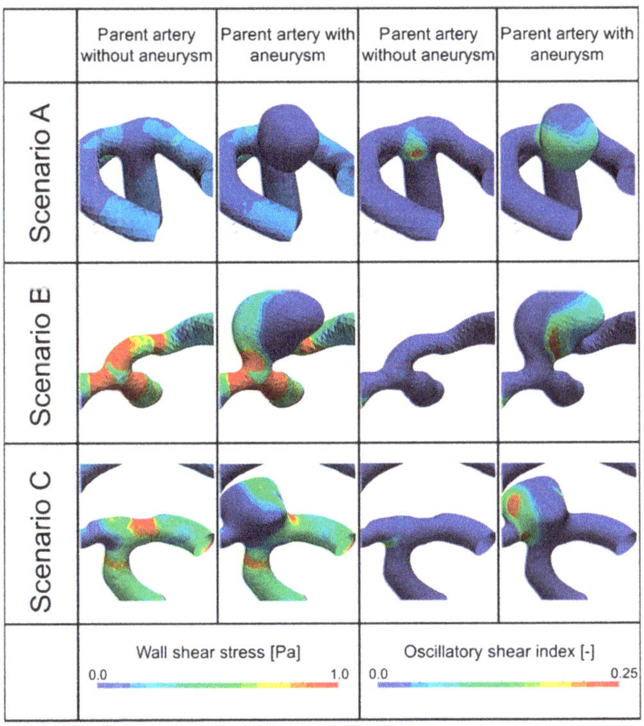

Figure 2. Hemodynamic scenarios. First two columns show the wall shear stress, the first column without the aneurysm sac and the second with the aneurysm sac; third and fourth columns show the oscillatory shear index OSI, the third column without the aneurysm sac and the fourth column with the aneurysm sac.

The results indicated that WSS and the OSI were reciprocally regulated. Table 2 shows the mean values of the three scenarios without an aneurysm sac. All three scenarios exhibited a significant difference ($p < 0.05$ in U-test), with scenario A clearly separating itself from the other two. A smaller yet still significant difference was found between scenarios B and C, with scenario C being in-between the two.

Table 2. Mean values of scenarios A, B, and C, as well as p-values between scenarios without aneurysms.

Young's Modulus		Mean Values			p-Values		
		A	B	C	A vs. B	A vs. C	B vs. C
2490 kPa	WSS [Pa]	0.261	1.772	1.176	1.90×10^{-4}	8.86×10^{-4}	3.82×10^{-2}
	OSI [-]	0.075	0.018	0.03	7.52×10^{-4}	2.88×10^{-3}	4.22×10^{-2}
5700 kPa	WSS [Pa]	0.259	1.768	1.164	1.86×10^{-4}	8.74×10^{-4}	3.73×10^{-2}
	OSI [-]	0.077	0.020	0.032	7.59×10^{-4}	2.92×10^{-3}	4.29×10^{-2}
500 kPa	WSS [Pa]	0.231	1.568	1.040	1.88×10^{-4}	8.81×10^{-4}	3.83×10^{-2}
	OSI [-]	0.084	0.020	0.034	7.56×10^{-4}	2.89×10^{-3}	4.25×10^{-2}

The change in Young's modulus in the structural mechanical part of the simulations from 2490 to 5700 kPa did not affect the hemodynamic part considerably in the geometries without an aneurysm sac. Lowering the value to 500 kPa slightly modified it. Statistical differences between the scenarios remained significant.

In the geometries with aneurysm sacs (second and fourth column in Figure 2), a similar, reciprocally regulated behavior of WSS and the OSI was observed. Additionally, the WSS was lowered, compared to the geometries without an aneurysm sac, approximately by a factor of 5–15, due to the growth of the sac, with an increase in the OSI by a factor of approximately 2–3 in those regions. In Scenario C, the aneurysm sac could be clearly divided into two separate regions, where either WSS was high and the OSI value was low, or vice versa. Aneurysm growth was directed primarily in the direction of low WSS and high OSI in all cases with an aneurysm sac.

Table 3 shows the mean values of aneurysms belonging to the three scenarios for the geometries with an aneurysm sac. A significant difference between the scenarios was evident (all p-values < 0.05). Also, here, Scenario A showed a strong difference compared to scenario B, with scenario C being in-between the two.

Table 3. Mean values of scenarios A, B, and C, as well as p-values between scenarios with aneurysms.

Young's Modulus		Mean Values			p-Values		
		A	B	C	A vs. B	A vs. C	B vs. C
2490 kPa	WSS [Pa]	0.025	0.39	0.193	3.00×10^{-3}	8.54×10^{-4}	1.83×10^{-2}
	OSI [-]	0.154	0.037	0.056	1.23×10^{-2}	3.72×10^{-3}	3.22×10^{-2}
5700 kPa	WSS [Pa]	0.034	0.441	0.243	1.98×10^{-3}	6.37×10^{-4}	1.13×10^{-2}
	OSI [-]	0.113	0.033	0.044	9.54×10^{-3}	2.27×10^{-3}	1.92×10^{-2}
500 kPa	WSS [Pa]	0.016	0.286	0.137	2.87×10^{-3}	7.23×10^{-4}	1.95×10^{-2}
	OSI [-]	0.241	0.050	0.078	1.33×10^{-2}	3.89×10^{-3}	3.12×10^{-2}

The change in Young's modulus from 2490 kPa to the higher value of 5700 kPa increased the average WSS in aneurysms and reduced the OSI. Introducing the lower value of 500 kPa lowered WSS and increased the OSI to a certain degree. Statistical differences between the scenarios remained significant.

Table 4 shows the distribution of scenarios in percentages amongst the patients with and without aneurysms. In geometries without aneurysms, scenarios B and C were more prominent with similar percentages, whereas scenario A was less likely. Strong contrast geometries with aneurysms showed a tendency towards scenario C. The percentage of scenario A was significantly increased, whereas scenario B dropped to approximately 11% of all cases. Despite the change in Young's modulus, all scenarios remained unaltered.

Table 4. Percentage of hemodynamic scenarios with and without aneurysms.

	A	B	C
without aneurysm	22.7%	34.1%	43.2%
with aneurysm	38.6%	11.4%	50.0%

Scenarios A and C did not change due to growth in any of the aneurysms. A very different behavior can be seen in geometries in scenario B. Although this scenario can be maintained in 33.42% of the cases, it can change to scenario A (46.65%), as well as to scenario C (19.93%). (Figure 3 shows illustrative cases).

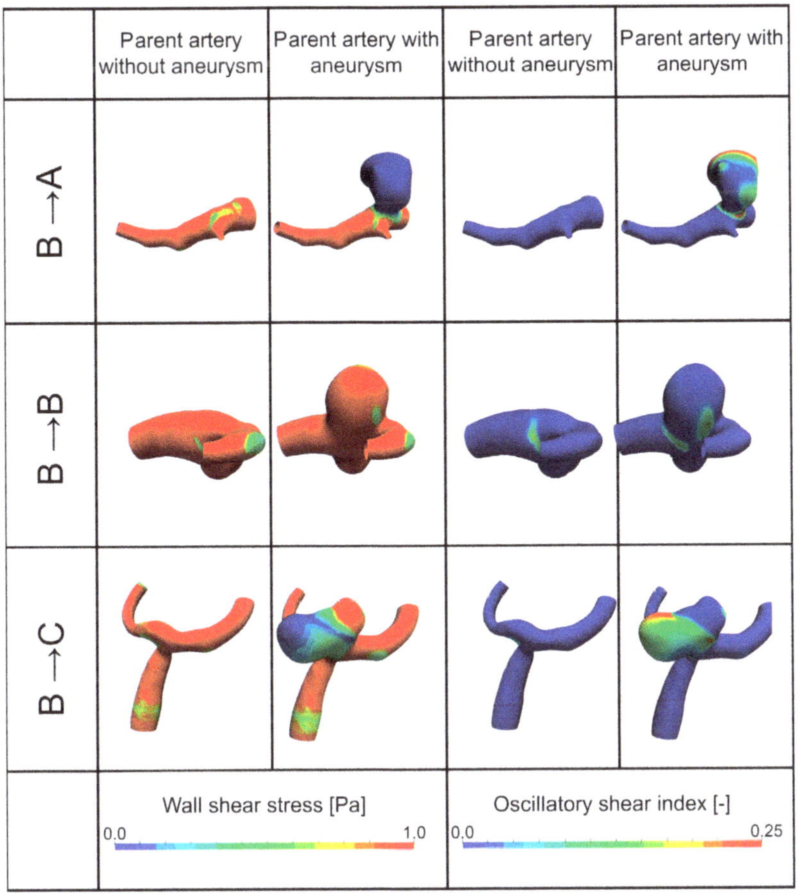

Figure 3. Change in hemodynamic features for scenario B. Individual rows show individual aneurysm geometries (row 1—scenario B to scenario A, row 2—scenario B remains scenario B, row 3—scenario B to scenario C); first two columns show the wall shear stress without the aneurysm sac (first column) and with the aneurysm sac (second column); third and fourth columns show the oscillatory shear index OSI without the aneurysm sac (third column) and with the aneurysm sac (fourth column).

3.2. Structural Mechanical Scenarios in the Parent Artery and Cerebral Aneurysm

Two scenarios (D and E) can be identified in the structural mechanical results; however, these scenarios did not fully correspond to the hemodynamic ones (A, B, and C). Thus, structural mechanics and hemodynamics were not directly correlated.

- **Scenario D** was characterized by regions with elevated equivalent wall stresses (MISES) (i.e., areas > ~70 kPa visible; see Figure 4, first row).
- **Scenario E** indicated regions with low equivalent wall stresses (i.e., areas mostly < ~50 kPa) in both the region of aneurysm onset and the aneurysm wall (see Figure 4, second row).

The aneurysm in the third row of Figure 4 showed a mixed behavior, where the parent vessel without a sac was characterized mostly by scenario E and the configuration with a sac by scenario D.

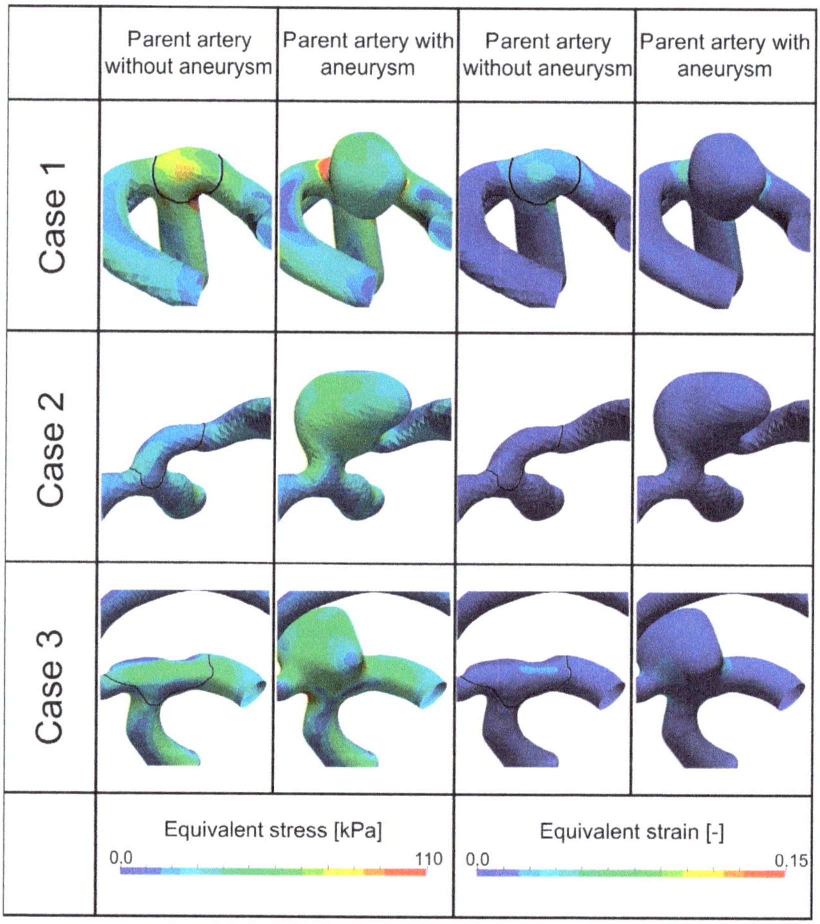

Figure 4. Structural dynamic features. The first two columns show the equivalent stress, first column without the aneurysm sac and the second column with the aneurysm sac; the third and fourth columns show the equivalent strain, the third column without the aneurysm sac and the fourth column with the aneurysm sac.

Equivalent strain values were relatively low (<0.1 [23]) in all geometries (except the simulation with low Young's modulus; see model limitations for more details). Tables 5 and 6 show the mean values of geometries without and with an aneurysm sac, respectively. The statistical difference in the conducted U-test was significant. There was increased stress, as well as strain, due to aneurysm growth.

Table 5. Mean values of scenarios D and E, as well as p-values between scenarios without aneurysms.

Young's Modulus		Mean Values		p-Value
		D	E	D vs. E
2490 kPa	MISES [kPa]	76.5	45.8	1.27×10^{-3}
	ES [-]	0.033	0.019	4.14×10^{-3}
5700 kPa	MISES [kPa]	77.3	46.3	1.65×10^{-3}
	ES [-]	0.014	0.008	4.89×10^{-3}
500 kPa	MISES [kPa]	77.0	46.2	1.33×10^{-3}
	ES [-]	0.167	0.095	4.43×10^{-3}

Table 6. Mean values of scenarios D and E, as well as p-values between scenarios with aneurysms.

Young's Modulus		Mean Values		p-Value
		D	E	D vs. E
2490 kPa	MISES [kPa]	83.6	49.0	1.55×10^{-4}
	ES [-]	0.103	0.046	1.38×10^{-3}
5700 kPa	MISES [kPa]	84.2	49.3	2.67×10^{-4}
	ES [-]	0.043	0.019	3.39×10^{-3}
500 kPa	MISES [kPa]	83.9	49.1	1.94×10^{-4}
	ES [-]	0.515	0.23	1.77×10^{-3}

The change in Young's modulus (see Tables 5 and 6) did not change the mean stress considerably, as due to the workflow in FSI, the force of the blood exerted by the blood pressure upon the vessel wall remained constant; however, the strain changed according to the linear material low in a mostly linear fashion.

The results suggested a certain dynamic between the two scenarios. In geometries without aneurysms, scenario E with lowered stress values was more prominent (see Table 7), whereas the initiation of an aneurysm clearly showed an increase in stress towards scenario D. Some Scenario E aneurysms (11.4%) remained in this scenario; however, most changed to scenario D. None of the geometries showed a decrease in stress after aneurysm growth (i.e., no change from scenario D towards E).

Table 7. Percentage of structural mechanic scenarios with and without aneurysms.

	D	E
without aneurysm	43.2%	56.8%
with aneurysm	88.6%	11.4%

4. Discussion

4.1. Hemodynamics

The role of WSS in the aneurysm initiation process has recently been discussed, with divergent results [9]. Kulcsar and Meng suggested that the combination of high WSS and high positive spatial WSS gradient (WSSG) might play a role in aneurysm formation [9,12]. According to Fujimura, the aneurysmal initiation area may correspond to the highest WSS divergence (WSSD point) [7]. Zimny et al. analyzed hemodynamic changes in patients with MCA aneurysms and postulated that a higher WSS may impact aneurysm formation, whereas WSSG may promote this process [8].

In this study, using the distribution of WSS, as well as the OSI, the main hemodynamic processes of aneurysm initiation could be identified. Scenario B resembled patterns identified in previously published studies [9]. Scenario A clearly showed low WSS values in the RAO, along with high OSI values. Interestingly, in this work, additional aneurysms with a complex hemodynamic behavior were presented in-between, as illustrated in Scenario C; certain parts of the region of aneurysm growth clearly showed low WSS values, and other regions showed high WSS values. However, we did not observe a specific low WSS/low OSI or high WSS/high OSI scenario.

Aneurysm initiation has been considered to be partially dependent on chronic inflammation in the vascular wall [7]. Our results may indicate that these processes might be triggered by high WSS conditions, as well as high OSI conditions. However, WSS and the OSI seem to be reciprocally regulated in this stage of the disease. Similarly, for aneurysm growth, Meng et al. postulated the "high-versus-low wall shear stress" controversy, indicating the complexity of this disease. Our results seem to suggest that one of these alternatives in one aneurysm does not rule the other out in another one. While low WSS may be associated with an inflammatory cell-mediated pathway, high WSS may lead to a mural cell-mediated pathology. Both pathways may trigger aneurysm growth and rupture [9]. However, our results suggest that these two pathways may play a role in aneurysm initiation and can coexist.

The investigation revealed a significant dynamic between identified scenarios. WSS did not increase in any of the investigated geometries but decreased after aneurysm initiation. The only change occurred in scenario B, where WSS levels were either maintained (scenario B→B in Figure 3), lowered (scenario B→A in Figure 3), or partially lowered (scenario B→C in Figure 3). Again, the OSI was regulated in an inverse way. Aneurysms with low WSS and a high OSI (scenario A) did not change this behavior due to aneurysm initiation, and a mixed distribution of WSS and OSI (scenario C) was maintained after the start of growth. Our results provide evidence that the inflammatory cell-mediated pathway with low WSS and a high OSI might be the more dominant one during aneurysm initiation.

The analysis of vessel wall stiffness (three different Young's moduli) strengthened our analysis. Changing the value from 2490 kPa [45] to the maximum value of 5700 kPa in [23] did not influence the hemodynamic behavior. Lowering the value to the lowest reported stiffness in [23] resulted in small changes; however, the identified behavior and dynamics of scenarios did not change.

4.2. Structural Mechanics

The structural mechanical behavior of the vessel and aneurysm wall appeared to be independent of the hemodynamics, showing two different scenarios (D and E). Although scenario D showed elevated stress values (>70–100 kPa), the stress level was still far away from the critical value of 421 kPa, as determined in [38], where rupture could be estimated. Similarly, in the other scenario with even lower stress values, rupture may not be expected.

Aneurysm initiation induced stress in the vessel wall in more than half of the investigated geometries. With the addition of cases with already elevated stress from the start, aneurysm initiation and growth clearly placed additional stress onto the vessel tissue rather than relieving it.

The ES in the geometries without and with an aneurysm sac were below 0.1. Cho et al. [23] provided a critical ES threshold value of 0.3, which was not reached in any of the geometries (with the exception of the simulations at a low Young's modulus and with an aneurysm sac; see model limitations). In hemodynamics, while the decreased pathway of wall shear stress seemed to be the more dominant one, in the vessel wall, stresses and strains seemed to increase due to aneurysm growth. Since both stress and strain values were significantly below the critical thresholds, as identified in [23,38], respectively, increasing the structural mechanical quantities could be considered a compromise in favor of the preferable reduction in WSS and increase in the OSI in hemodynamics.

The influence of stiffness can be clearly seen in the change in the equivalent strain. By changing the Young's modulus, the strain changed accordingly in an almost linear fashion. Stress values did not change, as they were defined by the FSI workflow via the force exerted by the blood pressure onto the vessel wall, which remained constant. The small change in strain for the geometries without an aneurysm sac resulted in a negligible or very small change in hemodynamics (see Tables 2 and 5). The increased change in strain for the geometries with aneurysms resulted in a corresponding increased modification in hemodynamics (see Tables 3 and 6). However, these changes could only be seen in the mean values, and the scenarios and their dynamics still remained unaltered.

Both the behaviors in stress and strain underline the fact that none of the aneurysms ruptured in reality. However, our results suggest that aneurysm initiation and growth are mainly associated with a reduction in WSS, along with an increase in stress in the vessel wall.

4.3. Model Limitations

Our investigation had certain limitations due to uncertainties in input data, which had to be approximated with certain assumptions. The assumption was made that during aneurysm development, the main shape of the artery does not change considerably (e.g., angle of outflow arteries, etc.). In the FSI simulations, an assumption regarding fixing the geometry must be made. Here, the blood vessel was fixed at the ends of the inflow vessel, as well as the outflow vessels. This does not correspond to real life, as the blood vessels are connected to other vessels. Additionally, the investigated parts may be in contact with parts of brain tissue as well. This contact was neglected in the simulations.

Parent vessels without aneurysms were created by manually removing the sac. Thus, this manual removal introduced a degree of subjective error. Therefore, extra attention was paid during aneurysm removal to minimize such subjective user error.

For the generation of the investigated scenarios, only unruptured but treated aneurysms were considered to avoid the influence of the change in shape due to rupture. In the next step, the influence of ruptured aneurysms will be investigated.

In this work, a constant vessel wall thickness of 0.3 mm was assumed [22]. This topic is currently under investigation, and further studies on wall thickness are needed in future steps to advance toward a more reliable description of aneurysm behavior.

Simulations with an aneurysm sac with the lowest reported value of Young's modulus in [23] showed increased strain values of >0.5, where the limits of the utilized linear elastic model were reached. This stiffness was considered to be a worst-case scenario for blood vessels. In future investigations, a non-linear approach will be utilized to better describe the material behavior at high strain values.

The data for the pulsatile blood flow was taken from experimental data found in the literature [36]. In experiments, systematic errors occur, which add additional uncertainty into the simulations. Since there was no information on the material properties for the tissues of the individual investigated aneurysms in this work, an assumption from literature was made for the Young's modulus of the material.

5. Conclusions

Our simulations suggest that hemodynamics, through the reciprocal regulation of WSS and OSI, are closely associated with aneurysm initiation and growth. Hemodynamics and structural mechanics appear to present separate and independent scenarios, with two hemodynamic scenarios remaining stable during growth, while the third showed a tendency towards change. Structural mechanics indicate increases in stress and strain as a result of aneurysm growth. It is important to note that our analysis was limited to unruptured aneurysms, which presents a limitation in fully understanding the rupture risk. Further, although 44 patients were carefully analyzed, we need to confirm these results in a prospective multi-center investigation. However, we believe our findings provide a solid foundation for future research aimed at predicting aneurysm rupture risk by considering their morphology, hemodynamics, and structural mechanics.

Author Contributions: Conceptualization: J.N. and M.G.; methodology: J.N., M.G., W.F., V.M.M., V.M., S.T., J.M., H.S., J.O., N.S. and P.-R.R.; data collection: M.G., W.F., V.M.M., V.M., S.T., H.S., J.O., N.S. and P.-R.R.; formal analysis and investigation: J.N. and M.G.; writing: J.N. and M.G.; funding acquisition: J.N., M.G., Z.M. and A.G.; resources: J.N., M.G., W.F., V.M.M., V.M., S.T., J.M., H.S., J.O., N.S. and P.-R.R.; supervision: J.N., M.G., Z.M. and A.G. All authors have read and agreed to the published version of the manuscript.

Funding: This work was supported by research subsidies granted by the government of Upper Austria via the Forschungsförderungsgesellschaft (Austrian Research Promotion Agency) [grant number 872604 (Project MEDUSA) and FO999895610 (Project ARES)]. RISC Software GmbH is a member of UAR (Upper Austrian Research) Innovation Network.

Institutional Review Board Statement: This study was approved by the local ethics committee (Ethikkommission der medizinischen Fakultät der Johannes Kepler Universität; EK Nr: 1129/2022), and the requirement for the acquisition of informed consent from patients was waived, owing to the retrospective nature of the research.

Informed Consent Statement: The requirement for the acquisition of informed consent from patients was waived, owing to the retrospective nature of the research.

Data Availability Statement: The data are not publicly available due to the fact that authors want to keep patient data private, however data can be made available upon request.

Conflicts of Interest: Author Jozsef Nagy was employed by the company eulerian-solutions e.U., Authors Wolfgang Fenz, Stefan Thumfart were employed by the company RISC Software GmbH. All authors certify that they have no affiliations with or involvement in any organization or entity with any financial interest (such as honoraria; educational grants; participation in speakers' bureaus; membership, employment, consultancies, stock ownership, or other equity interest; and expert testimony or patent-licensing arrangements) or non-financial interest (such as personal or professional relationships, affiliations, knowledge, or beliefs) in the subject matter or materials discussed in this manuscript. Generative AI was not used in the process of scientific writing.

References

1. Dhar, S.; Tremmel, M.; Mocco, J.; Kim, M.; Yamamoto, J.; Siddiqui, A.H.; Hopkins, L.N.; Meng, H. Morphology parameters for intracranial aneurysm rupture risk assessment. *Neurosurgery* **2008**, *63*, 185–197. [CrossRef] [PubMed]
2. Hackenberg, K.; Hänggi, D.; Etminan, N. Unruptured intracranial aneurysms contemporary data and management. *Stroke* **2018**, *49*, 2268–2275. [CrossRef] [PubMed]
3. Jirjees, S.; Htun, Z.M.; Aldawudi, I.; Katwal, P.C.; Khan, S. Role of Morphological and Hemodynamic Factors in Predicting Intracranial Aneurysm Rupture: A Review. *Cureus* **2020**, *12*, e9178. [CrossRef] [PubMed]
4. Detmer, F.J.; Chung, B.J.; Mut, F.; Pritz, M.; Slawski, M.; Hamzei-Sichani, F.; Kallmes, D.; Putman, C.; Jimenez, C.; Cebral, J.R. Development of a statistical model for discrimination of rupture status in posterior communicating artery aneurysms. *Acta Neurochir.* **2018**, *160*, 1643–1652. [CrossRef]
5. Jiang, P.; Liu, Q.; Wu, J.; Chen, X.; Li, M.; Li, Z.; Yang, S.; Guo, R.; Gao, B.; Cao, Y.; et al. A Novel Scoring System for Rupture Risk Stratification of Intracranial Aneurysms: A Hemodynamic and Morphological Study. *Front Neurosci.* **2018**, *12*, 596. [CrossRef]
6. Soldozy, S.; Norat, P.; Elsarrag, M.; Chatrath, A.; Costello, J.S.; Sokolowski, J.D.; Tvrdik, P.; Kalani, M.Y.S.; Park, M.S. The biophysical role of hemodynamics in the pathogenesis of cerebral aneurysm formation and rupture. *Neurosurg. Focus.* **2019**, *47*, E11. [CrossRef]
7. Fujimura, S.; Tanaka, K.; Takao, H.; Okudaira, T.; Koseki, H.; Hasebe, A.; Suzuki, T.; Uchiyama, Y.; Ishibashi, T.; Otani, K.; et al. Computational fluid dynamic analysis of the initiation of cerebral aneurysms. *J. Neurosurg.* **2022**, *137*, 335–343. [CrossRef]
8. Zimny, M.; Kawlewska, E.; Hebda, A.; Wolański, W.; Ładziński, P.; Kaspera, W. Wall shear stress gradient is independently associated with middle cerebral artery aneurysm development: A case-control CFD patient-specific study based on 77 patients. *BMC Neurol.* **2021**, *21*, 281. [CrossRef] [PubMed]
9. Meng, H.; Tutino, V.M.; Xiang, J.; Siddiqui, A. High WSS or Low WSS? Complex Interactions of Hemodynamics with Intracranial Aneurysm Initiation, Growth, and Rupture: Toward a Unifying Hypothesis. *AJNR Am. J. Neuroradiol.* **2014**, *35*, 1254–1262. [CrossRef]
10. Rajabzadeh-Oghaz, H.; Siddiqui, A.H.; Asadollahi, A.; Kolega, J.; Tutino, V.M. The association between hemodynamics and wall characteristics in human intracranial aneurysms: A review. *Neurosurg. Rev.* **2022**, *45*, 49–61. [CrossRef]
11. Villablanca, J.P.; Duckwiler, G.R.; Jahan, R.; Tateshima, S.; Martin, N.A.; Frazee, J.; Gonzalez, N.R.; Sayre, J.; Vinuela, F.V. Natural history of asymptomatic unruptured cerebral aneurysms evaluated at CT angiography: Growth and rupture incidence and correlation with epidemiologic risk factors. *Neuroradiology* **2013**, *269*, 258–265. [CrossRef] [PubMed]

12. Kulcsár, Z.; Ugron, A.; Marosfői, M.; Berentei, Z.; Paál, G.; Szikora, I. Hemodynamics of cerebral aneurysm initiation: The role of wall shear stress and spatial wall shear stress gradient. *AJNR Am. J. Neuroradiol.* **2011**, *32*, 587–594. [CrossRef]
13. Xiang, J.; Natarajan, S.K.; Tremmel, M.; Ma, D.; Mocco, J.; Hopkins, L.N.; Siddiqui, A.H.; Levy, E.I.; Meng, H. Hemodynamic-morphologic discriminants for intracranial aneurysm rupture. *Stroke* **2011**, *42*, 144–152. [CrossRef] [PubMed]
14. Jou, L.D.; Lee, D.H.; Morsi, H.; Mawad, M. Wall shear stress on ruptured and unruptured intracranial aneurysms at the internal carotid artery. *AJNR Am. J. Neuroradiol.* **2008**, *29*, 1761–1767. [CrossRef] [PubMed]
15. Shojima, M.; Oshima, M.; Takagi, K.; Torii, R.; Hayakawa, M.; Katada, K.; Morita, A.; Kirino, T. Magnitude and role of wall shear stress on cerebral aneurysm: Computational fluid dynamic study of 20 middle cerebral artery aneurysms. *Stroke* **2004**, *35*, 2500–2505. [CrossRef]
16. Boussel, L.; Rayz, V.; McCulloch, C.; Martin, A.; Acevedo-Bolton, G.; Lawton, M.; Higashida, R.; Smith, W.S.; Young, W.L.; Saloner, D. Aneurysm growth occurs at region of low wall shear stress: Patient-specific correlation of hemodynamics and growth in a longitudinal study. *Stroke* **2008**, *39*, 2997–3002. [CrossRef]
17. Acevedo-Bolton, G.; Jou, L.-D.; Dispensa, B.P.; Lawton, M.T.; Higashida, R.T.; Martin, A.J.; Young, W.L.; Saloner, D. Estimating the hemodynamic impact of interventional treatments of aneurysms: Numerical simulation with experimental validation: Technical case report. *Neurosurgery* **2006**, *59*, E429–E430. [CrossRef] [PubMed]
18. Castro, M.A.; Putman, C.M.; Sheridan, M.J.; Cebral, J.R. Hemodynamic patterns of anterior communicating artery aneurysms: A possible association with rupture. *AJNR Am. J. Neuroradiol.* **2009**, *30*, 297–302. [CrossRef]
19. Qian, Y.; Takao, H.; Umezu, M.; Murayama, Y. Risk analysis of unruptured aneurysms using computational fluid dynamics technology: Preliminary results. *AJNR Am. J. Neuroradiol.* **2011**, *32*, 1948–1955. [CrossRef]
20. Sugiyama, S.-I.; Meng, H.; Funamoto, K.; Inoue, T.; Fujimura, M.; Nakayama, T.; Omodaka, S.; Shimizu, H.; Takahashi, A.; Tominaga, T. Hemodynamic analysis of growing intracranial aneurysms arising from a posterior inferior cerebellar artery. *World Neurosurg.* **2012**, *78*, 462–468. [CrossRef]
21. Takao, H.; Murayama, Y.; Otsuka, S.; Qian, Y.; Mohamed, A.; Masuda, S.; Yamamoto, M.; Abe, T. Hemodynamic differences between unruptured and ruptured intracranial aneurysms during observation. *Stroke* **2012**, *43*, 1436–1439. [CrossRef] [PubMed]
22. Acosta, J.M.; Cayron, A.F.; Dupuy, N.; Pelli, G.; Foglia, B.; Haemmerli, J.; Allémann, E.; Bijlenga, P.; Kwak, B.R.; Morel, S. Effect of Aneurysm and Patient Characteristics on Intracranial Aneurysm Wall Thickness. *Front. Cardiovasc. Med.* **2021**, *8*, 775307. [CrossRef] [PubMed]
23. Cho, C.K.; Yang, H.; Kim, J.J.; Oh, J.H.; Kim, Y.B. Prediction of rupture risk in cerebral aneurysms by comparing clinical cases with fluid–structure interaction analyses. *Sci. Rep.* **2020**, *10*, 18237. [CrossRef] [PubMed]
24. Gasser, T.C.; Auer, M.; Labruto, F.; Swedenborg, J.; Roy, J. Biomechanical rupture risk assessment of abdominal aortic aneurysms: Model complexity versus predictability of finite element simulations. *Eur. J. Vasc. Endovasc. Surg.* **2010**, *40*, 176–185. [CrossRef] [PubMed]
25. Reeps, C.; Gee, M.; Maier, A.; Gurdan, M.; Eckstein, H.H.; Wall, W.A. The impact of model assumptions on results of computational mechanics in abdominal aortic aneurysm. *J. Vasc. Surg.* **2010**, *51*, 679–688. [CrossRef]
26. Rissland, P.; Alemu, Y.; Einav, S.; Ricotta, J.; Bluestein, D. Abdominal aortic aneurysm risk of rupture: Patient-specific FSI simulations using anisotropic model. *J. Biomech. Eng.* **2009**, *131*, 031001. [CrossRef]
27. Huang, Z.; Zeng, M.; Tao, W.G.; Zeng, F.Y.; Chen, C.Q.; Zhang, L.B.; Chen, F.H. A Hemodynamic Mechanism Correlating with the Initiation of MCA Bifurcation Aneurysms. *Am. J. Neuroradiol.* **2020**, *41*, 1217–1224. [CrossRef]
28. Bergman, T.L.; Lavine, A.S.; Incropera, F.P.; De Witt, D.P. *Fundamentals of Heat and Mass Transfer*; John Wiley & Sons: Hoboken, NJ, USA, 2018; ISBN 978-1-119-35388-1.
29. Çengel, Y.A.; Cimbala, J.M. *Fluid Mechanics: Fundamentals and Applications*, 4th ed.; McGraw-Hill Higher Education: Boston, MA, USA, 2019; ISBN 978-9-813-15788-0.
30. Guo, H.; Liu, J.F.; Li, C.H.; Wang, J.W.; Li, H.; Gao, B.L. Greater hemodynamic stresses initiate aneurysms on major cerebral arterial bifurcations. *Front. Neurol.* **2023**, *14*, 1265484. [CrossRef]
31. Guo, H.; Yang, S.T.; Wang, J.W.; Li, H.; Gao, B.L.; Li, C.H. High hemodynamic stresses induce aneurysms at internal carotid artery bends. *Medicine* **2023**, *102*, e34587. [CrossRef]
32. Geers, A.J.; Morales, H.G.; Larrabide, I.; Butakoff, C.; Bijlenga, P.; Frangi, A.F. Wall shear stress at the initiation site of cerebral aneurysms. *Biomech. Model. Mechanobiol.* **2017**, *16*, 97–115. [CrossRef]
33. Mantha, A.R.; Karmonik, C.; Benndorf, G.; Strother, C.; Metcalfe, R.W. Hemodynamics in a cerebral artery before and after the formation of an aneurysm. *Am. J. Neuroradiol.* **2006**, *27*, 1113–1118. [PubMed]
34. Baek, H.; Jayaraman, M.V.; Karniadakis, G.E. Wall shear stress and pressure distribution on aneurysms and infundibulae in the posterior communicating artery bifurcation. *Ann. Biomed. Eng.* **2009**, *37*, 2469–2487. [CrossRef] [PubMed]
35. Castro, M.A.; Putman, C.M.; Cebral, J.R. Computational analysis of anterior communicating artery aneurysm shear stress before and after aneurysm formation. *J. Phys. Conf. Ser.* **2011**, *332*, 012001. [CrossRef]
36. Lauric, A.; Hippelheuser, J.; Safain, M.G.; Malek, A.M. Curvature effect on hemodynamic conditions at the inner bend of the carotid siphon and its relation to aneurysm formation. *J. Biomech.* **2014**, *47*, 3018–3027. [CrossRef]
37. Shimogonya, Y.; Ishikawa, T.; Imai, Y.; Matsuki, N.; Yamaguchi, T. Can temporal fluctuation in spatial wall shear stress gradient initiate a cerebral aneurysm? A proposed novel hemodynamic index, the gradient oscillatory number (GON). *J. Biomech.* **2009**, *42*, 550–554. [CrossRef]

38. Cebral, J.R.; Sheridan, M.; Putman, C.M. Hemodynamics and bleb formation in intracranial aneurysms. *AJNR Am. J. Neuroradiol.* **2010**, *31*, 304–310. [CrossRef]
39. Nagy, J.; Maier, J.; Miron, V.; Fenz, W.; Major, Z.; Gruber, A.; Gmeiner, M. Methods, Validation and Clinical Implementation of a Simulation Method of Cerebral Aneurysms. *J. Biomed. Eng. Biosci.* **2023**, *10*, 10–19. [CrossRef]
40. Weller, H.G.; Tabor, G.; Jasak, H.; Fureby, C. A tensorial approach to computational continuum mechanics using object orientated techniques. *Comput. Phys.* **1998**, *12*, 620–631. [CrossRef]
41. Greenshields, C.J.; Weller, H.G. *Notes on Computational Fluid Dynamics: General Principles*; CFD Direct: Reading, UK, 2022; ISBN 978-1-3999-2078-0.
42. Cardiff, P.; Karač, A.; Jaeger, P.D.; Jasak, H.; Nagy, J.; Ivanković, A.; Tuković, Ž. An open-source finite volume toolbox for solid mechanics and fluid-solid interaction simulations. *arXiv* **2018**, arXiv:1808.10736v2. Available online: https://arxiv.org/abs/1808.10736 (accessed on 20 September 2024).
43. Blanco, P.; Müller, L.; Spence, J.D. Blood pressure gradients in cerebral arteries: A clue to pathogenesis of cerebral small vessel disease. *Stroke Vasc. Neurol.* **2017**, *2*, 108–117. [CrossRef]
44. Lorenzetti, F.; Suominen, S.; Tukianen, E. Evaluation of Blood Flow in Free Microvascular Flaps. *J. Reconstr. Microsurg.* **2001**, *17*, 163–167. [CrossRef] [PubMed]
45. Tóth, B.K. The Mechanical Interaction between the Red Blood Cells and the Blood Vessels. Ph.D. Thesis, University of Budapest, Budapest, Hungary, 2011.
46. Di Martino, E.S.; Guadagni, G.; Fumero, A.; Ballerini, G.; Spirito, R.; Biglioli, P.; Redaelli, A. Fluid-structure interaction within realistic three-dimensional models of the aneurysmatic aorta as a guidance to assess the risk of rupture of the aneurysm. *Med. Eng. Phys.* **2001**, *23*, 647–655. [CrossRef] [PubMed]
47. Lynch, S.; Nama, N.; Figueroa, C.A. Effects of non-Newtonian viscosity on arterial and venous flow and transport. *Sci. Rep.* **2022**, *12*, 20568. [CrossRef] [PubMed]

brain sciences

MDPI

Review

Characterizing the Microenvironment of Cerebral Arteriovenous Malformations to Test Novel Treatment Modalities

Kavin Wazhi [†], Fred C. Lam [†], Santosh Guru, Yusuke S. Hori, Deyaldeen AbuReesh, Lorelei Shoemaker, David J. Park and Steven D. Chang *

Department of Neurosurgery, Stanford University School of Medicine, Stanford, CA 94305, USA; kavin_wazhi@brown.edu (K.W.); fredlam@stanford.edu (F.C.L.); sg928@cam.ac.uk (S.G.); yshori@stanford.edu (Y.S.H.); abureesh@stanford.edu (D.A.); lshoe@stanford.edu (L.S.); djpark@stanford.edu (D.J.P.)

* Correspondence: sdchang@stanford.edu

† These authors contributed equally to this work.

Abstract

Brain arteriovenous malformations (bAVMs) consist of a tangled nidus of abnormal dilated vessels characterized by direct connections between arteries and veins that lack an intervening capillary bed, creating a high-to-low flow pressure system that is predisposed to spontaneous hemorrhage with significant associated neurologic morbidity and mortality. Treatment options for bAVMs include the following: surgical resection, intravascular embolization to obliterate blood flow through the AVM, and radiosurgery. Understanding the molecular mechanisms of bAVM formation and factors that predispose it to hemorrhage can lead to novel treatments that can improve the prognosis for patients. This review summarizes emerging insights into the complex and dynamic molecular mechanisms of bAVMs. Dysregulation in key VEGF, TGF-β/BMP9/10–ENG–ALK1–SMAD4, Notch, and MAPK/ERK signaling pathways drive abnormal angiogenesis in both syndromic and sporadic forms, with KRAS/BRAF/MAPK21 mutations specifically linked to the latter. Advances in bAVM-induced animal models have corroborated many of the genetic profiles found in humans, and they continue to provide novel insights into bAVM mechanisms. Collectively, these mechanistic findings are guiding translational advances, with targeted therapies and liquid biopsy approaches emerging as avenues for precision treatment and improved patient outcomes.

Keywords: brain arteriovenous malformations; radiosurgery; embolization; neurosurgery; organoids; animal models

1. Introduction

Brain arteriovenous malformations (bAVMs) are rare arteriovenous shunts, resulting from abnormal connections between cerebral arteries and veins that form a central nidus [1]. The prevalence of bAVMs is estimated to be approximately 10 to 18 per 100,000 adults [2,3]. The most common symptomatic manifestations of bAVM are intracranial hemorrhages followed closely by seizures; 11% of intracranial hemorrhages have a one-month case fatality while there is an approximate 8% risk of seizures five years post-diagnosis [1]. These risk factors make it critical to efficiently and effectively treat bAVMs. Current standard of care options to treat bAVMs include the following: microsurgery, embolization, and stereotactic radiosurgery (SRS) [4]. Each of these treatment options has its own series of risks and benefits in terms of patient experience and post-treatment outcomes.

Microsurgery ensures a high chance of bAVM obliteration coupled with low post-op hemorrhage occurrence with rates of 96% and 0.18% per 100 person-years, respectively [1]. However, microsurgery mandates an open craniotomy, requiring the bAVM to be in an area with an appropriate access corridor; microsurgery is also typically associated with longer hospital stays and recovery. The alternative option of vascular embolization provides far more flexibility in its use by combining various treatment modalities to achieve safer obliteration in certain cases. Lone embolization results in a lower rate of obliteration at 13% per 100 person-years, with neurological complications and hemorrhages occurring at rates of 6.6% and 1.7% per 100 person-years, respectively [1]. SRS, on the whole, tends to garner results in between that of microsurgery and embolization, with an obliteration rate and hemorrhage rate of 38% per 100 person-years and 1.7%, respectively [5]. A benefit of SRS is its minimal invasiveness and convenience for patients, but there is a latency period where the bAVM is not obliterated post-SRS, resulting in hemorrhage risk. Given these accumulated risks, there is an unmet need to gain a deeper understanding of the interactions within the microenvironment of bAVMs that predispose bAVMs to hemorrhage and rebleeding, as a means to develop strategies to reduce rupture risk.

Brain AVMs were traditionally thought to be congenital lesions arising from aberrant vasculogenesis during the fourth and eighth weeks of gestation. However, there have been few reported cases of fetal bAVMs, and with noted recurrence after surgical resection and remodeling over time [6,7], as well as reports of post-traumatic [8] and post-infectious bAVMs [9]. These observations suggest more dynamic and complex mechanisms at play. Similarly, there exists a "second hit" hypothesis, in which patients develop bAVMs after cerebral aneurysm occlusion, SRS treatments, hemorrhagic strokes, the growth of brain tumors, or encephalitic demyelinating lesions, further exemplifying the dynamic interactions between the local microenvironment of the brain that trigger bAVM formation [10]. We herein review the current understanding of the molecular biology driving bAVM formation, the signaling pathways and genes that are affected that lead to bAVM hemorrhage, and the novel therapeutic avenues of research that intend to decrease hemorrhage risk.

2. The Physiology of Brain Arteriovenous Malformation Formation

2.1. Angiogenesis

A recently published single-cell atlas, comparing normal human brain vasculature compared to surgically resected human bAVMs, reported differential gene expression across 15 major cell populations [11]. Similarly to previously published gene signatures, the study identified enriched vascular cell signatures, including the following: endothelial cells (*CLDN5*), pericytes (*KCNJ8*), smooth muscle cells (*MYH11*), and perivascular fibroblasts (*DCN*). The study also identified differential gene expression signatures to the following four arteriovenous segments: arteries, capillaries, venues, and veins. Brain AVM endothelial cells (ECs) were enriched in *TXNIP*, a regulator of glucose metabolism and oxidative stress [12], reflecting the increased metabolic state of bAVM arterial endothelial cells. Other genes that were enriched in human endothelial AVM zonations included *VEGF* in the arteries, *MFSD2A* in the capillaries, and *ACKR1* in the veins [13–15]. Taken together, this study identified distinct, conserved clusters of genes in the endothelial arteriovenous zonations in human bAVMs.

Data from animal and human studies support dysregulated angiogenesis as playing a role in the formation of bAVMs. Human bAVM ECs have upregulation of the VEGF and TGFβ pathways, and increased EC turnover. The localized injection of adeno-associated viral vector expressing *VEGF* (*AAV-VEGF*) into the brains of adult transgenic mice deficient in *Eng* or *Acvrl* induced focal angiogenesis, while the embryonic deletion of *Eng* caused postnatal formation of brain, spinal cord, and intestinal AVMs [16]. Endoglin expression was found in the endothelium and adventitial layer of arteries and arterioles, with expression in the mesenchymal cells of the adventitia and perivascular connective tissue in the arterialized veins of sporadic human bAVMs [17]. However, unlike hereditary hemorrhagic telangiectasia (HHT) type 1 bAVMs, in which endoglin expression is reduced, levels of endoglin were found to be normal with increased numbers of endoglin-positive endothelial and adventitial cells. Endoglin expression was also seen in fibroblasts in the perivascular stroma, suggesting an active role in vascular remodeling in response to increased blood flow and shear stress [17]. In addition, an intronic variant of *ACVRL-1*, IVS3-35A>G has been found to be associated with bAVMs [18,19], further implicating the TGFβ pathway in the physiology of bAVM formation.

2.2. *Pathophysiology of Syndromic-Related Brain Arteriovenous Malformations*

2.2.1. Hereditary Hemorrhagic Telangiectasias

The majority of bAVMs are sporadic, with only approximately 5% of patients associated with genetic syndromes, such as hereditary hemorrhagic telangiectasia (HHT) and/or capillary malformations-arteriovenous malformations (CM-AVM) [20]. HHT (also known as Osler–Weber–Rendu syndrome) is characterized by mucocutaneous telangiectasias and AVMs. However, the familial germline mutations in the genes underlying these syndromes have shed important insights into the signaling pathways and networks that contribute to the pathophysiology of bAVM formation. These families of genes include the following: transforming growth factor-β (*TGF-β*), endoglin (*ENG*), activin receptor-like kinase (*ALK1*), *SMAD*, *KRAS*, and *MAPK* [20], and are involved in the regulation of angiogenesis [21] (Figure 1). Approximately 5–20% of HHT patients have at least one bAVM, with multiple bAVMs being a predictive factor of HHT [22–24]. HHT-associated bAMVs tend to have a smaller nidus than sporadic bAVMs, with no statistical significance in age at diagnosis, prevalence of intracranial hemorrhage (ICH), or age at first ICH [25]. There are three types of HHT, characterized by mutations in members of the TGFβ/BMP signaling pathway: (1) type 1 results from loss-of-function (LoF) mutations in one copy of endoglin (*ENG*) [26,27]; (2) type 2 results from LoF mutations in activin A receptor like type 1 (*ACVRL1* or *ALK1+/−*) [28]; and (3) mutations in *SMAD4* cause a combined syndrome of juvenile polyposis and HHT (JP-HHT), accounting for 2% of HTT cases [29] (Figure 1).

2.2.2. Wyburn–Mason Syndrome

Wyburn–Mason syndrome (WMS), also known as Bonnet–Dechaume–Blanc syndrome, is a rare non-hereditary congenital neurocutaneous disorder characterized by AVMs. WMS lesions typically affect the skin, retina, and brain; the resulting bAVMs tend to be ipsilateral, with the midbrain most affected [30]. An embryonic defect is thought to result in the spread of vascular lesions that involve both the developing optic cup and anterior neural tube [30–32]. The specific genetic and molecular mechanisms underpinning WMS are not yet understood, and current clinical practices in treating associated bAVMs resembles that of sporadic bAVMs [30,31].

2.2.3. Sturge–Weber Syndrome

The presence of bAVM in patients with Sturge–Weber syndrome (SWS) are limited to a few exceptional cases [33]. SWS typically presents as facial cutaneous vascular malformations (port-wine stains), with the presence of port-wine stains underlying greater risk in ocular and neurological disorders [34,35]. Brain involvement in SWS patients is typically marked with leptomeningeal vascular malformation [36]. Recurrent somatic mosaic of the R183Q mutation in GNAQ was found to be the major determining factor in the development of SWS [34,36]. The R183Q GNAQ mutation is thought to hyperactivate the downstream Ras/Raf/MEK/ERK and mTOR pathways, resulting in SWS [36]. Increases in levels of Angiopoietin-2 from the GNAQ mutation have been implicated in the formation of capillary malformations associated with SWS [37]. Despite our growing understanding of the mechanisms contributing to SWS, the mechanistic link between bAVM occurrence with SWS remains a mystery. One paper has pointed to the theory that the R183Q-GNAQ mutation may disrupt arteriovenous specification through Notch signaling in the formation of malformed episcleral vasculature, but direct links to bAVMs remain speculative [37].

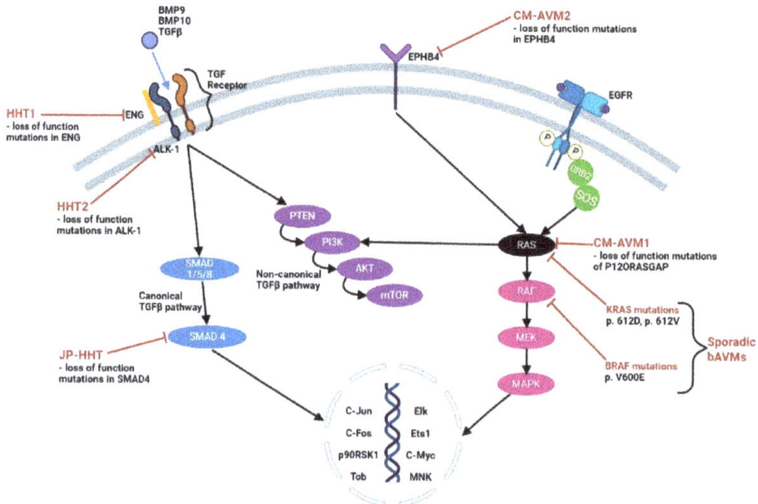

Figure 1. Signaling pathways involved in the formation of sporadic and syndromic brain AVMs. Abbreviations: BMP9 = bone morphogenic protein 9; BMP10 = bone morphogenic protein 10; TGFβ = transforming growth factor beta; ENG = endoglin; TGF = transforming growth factor; HHT1, HHT2 = hereditary hemorrhagic telangiectasia type 1, type 2; ALK-1 = activin A receptor-like type 1; SMAD 1, 4, 5, 8 = mothers against decapentaplegic homolog 1, 4, 5, 8; JP-HHT = juvenile polyposis/hereditary hemorrhagic telangiectasia; PTEN = phosphatase and tensin homolog; PI3K = phosphatidylinositol-3-kinase; AKT = protein kinase B; mTOR = mammalian target of rapamycin; C-Jun = transcription factor Jun; C-Fos = protein C-Fos; p90RSK1 = 90 kilodalton protein ribosomal protein S6 kinase 1; Tob = Tob protein; Elk = transcription factor Elk; Ets1 = transcription factor Ets1; C-Myc = proto-oncogene c-Myc; MNK = mitogen activated protein kinase-interacting kinases; CV-AVM1, 2 = capillary malformation-arteriovenous malformation types 1 and 2; EPHB4 = Ephrin B4; EGFR = epidermal growth factor receptor; GRB2 = growth factor receptor-bound protein 2; SOS = son of sevenless; RAS = RAS protein; RAF = RAF protein; MEK = mitogen-activated protein kinase kinase; MAPK = mitogen activated protein kinase; P120RASGAP = p120 RAS guanosine triphosphatase activating protein; KRAS = Kirsten rat sarcoma virus oncogene; BRAF = B-Raf proto-oncogene; and bAVMs = brain arteriovenous malformations.

2.3. Pathophysiology of Sporadic Brain Arteriovenous Malformations

Much of the pathophysiology of bAVM formation can be derived from understanding the pathways that drive the normal development of the vascular system. Fibroblast growth factor (FGF) drives the differentiation of mesodermal progenitors into hemangioblasts, which are thought to be the precursor cells of endothelial precursor cells (EPCs) and hematopoietic stem cells (HSCs) [38,39]. The differentiation of EPCs into ECs is an essential step in vasculogenesis. EPCs and HSCs form blood islands under vascular endothelial growth factor (VEGF) signaling [40]. Angiogenesis (the formation of new blood vessels from pre-existing vessels), is also under the influence of VEGF signaling. Sprouting angiogenesis requires proteolysis of laminin and type IV collagen in endothelial basement membranes, a process that is initiated by matrix metalloproteinases (MMPs), heparanases, cathepsins, and the urokinase plasminogen activator [41–43]. The formation of a mature, organized, vascular network depends on the inhibitory signaling via plasminogen activator inhibitor-1 (PAI-1) and the tissue inhibitors of metalloproteinases (TIMPs) [44], which lead to the release of angiogenic factors such as VEGF, FGF, and chemokines, and anti-angiogenic molecules to complete angiogenesis [45]. Human and animal studies support the role of dysregulated angiogenesis as involving the TGFβ and VEGF pathways [46]. Further dysregulation of cell proliferation and endothelial cell migration also leads to elevated angiogenic signaling [47].

An early hypothesis explaining the sporadic formation of bAVMs postulates that a hypoxic event occurs in the surrounding brain tissues, leading to the upregulation and overexpression of VEGF [48]. This hypothesis is supported by the findings that VEGF is overexpressed in tissues adjacent to bAVMs [49–51] and in peripheral blood samples [52,53]. Hypoxia inducible factor 1 (HIF-1) is normally undetectable in oxygenated tissues; however, its expression is increased in hypoxic conditions providing a feedback loop leading to the increased expression of VEGF and its receptors [48]. Another condition that leads to the concomitant upregulation of HIF-1 and VEGF is intracranial venous hypertension [54,55], which has been shown to induce high expression of VEGF in blood vessel endothelium in rodents [56]. The upregulation of VEGF creates a positive feedback loop leading to the increased expression of metalloproteinases MMP-2 and MMP-9 in bAVMs, and of cerebral cavernous malformations [57,58]. The glycoprotein carcinoembryonic antigen-related cell adhesion molecule 1, which is involved in angiogenesis and cell proliferation, has been previously linked to bAVM rupture in male patients [59].

Abnormally elevated levels of inflammatory and immune cells have also been associated in both unruptured and ruptured bAVMs, including perinidal macrophages [60], neutrophils, and T lymphocytes [61]. Cx3cr1+ microglia and Ccr2+ macrophages are present in bAVMs in *Alk1* knockout mice [62]. Similarly, astrocytes and endothelial cells upregulate the expression of glutamate transporter 1 (GLUT1) in AVM nidus vessels compared to control vessels [63]. Whole exome sequencing of endothelial cells from resected bAVMs has shown them to harbor activating somatic *KRAS* G12D or G12V, *BRAF*, and *MAP2K1/MEK* mutations [64–68]. The upregulation of MEK/ERK activity can also be detected in bAVM tissues that do not harbor KRAS mutations, suggesting the central roles of mitogenic pathways in the pathophysiology of sporadic bAVM formation [64] (Figure 1).

While activating somatic mutations in *KRAS*, *BRAF*, and *MAP2K1* have been implicated in aberrant MAPK signaling in bAVM pathogenesis, studies also suggest the involvement of broader dysregulation of endothelial developmental programs. Human bAVM tissue has been found to aberrantly express genes implicated in venous and lymphatic specification, such as *COUP-TFII*, *PROX1*, *SOX18* that were co-expressed in PECAM+ ECs which correlated with upregulated cellular proliferation [69]. The mixed venous/lymphatic identity of the bAVM endothelium implies that, in its development, the bAVM undergoes a reprogramming of endothelial identity [69]. This reprogramming of endothelial identity observed in bAVMs may only reflect one part of a broader endothelial plasticity. Novel research suggests that endothelial–mesenchymal transition (End-MT) signaling may play a role in bAVM pathophysiology. A study by Shoemaker and colleagues reported that compared to normal brain tissue, bAVM tissue expressed End MT associated transcription factors like KLF4, SNAI1, and SNAI2 along with key mesenchymal markers Vimentin, ACTA2, and S100A4 at much greater levels [70]. Additionally, the strong collagen deposition and high expression of PAI-1 throughout the bAVM tissue further implicates the process of End-MT in vessel remodeling and lesion maintenance [70]. Collectively, Shoemaker's studies reveal that dysregulated endothelial identity and plasticity, rather than genetic mutation alone, could underlie the maladaptive remodeling characteristic of bAVMs. We have summarized the genes involved in the formation of bAVMs in Table 1 for our readers.

Table 1. Genes implicated in the development of brain arteriovenous malformations and their mechanisms of action.

Study	Genes	Mechanism of Action
Fish et al., 2020 [71]	*MEK-ERK*	Upstream KRAS activation increases MEK kinase activation.
Giarretta et al., 2021 [72]; Shoemaker et al., 2014 [69]	*Shh* *COUP-TFII*	Induced AVM-like properties of vessels. Gli1 and COUP-TFII.
Wang et al., 2023 [73]	*ACVRL1*	Mutation linked to HHT. Found links to sporadic bAVMs.
Mansur and Radovanovic, 2023 [74]; Pérez-Alfayate et al., 2022 [75]	*VEGF*	Upregulated signaling in HHT activates MAPK-ERK pathway. Role in endothelial cell function.
Mansur and Radovanovic, 2023 [74]; Wang et al., 2023 [73]; Pan et al., 2021 [76]; Pérez-Alfayate et al., 2022 [75]; Goss et al., 2019 [77]; Fish et al., 2020 [71]; Nikolaev et al., 2018 [64]	*KRAS*	Increased downstream ERK phosphorylation and angiogenic signaling. Enhanced cell migratory behavior. Somatic KRAS activating mutations: KRAS G12V, KRAS G12D, KRAS G12C, and BRAF. Altered endothelial morphogenesis and growth dynamics.
Murphy et al., 2008 [78]; ZhuGe et al., 2009 [79]; Li et al., 2014 [80]; Pérez-Alfayate et al., 2022 [75];	*NOTCH*	Abnormal gain or loss of NOTCH function. Increased expression of NOTCH-1 and downstream target HES-1 are observed in human bAVM tissue compared to control vessels. *Alk1* knockout mice have decreased Notch signaling. Connects Alk1 and Notch signaling during vascular morphogenesis. Abnormal NOTCH-1 expression in bAVM hemorrhage.
Zhang et al., 2016 [53]; Mansur and Radovanovic, 2023 [74]; Pan et al., 2021 [20]	*Alk1*	$Cx3cr1^+$ microglia and $Ccr2^+$ macrophages are present in AVM lesions of an *Alk1* deficient mouse model. LOF mutation in HHT patients.
Wang et al., 2023 [73]; Xu et al., 2023 [81]	*TGF-β*	Mutated in ECs, essential for bAVM initiation. Low doses TGF-β stimulate proliferation and migration of ECs through ALK1. High doses of TGF-β result in quiescent endothelium. End-MT in bAVM tissues.

Table 1. *Cont.*

Study	Genes	Mechanism of Action
Mansur and Radovanovic, 2023 [74]; Wang et al., 2023 [73]	*RAS-MAPK Ex. RASA1*	Mutated in ECs, essential for bAVM initiation. LOF mutation in *RASA1* specifically causes abnormal activation of RAS-MAPK pathway and increases cellular proliferation, growth, differentiation, motility.
Mansur and Radovanovic, 2023 [74]; Pan et al., 2021 [20]; Pérez-Alfayate et al., 2022 [75]	*Endoglin (ENG)*	LOF mutations. ENG is a receptor for TGF-β and BMPs which are predominantly expressed in ECs. LOF undoes BMP/Alk1 signal cascade which suppresses endothelial cell migration and proliferation.
Wang et al., 2023 [73]; Pan et al., 2021 [20]	*SMAD4*	LOF mutation in HHT patients. Linked to juvenile polyposis.
Mansur and Radovanovic, 2023 [74]; Xu et al., 2023 [81]	*BMP9, BMP10*	Mutated in HHT patients. Plays important role in EC function and angiogenesis. BMP9 and BMP10 are probably the natural ligands for the ENG/ALK1 signaling pathway.
Winkler et al., 2022 [82]	*PLVAP, ANGPT2*	Marker of fenestrated endothelium normally confined to developmental angiogenesis, the brain's circumventricular organs and choroid plexus.
Adhicary et al., 2023 [83]	*Rbpj*	GTPase-mediated cellular function in brain ECs. Deficient expression increased Cdc-42 activity in isolated ECs. Disrupted cell polarity and focal adhesion properties.
Hermanto et al., 2016 [84]; Shoemaker et al., 2014 [69]	*Sox17*	Downstream pathways implicated in bAVM. High expression in thick-walled veins and arteries.

Abbreviation: ACVRL1 = activin A receptor-like type 1; ALK1 = activin receptor-like kinase 1; ANGPT2 = angiopoietin 2; AVM = arteriovenous malformation; bAVM = brain arteriovenous malformation; BMP9/10 = bone morphogenetic proteins 9 and 10; BRAF = v-raf murine sarcoma viral oncogene homolog B1; Cdc42 = cell division control protein 42 homolog; Cx3cr1 = C-X3-C motif chemokine receptor 1; Ccr2 = C-C motif chemokine receptor 2; COUP-TFII = chicken ovalbumin upstream promoter transcription factor II; ECs = endothelial cells; ENG = endoglin; ERK = extracellular signal-regulated kinase; HES1 = hairy and enhancer of split 1; HHT = hereditary hemorrhagic telangiectasia; KRAS = Kirsten rat sarcoma viral oncogene homolog; LOF = loss of function; MAPK = mitogen-activated protein kinase; MEK = MAPK/ERK kinase; NOTCH = neurogenic locus notch homolog protein; PLVAP = plasmalemma vesicle-associated protein; RAS = rat sarcoma viral oncogene homolog; RASA1 = RAS p21 protein activator 1; RAS-MAPK = rat sarcoma–mitogen-activated protein kinase; Shh = sonic hedgehog; SMAD = mothers against decapentaplegic homolog; Sox17 = SRY-box transcription factor 17; TGF-β = transforming growth factor beta; and VEGF = vascular endothelial growth factor.

The recent single-cell analysis of human bAVM samples by Winkler and colleagues further exemplifies the diverse cellular make-up of bAVMs, identifying spatially distinct

CLDN5+ endothelial cells, TAGLN+ smooth muscle cells, CCL19+ fibromyocytes, and COL1A2+ perivascular fibroblasts [11]. Clusters of myeloid cells, vessel-associated microglia, dendritic cells, perivascular macrophages, monocytes, CD4+ and CD8+ T cells, regulatory T cells, B cells, and natural killer cells were also found to be infiltrated into the perivascular space and adjacent brain that was surrounding the AVMs. Vessel-associated CD11c+ antigen-presenting cells, IBA1+P2RY12- macrophages, and IBA1+P2RY12+ microglia were also found infiltrated into the bAVM vasculature. Finally, AIF1+P2RY12- monocytes were over-represented in ruptured AVMs, suggesting the upregulation of the immune system associated with AVM hemorrhage. Taken together, these studies reveal an intricate and dynamic cellular microenvironment that is associated with bAVMs, which helps to remodel the surrounding brain milieu following bAVM rupture. We have summarized these cell types for our readers in Table 2.

Table 2. Cell types associated with the brain arteriovenous malformation microenvironment and their molecular roles.

Studies	Cell Type	Role in AVM Biology
Winkler et al., 2022 [11]; Wang et al., 2023 [73]	Macrophages	Perivascular macrophages (28.3% of bAVMs), $IBA1^{+}P2RY12^{-}$ MΦ. Significantly increased in bAVM tissue.
Winkler et al., 2022 [11]	Monocytes	$AIF1^{+}$-$P2RY12^{-}$ monocytes over-represented in ruptured bAVMs.
Winkler et al., 2022 [11]	Microglia	Discrete areas have numerous IBA1+ PSRY12+ monocytes.
Wang et al., 2023 [73]	Neutrophils	Significantly increased in bAVM tissue.
Winkler et al., 2022 [11]; Shabani et al., 2022 [85]	T lymphocytes	CD4+, CD8+, Tregs found in immune cell clusters associated with cerebrovasculature. Predominant detection in unruptured bAVM tissue.
Winkler et al., 2022 [11]	Natural killer cells	Found in immune cell clusters associated with cerebrovasculature.
Winkler et al., 2022 [11]	Plasmacytoid Dendritic Cells	Found in immune cell clusters associated with cerebrovasculature.
Tu et al., 2025 [86]; Shabani et al., 2022 [85]; Thomas et al., 2021 [87]	Astrocytes	Promotion of angiogenesis and vascular instability (hemorrhagic risk). Aberrant expressions of ALDH1A2 and CYR61 in abnormal neighboring astrocytes.
Winkler et al., 2022 [11]; Mansur and Radovanovic, 2023 [74]; Nikolaev et al., 2018 [64]; Shabani et al., 2022 [85]	Endothelial Cells	$CLDN5^{+}$ within bAVM cell population. Clusters with suppressed venule and capillary cell identities. Alk1, Eng, and SMAD transcription factors work to suppress migration. VEGF and ET-1. KRAS mutations.
Winkler et al., 2022 [11]	Fibromyocytes	$CCL19^{+}$ within bAVM cell population.
Winkler et al., 2022 [11]	Smooth Muscle Cells	$TAGLN^{+}$ within bAVM cell population.
Winkler et al., 2022 [11]	Perivascular Fibroblasts	$COL1A2^{+}$ within bAVM cell population.

Table 2. *Cont.*

Studies	Cell Type	Role in AVM Biology
Winkler et al., 2022 [11]; Pan et al., 2021 [76]; Nakisli et al., 2023 [88]; Shabani et al., 2022 [85]	Mural Cells	*KCNJ8+* Pericyte number and coverage reduced. PDGF-B/PDGFR-disruption. Notch signaling pathway. BMP/ALK/SMAD pathway. RAS/MAPK pathway.
Winkler et al., 2022 [11]	Perivascular Fibroblasts	*DCN*$^+$ *APOD*$^+$
Shoemaker et al., 2020 [70]; Xu et al., 2023 [81]	Mesenchymal Cells	The result of endothelial–mesenchymal transition signaling within bAVMs.

Abbreviations: ALDH1A2 = aldehyde dehydrogenase 1 family member A2; ANGPT2 = angiopoietin 2; APO D = apolipoprotein D; AVM = arteriovenous malformation; bAVM = brain arteriovenous malformation; BMP = bone morphogenetic protein; CD4+ = cluster of differentiation 4 positive; CD8+ = cluster of differentiation 8 positive; CLDN5 = claudin-5; COL1A2 = collagen type I alpha 2 chain; CCL19 = C-C motif chemokine ligand 19; CYR61 = cysteine-rich angiogenic inducer 61; DCN = decorin; ECs = endothelial cells; ENG = endoglin; ET-1 = endothelin-1; HHT = hereditary hemorrhagic telangiectasia; IBA1 = ionized calcium-binding adaptor molecule 1; KRAS = Kirsten rat sarcoma viral oncogene homolog; MAPK = mitogen-activated protein kinase; MΦ = macrophage; PDGF-B = platelet-derived growth factor subunit B; PDGFR = platelet-derived growth factor receptor; P2RY12 = purinergic receptor P2Y12; SMAD = mothers against decapentaplegic homolog; TAGLN = transgelin; TGF-β = transforming growth factor beta; and VEGF = vascular endothelial growth factor.

2.4. Pathophysiology of Acquired Brain Arteriovenous Malformations

The hypothesis that bAVMs can be acquired comes from isolated reports of de novo cases [8,89], recurrences in pediatric patients after surgical resections [90–92], and remodeling throughout the post-resection follow-up period [93,94]. Lasjaunais and colleagues postulated that bAVMs were an indirect sequelae of other intracranial pathologies leading to remodeling of the capillarovenous junction to form secondary acquired bAVMs [95]. Similarly, patients who acquired bAVMs after stereotactic radiotherapy treatments, hemorrhagic and ischemic stroke, traumatic brain injury, cerebral aneurysm occlusion, brain tumors, or demyelinating encephalitic lesions, are thought to develop bAVMs via a "second hit" phenomenon [10].

3. Animal Models of Brain AVMs

Studies have shown that adenovirus Cre recombinase transgenic mice with heterozygous and homozygous *Alk1* or *Eng* mutations show different vascular phenotypes. In the brains of *Eng*-floxed mice, the homozygous deletion of *Eng* led to a severe vascular dysplasia phenotype in mice treated with VEGF compared to heterozygous *Eng* mice [96]. Inducible *Eng*- or *Alk1*-conditional knockouts, specifically in brain ECs but not in pericytes or macrophages, led to the formation of bAVMs in adult mice, suggesting that there is a cell-specific lineage in bAVM pathogenesis [16,97]. Interestingly, *Eng* or *Alk1* mutations in a small portion of ECs and in bone-marrow-derived ECs were also sufficient to cause bAMV formation, confirming a central role for ECs in bAVM pathogenesis [96,98,99]. Kim and colleagues demonstrated that the over-expression of *Alk1* can rescue the AVM phenotypes in *Alk1*- and *Eng*-inducible knock out mice via normalizing the expression of the *Notch* and *Smad* pathway genes in *Eng*-deficient ECs [100]. Activation of Notch1 and Notch4 in ECs of mouse brains induced bAVM formation [78,101]. Inhibition of Notch signaling via the deletion of the recombination signal binding protein for immunoglobulin kappa J region (*Rbpj*) in ECs of postnatal mice also led to bAVM formation [102], while *Alk1* knockout mice have endogenously decreased Notch signaling, suggesting an intimate connection between *Alk1* and *Notch* involvement in vasculogenesis [103]. The over-expression of soluble ENG has been shown to cause bAVM formation in mice. Soluble ENG binds to bone morphogenic protein type 9 (BMP9), inhibiting blood vessel formation and causing bAVM inflammation [104,105]. Inhibiting BMP9 and BMP10 induces AVMs in the retina [106], and studies suggest that BMP9 and BMP10 are likely natural ligands for the ENG/ALK1 signaling pathway [107], thereby suggesting that the BMP9/10-ENG-ALK1-SMAD4 pathway plays a role in bAVM formation in HHT patients [108,109].

Sporadic bAVMs have been formed in mice by generating EC-specific *Kras* G12D or G12V gain-of-function mutations [71], while the adenovirus-associated viral vector infection of *Kras* G12D into the brain ECs of mice also promotes the development of bAVMs via the activation of the mitogen-activated protein kinase (MAPK) pathway [110]. In the same study in which Fish and colleagues were able to generate bAVM in mice by introducing EC-specific *Kras* G12D or G12V mutations, they also generated bAVM using the same technique in zebrafish and were able to show that zebrafish embryos harboring the EC-specific *Kras* G12V mutation had a higher incidence of cranial hemorrhage, which was not seen in the embryos expressing wild-type Kras [71]. This correlates well with the findings of somatic mutations in members of the KRAS/MAPK pathways in human sporadic bAVM and peripheral AVM samples [64,66–68,77,111].

Murphy and colleagues expressed constitutively active *int3*, the murine homolog of Notch4, in ECs of tetracycline-regulated transgenic mice [78]. Mutant mice died between 2 and 5 weeks of age, with signs of neurological dysfunction including ataxia and seizures, which were evident in approximately 25% of the mice. The histology of the mutant brains demonstrated visual evidence of intracranial hemorrhage occurring most often in the cerebellum, followed by the neocortex, but never in the brainstem. Underlying the areas of hemorrhage were enlarged and tangled vessels, resembling bAVMs. Leveraging their Tet-on/off transgenic system to repress endothelial *int3* expression, the authors were able to reverse the neurological deficits in postnatal day 20- or day 21-old mice, further supporting the role of Notch expression in the pathophysiology of bAVMs [78]. We have summarized current animal models of bAVMs in Table 3.

Table 3. Animal models of brain arteriovenous malformations.

Animal Model	Features
$Eng^{f/f}$ mice [96]	- Ad-Cre-treated brains have *Eng*-null ECs. - VEGF induced more severe vascular dyplasia in Ad-Cre-treated brains of $Eng^{f/f}$ mice compared with $Eng^{+/-}$ mice.
Eng or *Alk1* conditional knockout mice [16,112]	- Inducible conditional knockout of *Eng* or *Alk1*, specifically in brain ECs but not in pericytes or macrophages. - Leads to focal angiogenic stimulation in the brains of mice.
Eng or *Alk1* conditional knockout mice [100]	- Showed that over-expression of *Alk1* can rescue the AVM phenotype via normalizing expression of Notch and Smad pathways gene in *Eng*-deficient ECs.

Table 3. *Cont.*

Animal Model	Features
Kras^{G12D} or *Kras*^{G12V} transgenic mice [71,110]	- Brain EC-specific *Kras* G12D or G12V gain-of-function mutations in mice lead to formation of bAVMs. - Adenovirus-associated viral vector infection of *Kras* G12D into brain ECs of mice promotes bAVM formation via activation of the mitogen-activated protein kinase (MAPK) pathway. - 50% of mice developed bAVM which may not necessarily require physiological angiogenesis during early development.
Int3 transgenic mice [78]	- Constitutive expression of *int3*, the murine homolog of *Notch4*, in brain ECs of tetracycline-regulated transgenic mice leads to formation of dilated and tangled brain vessels that hemorrhage. - Repression of endothelial *int3* expression in P20- or P21-day-old mice reverses neurological deficits.
Kras^{G12D} zebrafish [71]	- Constitutively active *Kras* G12D into ECs. - 50% of zebrafish developed AV shunts. - NOT completely representative of human bAVMs. - Established shunts were reversed by pharmacological MEK inhibition but refractory to PI3K inhibition.

Abbreviations: Ad-Cre = adenovirus–Cre recombinase; ALK1 = activin receptor-like kinase 1; AVM = arteriovenous malformation; bAVM = brain arteriovenous malformation; ECs = endothelial cells; ENG = endoglin; HHT = hereditary hemorrhagic telangiectasia; Int3 = intracellular domain of Notch4 (murine homolog of Notch4); KRAS = Kirsten rat sarcoma viral oncogene homolog; MAPK = mitogen-activated protein kinase; P20/P21 = postnatal day 20/postnatal day 21; SMAD = mothers against decapentaplegic homolog; and VEGF = vascular endothelial growth factor.

4. Targeted Therapeutic Approaches for the Treatment of AVMs

Brain AVMs are currently treated with surgery, radiosurgery, or embolization (Figure 2). Each of these modalities have their pros and cons, and their inherent risks and benefits. A large registry of 1010 bAVM patients from The Treatment of Brain Arteriovenous Malformation Study were stratified to surgery, endovascular therapy, or radiosurgery [113]. In total, 229 out of 512 bAVM patients were selected for surgery, with the goal of cure. Surgical cure was achieved in 88% of patients. At the mean time of follow-up, 12% of patients reached the primary safety outcome, with serious adverse events occurring in 21% of patients. Permanent treatment-related complications occurred in 4% of patients, the majority of whom had complications from preoperative embolization; however, one should take care in interpreting these results as there is considerable patient variability with low- and high-grade bAVMs, and the jury is still out regarding whether low-grade, unruptured, bAVMs should be observed rather than subjected to surgery [113]. Similarly, a recent retrospective study of 262 adult patients with unruptured bAVMs, who underwent upfront SRS, reported higher rates of post-treatment hemorrhage, with larger bAVM volumes only among patients with a diffuse nidus compared to those with a compact nidus, exceeding the 2.2% annual rate of post-SRS hemorrhage, suggesting that studying the cytoarchitecture of the bAVM nidus could mitigate post-treatment complications [114]. Finally, recently published consensus guidelines from the ARISE I Consortium (Aneurysm/bAVM/chronic subdural hematoma Roundtable Discussion with Industry and Stroke Experts) recognized the need to improve bAVM characterization, genetic evaluation, and phenotyping in a multidisciplinary manner, with collaborative research efforts to improve outcomes for bAVM patients [4]. As a proper review of these conventional approaches exceeds the scope of this review, we will focus on how investigators have leveraged the understanding of the biological drivers of bAVM formation to run clinical trials using targeted pharmacological therapies. Several of these trials are not specifically aimed at the treatment of bAVMs but are still informative with regard to how pharmacological therapies might be translated into viable strategies for bAVM treatment.

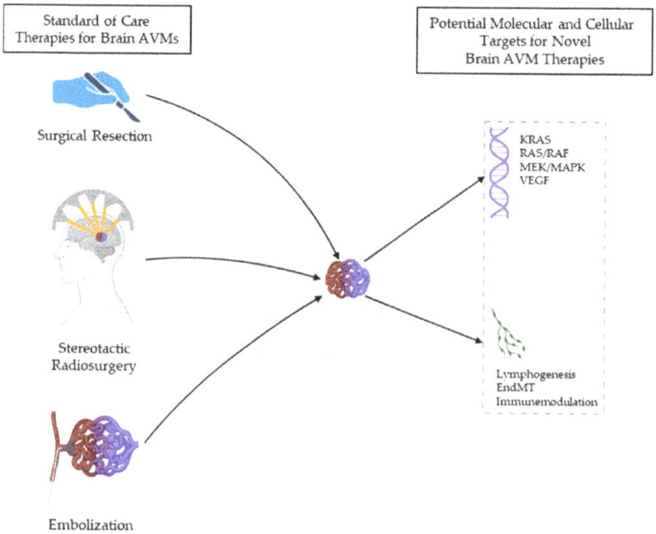

Figure 2. Schematic of the standard of care and potential novel targets for brain AVM therapies. Abbreviations: KRAS = Kirsten rat sarcoma virus oncogene; RAF = RAF protein; MEK = mitogen-activated protein kinase kinase; MAPK = mitogen activated protein kinase; and AVMs = arteriovenous malformations.

Early trials targeting upstream angiogenic stimulus using tetracycline derivatives, bevacizumab to reduce angiogenic activity, and thalidomide delivered mixed results, with dose-limited patient toxicities to tetracylines [115], with minimal clinical effects on angiogenic activity despite serum reductions in VEGF levels in patients with AVMs treated with bevacizumab [116]. Surprisingly, the drug thalidomide, which was initially prescribed to pregnant women to treat morning sickness in the early 1960s but was discontinued due to teratogenicity, has been found to have anti-angiogenic properties through cytokine inhibition, and the inhibition of TGFα and nitric oxide [117]. In a prospective observational study of 18 patients with severe symptomatic extracranial AVMs treated with thalidomide, all patients experienced reduction in pain, and decreased bleeding and ulceration [118]. Of the twelve patients who stopped treatment due to clinical improvement, eight remained stable, and four had a recurrence of their AVMs within the first year. Adverse events following dose escalation included asthenia, erythroderma, and cerebral infarct (which may have been unrelated to thalidomide drug effect). These initially promising results in treating extracranial AVM patients with thalidomide opens up potential avenues of translation for use in bAVM patients, but further research using preclinical animal models of bAVMs to determine safety would be warranted.

Isolated case reports of using the MEK inhibitor trametinib to target the KRAS/MEK/MAPK pathway as a driver of sporadic AVM formation in the pediatric population with severe extracranial AVMs have reported a good clinical effect [119,120]. One patient also had a spinal intramedullary AVM that responded well to trametinib, with reduced shunting and no reported serious adverse events, opening the door for its potential use in treating intracranial AVMs [121]. A phase II European safety and efficacy trial of trametinib called TRAMAV is currently recruiting adult patients with severe extracranial AVMs (EudraCT: 2019-003573-26). A prospective trial is also currently ongoing in Toronto, Canada, studying the safety and efficacy of MEK inhibition for compassionate use in patients with palliative extra- and intracranial AVMs [74]. These promising results using targeted therapies open avenues of clinical investigation that combine novel and existing treatment modalities to enable more effective treatment outcomes for bAVM patients. We also recognize recently published excellent reviews on the genetic insights, advances in treatments, and emerging therapies for bAVMs to give our readers further references to enrich their learning [122–125].

5. Future Directions

The ability to perform deep sequencing and multi-omic analysis of clinical samples have garnered our ability to gain further insights into the biology of bAVMs. A recent study by Scimone and colleagues conducted differential methylome analysis on ECs from human bAVM samples and compared them to human cerebral microvascular ECs. This study uncovered novel methylated gene loci involved in EC adhesion and crosstalk between EC and vascular smooth muscle cell networks [126]. Not only did this study recapitulate known loci linked to bAVM formation such as *KRAS* and *RBPJ*, but it also identified aberrant methylation patterns at several long non-coding RNA genes targeting transcription factors expressed in neurovascular development, and differential CHG methylated gene clustered in pathways related to EC homeostasis, which point towards more complex mechanisms other than EC dysfunction as a driver of bAVM formation.

A recent study of a single-cell atlas of normal and malformed human brain vasculature by Winkler and colleagues elegantly characterized the immune microenvironment in response to AVM rupture, identifying distinct immune cell clusters including *GPNMB*+ monocytes as key players in the depletion of stabilizing smooth muscle cells in AVMs that have bled [11]. They were also able to spatially define cellular and gene expression signatures involving endothelial cell transformations localized to areas around the AVM nidus, and identify clusters of cerebrovascular-derived inflammatory and immune cells associated with sites of hemorrhage, which could lead to novel avenues of therapeutic targeting.

A group from Italy recently reported the use of cell-free DNA next-generation sequencing of liquid biopsy plasma samples to detect mutational burdens in patients with cutaneous AVMs, as a less invasive alternative that avoids morbidities associated with direct lesional sampling [127]. To increase sample sensitivity, they sampled blood from patients at the time of angiography and compared this alongside paired blood from a peripheral blood draw, and were able to detect known mutations in the isolated cell-free DNA sampled from the efferent draining vein. A study by Zenner and colleagues also reported the safety and efficacy of liquid biopsy sampling of peripheral AVMs and venous malformations in detecting driver mutations [128]. Lastly, Winkler and colleagues at the University of San Francisco proposed the "endoluminal biopsy" technique whereby DNA is isolated from the endovascular coil that is placed next to the wall of the AVM vessel lumen prior to a planned endovascular treatment session. The retrieval of the coil following the procedure allowed for the genomic sampling of AVM cells that can be processed for downstream next-generation sequencing, allowing them to identify *KRAS* mutations in four patients with bAVMs [82]. This endoluminal sampling technique could further open avenues of investigation to gain a deeper understanding of the evolving biology of bAVMs and to identify novel targeted therapies that could improve the outcomes of bAVM patients.

Finally, investigators are developing three-dimensional (3D) blood vessel organoids (BVOs) to enable high-throughput screening methods to discover novel treatments for neurovascular disorders. Several 3D vascular organoid models have been developed using human-derived fibroblasts and reprogrammed human pluripotent stem cells (hiPSCs) to mimic different organ systems, including that of the cardiovascular [129], pulmonary [130], gastrointestinal [131], and brain [132]. Oh and colleagues recently utilized 3D BVOs from ECs and compared their gene expression profiles to those of human AVM tissues [133]. Their AVM organoids expressed significantly higher levels of expression of CD31, phalloidin, the angiogenesis-associated gene *FSTL1*, and has-mir-135b-5p, a small RNA related to AVMs. *CSPG4*, a capillary-related gene, exhibited the lowest expression in the 3D AVM organoids. Nikolova and colleagues compiled a comprehensive single-cell genomic atlas of developing hBVOs on the backdrop of genetic and environmental perturbation screens to assess the fate and state landscape of their 3D models of human vasculature [134]. Their hBVOs formed vascular networks of PDGFR-β+, CD31+ ECs, which matured to form vessel lumens. Whilst the goal was to develop diabetic hBVOs that would allow them to study diabetic vasculopathy and not AVM disease, their tunable platform demonstrates the promise in adopting 3D hBVO technology to study neurovascular pathologies. Salewskij and Penninger recently developed self-organizing human capillary blood vessel organoids that recapitulate key processes of vasculogenesis and angiogenesis [135]. One key limitation of these 3D hBVOs is lack of perfusion in vitro, which may be achieved only if transplanted into an animal host for in vivo vascularization and perfusion. This in vivo implantation process unfortunately adds significant experimental costs, precludes high-throughput screening, and introduces potential species-specific effects. Cai and colleagues recently published an elegant study generating 3D vascular network-inspired diffusible (VID) scaffolds of functional midbrain organoids, which were used to test pharmacological responses and neuronal activity changes to fentanyl exposure [136]. These VID scaffolds deliver medium-carrying nutrients, oxygen, and signaling molecules to the organoids with tunable delivery to engineered neural organoids (ENO), leading to reduced apoptosis, stress, and sustained neurogenesis with region-specific functional differentiation. This is in comparison to conventional neural organoids, which developed hypoxic and necrotic cores. Even though this 3D ENO system was not designed with the intent to study the interactions of the neuronal environment around AVMs, the ability to develop 3D vascular networks around functional neural organoids holds promise in their adaptability to study neurovascular disorders. Finally, Kistemaker and colleagues hint at the possibility of the incorporation of hBVOs into a microfluidic chip platform, which could introduce laminar flow and shear stress into the hBVO vasculature to overcome the current limitations of in vitro perfusion, and improve functionality of these hBVO models [137].

6. Conclusions

In summary, advances in the understanding of the molecular drivers of non-syndromic and syndromic bAVM formation have allowed for the development of preclinical bAVM models which can be leveraged for translational research. Taken together, these advances hold promise in further characterizing the pathophysiology of bAVMs and offering novel treatment options to decrease the annual hemorrhage rates and subsequent neurological sequelae of bAVM patients.

Author Contributions: Conceptualization, K.W. and F.C.L.; methodology, K.W., F.C.L., and L.S.; resources, K.W., S.G., F.C.L., L.S., D.J.P., and S.D.C.; data curation, K.W. and F.C.L.; writing—original draft preparation, K.W., F.C.L., and S.G.; writing—review and editing, K.W., S.G., F.C.L., Y.S.H.,

D.A., L.S., D.J.P., and S.D.C.; supervision, D.J.P. and S.D.C. All authors have read and agreed to the published version of the manuscript.

Funding: This research received no external funding.

Institutional Review Board Statement: Ethical review and approval were waived for this study, due to the descriptive nature of this review not affecting nor involving the well-being of human subjects.

Informed Consent Statement: Patient consent was waived due to all images being stripped of all patient identifiers.

Data Availability Statement: No new data were created or analyzed in this study.

Conflicts of Interest: The authors declare no conflicts of interest.

References

1. Chen, C.J.; Ding, D.; Derdeyn, C.P.; Lanzino, G.; Friedlander, R.M.; Southerland, A.M.; Lawton, M.T.; Sheehan, J.P. Brain arteriovenous malformations: A review of natural history, pathobiology, and interventions. *Neurology* **2020**, *95*, 917–927. [CrossRef]
2. Al-Shahi, R.; Fang, J.S.; Lewis, S.C.; Warlow, C.P. Prevalence of adults with brain arteriovenous malformations: A community based study in Scotland using capture-recapture analysis. *J. Neurol. Neurosurg. Psychiatry* **2002**, *73*, 547–551. [CrossRef]
3. Berman, M.F.; Sciacca, R.R.; Pile-Spellman, J.; Stapf, C.; Connolly, E.S., Jr.; Mohr, J.P.; Young, W.L. The epidemiology of brain arteriovenous malformations. *Neurosurgery* **2000**, *47*, 389–396; discussion 397. [CrossRef] [PubMed]
4. Samaniego, E.A.; Dabus, G.; Meyers, P.M.; Kan, P.T.; Frosen, J.; Lanzino, G.; Welch, B.G.; Volovici, V.; Gonzalez, F.; Fifi, J.; et al. Most Promising Approaches to Improve Brain AVM Management: ARISE I Consensus Recommendations. *Stroke* **2024**, *55*, 1449–1463. [CrossRef]
5. Daou, B.J.; Palmateer, G.; Thompson, B.G.; Maher, C.O.; Hayman, J.A.; Lam, K.L.; Wahl, D.R.; Kim, M.; Pandey, A.S. Stereotactic Radiosurgery for Brain Arteriovenous Malformations: Evaluation of Obliteration and Review of Associated Predictors. *J. Stroke Cerebrovasc. Dis.* **2020**, *29*, 104863. [CrossRef]
6. Morales-Valero, S.F.; Bortolotti, C.; Sturiale, C.; Lanzino, G. Are parenchymal AVMs congenital lesions? *Neurosurg. Focus* **2014**, *37*, E2. [CrossRef]
7. Walcott, B.P.; Winkler, E.A.; Zhou, S.; Birk, H.; Guo, D.; Koch, M.J.; Stapleton, C.J.; Spiegelman, D.; Dionne-Laporte, A.; Dion, P.A.; et al. Identification of a rare BMP pathway mutation in a non-syndromic human brain arteriovenous malformation via exome sequencing. *Hum. Genome Var.* **2018**, *5*, 18001. [CrossRef]
8. Nagai, Y.; Anan, M.; Fujiki, M. Cerebral Arteriovenous Malformations as Acquired Lesions: Case Reports and Review of the Literature. *J. Stroke Cerebrovasc. Dis.* **2020**, *29*, 105157. [CrossRef]
9. Park, H.; Koh, E.J.; Lee, E.J.; Cheon, J.E.; Kim, S.K. An acquired cerebral arteriovenous malformation after brain abscess treatment: Case report and a review of the literature. *Childs Nerv. Syst.* **2021**, *37*, 2923–2926. [CrossRef]
10. Florian, I.A.; Beni, L.; Moisoiu, V.; Timis, T.L.; Florian, I.S.; Balasa, A.; Berindan-Neagoe, I. 'De Novo' Brain AVMs-Hypotheses for Development and a Systematic Review of Reported Cases. *Medicina* **2021**, *57*, 201. [CrossRef]
11. Winkler, E.A.; Kim, C.N.; Ross, J.M.; Garcia, J.H.; Gil, E.; Oh, I.; Chen, L.Q.; Wu, D.; Catapano, J.S.; Raygor, K.; et al. A single-cell atlas of the normal and malformed human brain vasculature. *Science* **2022**, *375*, eabi7377. [CrossRef] [PubMed]
12. Li, X.; Kover, K.L.; Heruth, D.P.; Watkins, D.J.; Guo, Y.; Moore, W.V.; He, L.G.; Zang, M.; Clements, M.A.; Yan, Y. Thioredoxin-interacting protein promotes high-glucose-induced macrovascular endothelial dysfunction. *Biochem. Biophys. Res. Commun.* **2017**, *493*, 291–297. [CrossRef] [PubMed]
13. Vanlandewijck, M.; He, L.; Mae, M.A.; Andrae, J.; Ando, K.; Del Gaudio, F.; Nahar, K.; Lebouvier, T.; Lavina, B.; Gouveia, L.; et al. A molecular atlas of cell types and zonation in the brain vasculature. *Nature* **2018**, *554*, 475–480. [CrossRef]
14. Chen, M.B.; Yang, A.C.; Yousef, H.; Lee, D.; Chen, W.; Schaum, N.; Lehallier, B.; Quake, S.R.; Wyss-Coray, T. Brain Endothelial Cells Are Exquisite Sensors of Age-Related Circulatory Cues. *Cell Rep.* **2020**, *30*, 4418–4432.e4. [CrossRef]
15. Kalucka, J.; de Rooij, L.; Goveia, J.; Rohlenova, K.; Dumas, S.J.; Meta, E.; Conchinha, N.V.; Taverna, F.; Teuwen, L.A.; Veys, K.; et al. Single-Cell Transcriptome Atlas of Murine Endothelial Cells. *Cell* **2020**, *180*, 764–779.e20. [CrossRef]
16. Choi, E.J.; Chen, W.; Jun, K.; Arthur, H.M.; Young, W.L.; Su, H. Novel brain arteriovenous malformation mouse models for type 1 hereditary hemorrhagic telangiectasia. *PLoS ONE* **2014**, *9*, e88511. [CrossRef]
17. Matsubara, S.; Bourdeau, A.; terBrugge, K.G.; Wallace, C.; Letarte, M. Analysis of endoglin expression in normal brain tissue and in cerebral arteriovenous malformations. *Stroke* **2000**, *31*, 2653–2660. [CrossRef]

18. Pawlikowska, L.; Tran, M.N.; Achrol, A.S.; Ha, C.; Burchard, E.; Choudhry, S.; Zaroff, J.; Lawton, M.T.; Castro, R.; McCulloch, C.E.; et al. Polymorphisms in transforming growth factor-beta-related genes ALK1 and ENG are associated with sporadic brain arteriovenous malformations. *Stroke* **2005**, *36*, 2278–2280. [CrossRef]
19. Simon, M.; Franke, D.; Ludwig, M.; Aliashkevich, A.F.; Koster, G.; Oldenburg, J.; Bostrom, A.; Ziegler, A.; Schramm, J. Association of a polymorphism of the ACVRL1 gene with sporadic arteriovenous malformations of the central nervous system. *J. Neurosurg.* **2006**, *104*, 945–949. [CrossRef]
20. Pan, P.; Weinsheimer, S.; Cooke, D.; Winkler, E.; Abla, A.; Kim, H.; Su, H. Review of treatment and therapeutic targets in brain arteriovenous malformation. *J. Cereb. Blood Flow. Metab.* **2021**, *41*, 3141–3156. [CrossRef]
21. Vetiska, S.; Walchli, T.; Radovanovic, I.; Berhouma, M. Molecular and genetic mechanisms in brain arteriovenous malformations: New insights and future perspectives. *Neurosurg. Rev.* **2022**, *45*, 3573–3593. [CrossRef]
22. Bharatha, A.; Faughnan, M.E.; Kim, H.; Pourmohamad, T.; Krings, T.; Bayrak-Toydemir, P.; Pawlikowska, L.; McCulloch, C.E.; Lawton, M.T.; Dowd, C.F.; et al. Brain arteriovenous malformation multiplicity predicts the diagnosis of hereditary hemorrhagic telangiectasia: Quantitative assessment. *Stroke* **2012**, *43*, 72–78. [CrossRef]
23. Corti, P.; Young, S.; Chen, C.Y.; Patrick, M.J.; Rochon, E.R.; Pekkan, K.; Roman, B.L. Interaction between alk1 and blood flow in the development of arteriovenous malformations. *Development* **2011**, *138*, 1573–1582. [CrossRef] [PubMed]
24. Fulbright, R.K.; Chaloupka, J.C.; Putman, C.M.; Sze, G.K.; Merriam, M.M.; Lee, G.K.; Fayad, P.B.; Awad, I.A.; White, R.I., Jr. MR of hereditary hemorrhagic telangiectasia: Prevalence and spectrum of cerebrovascular malformations. *AJNR Am. J. Neuroradiol.* **1998**, *19*, 477–484. [PubMed]
25. Nishida, T.; Faughnan, M.E.; Krings, T.; Chakinala, M.; Gossage, J.R.; Young, W.L.; Kim, H.; Pourmohamad, T.; Henderson, K.J.; Schrum, S.D.; et al. Brain arteriovenous malformations associated with hereditary hemorrhagic telangiectasia: Gene-phenotype correlations. *Am. J. Med. Genet. A* **2012**, *158A*, 2829–2834. [CrossRef] [PubMed]
26. McAllister, K.A.; Grogg, K.M.; Johnson, D.W.; Gallione, C.J.; Baldwin, M.A.; Jackson, C.E.; Helmbold, E.A.; Markel, D.S.; McKinnon, W.C.; Murrell, J.; et al. Endoglin, a TGF-beta binding protein of endothelial cells, is the gene for hereditary haemorrhagic telangiectasia type 1. *Nat. Genet.* **1994**, *8*, 345–351. [CrossRef]
27. Vincent, P.; Plauchu, H.; Hazan, J.; Faure, S.; Weissenbach, J.; Godet, J. A third locus for hereditary haemorrhagic telangiectasia maps to chromosome 12q. *Hum. Mol. Genet.* **1995**, *4*, 945–949. [CrossRef]
28. Johnson, D.W.; Berg, J.N.; Gallione, C.J.; McAllister, K.A.; Warner, J.P.; Helmbold, E.A.; Markel, D.S.; Jackson, C.E.; Porteous, M.E.; Marchuk, D.A. A second locus for hereditary hemorrhagic telangiectasia maps to chromosome 12. *Genome Res.* **1995**, *5*, 21–28. [CrossRef]
29. Gallione, C.J.; Richards, J.A.; Letteboer, T.G.; Rushlow, D.; Prigoda, N.L.; Leedom, T.P.; Ganguly, A.; Castells, A.; Ploos van Amstel, J.K.; Westermann, C.J.; et al. SMAD4 mutations found in unselected HHT patients. *J. Med. Genet.* **2006**, *43*, 793–797. [CrossRef]
30. Shameem, Y.; Irshad, S.; Mirza, N.; Hassan, N. Wyburn-Mason Syndrome: A Narrative Review. *Cureus* **2024**, *16*, e68070. [CrossRef]
31. So, J.M.; Mishra, C.; Holman, R.E. *Wyburn-Mason Syndrome*; StatPearls: Treasure Island, FL, USA, 2025.
32. Vanaman, M.J.; Hervey-Jumper, S.L.; Maher, C.O. Pediatric and inherited neurovascular diseases. *Neurosurg. Clin. N. Am.* **2010**, *21*, 427–441. [CrossRef]
33. Kasasbeh, A.S.; Kalaria, A.; Comi, A.M.; Lo, W.; Lin, D.D.M. Atypical Intracerebral Developmental Venous Anomalies in Sturge-Weber Syndrome: A Case Series and Review of Literature. *Pediatr. Neurol.* **2020**, *104*, 54–61. [CrossRef]
34. Nakashima, M.; Miyajima, M.; Sugano, H.; Iimura, Y.; Kato, M.; Tsurusaki, Y.; Miyake, N.; Saitsu, H.; Arai, H.; Matsumoto, N. The somatic GNAQ mutation c.548G>A (p.R183Q) is consistently found in Sturge-Weber syndrome. *J. Hum. Genet.* **2014**, *59*, 691–693. [CrossRef] [PubMed]
35. Sudarsanam, A.; Ardern-Holmes, S.L. Sturge-Weber syndrome: From the past to the present. *Eur. J. Paediatr. Neurol.* **2014**, *18*, 257–266. [CrossRef]
36. Yeom, S.; Comi, A.M. Updates on Sturge-Weber Syndrome. *Stroke* **2022**, *53*, 3769–3779. [CrossRef] [PubMed]
37. Huang, L.; Sun, H.; Liu, Y.; Xu, L.; Hu, M.; Yang, Y.; Wang, N.; Wu, Y.; Guo, W. GNAQ R183Q somatic mutation contributes to aberrant arteriovenous specification in Sturge-Weber syndrome through Notch signaling. *FASEB J.* **2023**, *37*, e23148. [CrossRef] [PubMed]
38. Krah, K.; Mironov, V.; Risau, W.; Flamme, I. Induction of vasculogenesis in quail blastodisc-derived embryoid bodies. *Dev. Biol.* **1994**, *164*, 123–132. [CrossRef]
39. Yamaguchi, T.P.; Dumont, D.J.; Conlon, R.A.; Breitman, M.L.; Rossant, J. flk-1, an flt-related receptor tyrosine kinase is an early marker for endothelial cell precursors. *Development* **1993**, *118*, 489–498. [CrossRef]
40. Conway, E.M.; Collen, D.; Carmeliet, P. Molecular mechanisms of blood vessel growth. *Cardiovasc. Res.* **2001**, *49*, 507–521. [CrossRef]
41. Moses, M.A. The regulation of neovascularization of matrix metalloproteinases and their inhibitors. *Stem Cells* **1997**, *15*, 180–189. [CrossRef]

42. Eelen, G.; Treps, L.; Li, X.; Carmeliet, P. Basic and Therapeutic Aspects of Angiogenesis Updated. *Circ. Res.* **2020**, *127*, 310–329. [CrossRef]
43. Siefert, S.A.; Sarkar, R. Matrix metalloproteinases in vascular physiology and disease. *Vascular* **2012**, *20*, 210–216. [CrossRef]
44. Brew, K.; Dinakarpandian, D.; Nagase, H. Tissue inhibitors of metalloproteinases: Evolution, structure and function. *Biochim. Biophys. Acta* **2000**, *1477*, 267–283. [CrossRef]
45. Rundhaug, J.E. Matrix metalloproteinases and angiogenesis. *J. Cell Mol. Med.* **2005**, *9*, 267–285. [CrossRef]
46. Wang, K.; Zhao, S.; Liu, B.; Zhang, Q.; Li, Y.; Liu, J.; Shen, Y.; Ding, X.; Lin, J.; Wu, Y.; et al. Perturbations of BMP/TGF-beta and VEGF/VEGFR signalling pathways in non-syndromic sporadic brain arteriovenous malformations (BAVM). *J. Med. Genet.* **2018**, *55*, 675–684. [CrossRef] [PubMed]
47. Ferreira, R.; Santos, T.; Amar, A.; Tahara, S.M.; Chen, T.C.; Giannotta, S.L.; Hofman, F.M. MicroRNA-18a improves human cerebral arteriovenous malformation endothelial cell function. *Stroke* **2014**, *45*, 293–297. [CrossRef] [PubMed]
48. Ng, I.; Tan, W.L.; Ng, P.Y.; Lim, J. Hypoxia inducible factor-1alpha and expression of vascular endothelial growth factor and its receptors in cerebral arteriovenous malformations. *J. Clin. Neurosci.* **2005**, *12*, 794–799. [CrossRef]
49. Sonstein, W.J.; Kader, A.; Michelsen, W.J.; Llena, J.F.; Hirano, A.; Casper, D. Expression of vascular endothelial growth factor in pediatric and adult cerebral arteriovenous malformations: An immunocytochemical study. *J. Neurosurg.* **1996**, *85*, 838–845. [CrossRef]
50. Koizumi, T.; Shiraishi, T.; Hagihara, N.; Tabuchi, K.; Hayashi, T.; Kawano, T. Expression of vascular endothelial growth factors and their receptors in and around intracranial arteriovenous malformations. *Neurosurgery* **2002**, *50*, 117–124; discussion 124–126. [CrossRef]
51. Han, C.; Choe, S.W.; Kim, Y.H.; Acharya, A.P.; Keselowsky, B.G.; Sorg, B.S.; Lee, Y.J.; Oh, S.P. VEGF neutralization can prevent and normalize arteriovenous malformations in an animal model for hereditary hemorrhagic telangiectasia 2. *Angiogenesis* **2014**, *17*, 823–830. [CrossRef]
52. Sandalcioglu, I.E.; Wende, D.; Eggert, A.; Muller, D.; Roggenbuck, U.; Gasser, T.; Wiedemayer, H.; Stolke, D. Vascular endothelial growth factor plasma levels are significantly elevated in patients with cerebral arteriovenous malformations. *Cerebrovasc. Dis.* **2006**, *21*, 154–158. [CrossRef]
53. Kim, G.H.; Hahn, D.K.; Kellner, C.P.; Hickman, Z.L.; Komotar, R.J.; Starke, R.M.; Mack, W.J.; Mocco, J.; Solomon, R.A.; Connolly, E.S., Jr. Plasma levels of vascular endothelial growth factor after treatment for cerebral arteriovenous malformations. *Stroke* **2008**, *39*, 2274–2279. [CrossRef] [PubMed]
54. Lawton, M.T.; Jacobowitz, R.; Spetzler, R.F. Redefined role of angiogenesis in the pathogenesis of dural arteriovenous malformations. *J. Neurosurg.* **1997**, *87*, 267–274. [CrossRef] [PubMed]
55. Zhu, Y.; Lawton, M.T.; Du, R.; Shwe, Y.; Chen, Y.; Shen, F.; Young, W.L.; Yang, G.Y. Expression of hypoxia-inducible factor-1 and vascular endothelial growth factor in response to venous hypertension. *Neurosurgery* **2006**, *59*, 687–696; discussion 96. [CrossRef] [PubMed]
56. Kojima, T.; Miyachi, S.; Sahara, Y.; Nakai, K.; Okamoto, T.; Hattori, K.; Kobayashi, N.; Negoro, M.; Yoshida, J. The relationship between venous hypertension and expression of vascular endothelial growth factor: Hemodynamic and immunohistochemical examinations in a rat venous hypertension model. *Surg. Neurol.* **2007**, *68*, 277–281; discussion 81. [CrossRef]
57. Hashimoto, T.; Wen, G.; Lawton, M.T.; Boudreau, N.J.; Bollen, A.W.; Yang, G.Y.; Barbaro, N.M.; Higashida, R.T.; Dowd, C.F.; Halbach, V.V.; et al. Abnormal expression of matrix metalloproteinases and tissue inhibitors of metalloproteinases in brain arteriovenous malformations. *Stroke* **2003**, *34*, 925–931. [CrossRef]
58. Bicer, A.; Guclu, B.; Ozkan, A.; Kurtkaya, O.; Koc, D.Y.; Necmettin Pamir, M.; Kilic, T. Expressions of angiogenesis associated matrix metalloproteinases and extracellular matrix proteins in cerebral vascular malformations. *J. Clin. Neurosci.* **2010**, *17*, 232–236. [CrossRef]
59. Neyazi, B.; Herz, A.; Stein, K.P.; Gawish, I.; Hartmann, C.; Wilkens, L.; Erguen, S.; Dumitru, C.A.; Sandalcioglu, I.E. Brain arteriovenous malformations: Implications of CEACAM1-positive inflammatory cells and sex on hemorrhage. *Neurosurg. Rev.* **2017**, *40*, 129–134. [CrossRef]
60. Nakamura, Y.; Sugita, Y.; Nakashima, S.; Okada, Y.; Yoshitomi, M.; Kimura, Y.; Miyoshi, H.; Morioka, M.; Ohshima, K. Alternatively Activated Macrophages Play an Important Role in Vascular Remodeling and Hemorrhaging in Patients with Brain Arteriovenous Malformation. *J. Stroke Cerebrovasc. Dis.* **2016**, *25*, 600–609. [CrossRef]
61. Guo, Y.; Tihan, T.; Kim, H.; Hess, C.; Lawton, M.T.; Young, W.L.; Zhao, Y.; Su, H. Distinctive distribution of lymphocytes in unruptured and previously untreated brain arteriovenous malformation. *Neuroimmunol. Neuroinflamm.* **2014**, *1*, 147–152. [CrossRef]
62. Zhang, R.; Han, Z.; Degos, V.; Shen, F.; Choi, E.J.; Sun, Z.; Kang, S.; Wong, M.; Zhu, W.; Zhan, L.; et al. Persistent infiltration and pro-inflammatory differentiation of monocytes cause unresolved inflammation in brain arteriovenous malformation. *Angiogenesis* **2016**, *19*, 451–461. [CrossRef]

63. Thomas, J.M.; Surendran, S.; Abraham, M.; Sasankan, D.; Bhaadri, S.; Rajavelu, A.; Kartha, C.C. Gene expression analysis of nidus of cerebral arteriovenous malformations reveals vascular structures with deficient differentiation and maturation. *PLoS ONE* **2018**, *13*, e0198617. [CrossRef] [PubMed]
64. Nikolaev, S.I.; Vetiska, S.; Bonilla, X.; Boudreau, E.; Jauhiainen, S.; Rezai Jahromi, B.; Khyzha, N.; DiStefano, P.V.; Suutarinen, S.; Kiehl, T.R.; et al. Somatic Activating KRAS Mutations in Arteriovenous Malformations of the Brain. *N. Engl. J. Med.* **2018**, *378*, 250–261. [CrossRef] [PubMed]
65. Oka, M.; Kushamae, M.; Aoki, T.; Yamaguchi, T.; Kitazato, K.; Abekura, Y.; Kawamata, T.; Mizutani, T.; Miyamoto, S.; Takagi, Y. KRAS G12D or G12V Mutation in Human Brain Arteriovenous Malformations. *World Neurosurg.* **2019**, *126*, e1365–e1373. [CrossRef] [PubMed]
66. Priemer, D.S.; Vortmeyer, A.O.; Zhang, S.; Chang, H.Y.; Curless, K.L.; Cheng, L. Activating KRAS mutations in arteriovenous malformations of the brain: Frequency and clinicopathologic correlation. *Hum. Pathol.* **2019**, *89*, 33–39. [CrossRef]
67. Hong, T.; Yan, Y.; Li, J.; Radovanovic, I.; Ma, X.; Shao, Y.W.; Yu, J.; Ma, Y.; Zhang, P.; Ling, F.; et al. High prevalence of KRAS/BRAF somatic mutations in brain and spinal cord arteriovenous malformations. *Brain* **2019**, *142*, 23–34. [CrossRef]
68. Al-Olabi, L.; Polubothu, S.; Dowsett, K.; Andrews, K.A.; Stadnik, P.; Joseph, A.P.; Knox, R.; Pittman, A.; Clark, G.; Baird, W.; et al. Mosaic RAS/MAPK variants cause sporadic vascular malformations which respond to targeted therapy. *J. Clin. Investig.* **2018**, *128*, 1496–1508. [CrossRef]
69. Shoemaker, L.D.; Fuentes, L.F.; Santiago, S.M.; Allen, B.M.; Cook, D.J.; Steinberg, G.K.; Chang, S.D. Human brain arteriovenous malformations express lymphatic-associated genes. *Ann. Clin. Transl. Neurol.* **2014**, *1*, 982–995. [CrossRef]
70. Shoemaker, L.D.; McCormick, A.K.; Allen, B.M.; Chang, S.D. Evidence for endothelial-to-mesenchymal transition in human brain arteriovenous malformations. *Clin. Transl. Med.* **2020**, *10*, e99. [CrossRef]
71. Fish, J.E.; Flores Suarez, C.P.; Boudreau, E.; Herman, A.M.; Gutierrez, M.C.; Gustafson, D.; DiStefano, P.V.; Cui, M.; Chen, Z.; De Ruiz, K.B.; et al. Somatic Gain of KRAS Function in the Endothelium Is Sufficient to Cause Vascular Malformations That Require MEK but Not PI3K Signaling. *Circ. Res.* **2020**, *127*, 727–743. [CrossRef]
72. Giarretta, I.; Sturiale, C.L.; Gatto, I.; Pacioni, S.; Gaetani, E.; Porfidia, A.; Puca, A.; Palucci, I.; Tondi, P.; Olivi, A.; et al. Sonic hedgehog is expressed in human brain arteriovenous malformations and induces arteriovenous malformations in vivo. *J. Cereb. Blood Flow. Metab.* **2021**, *41*, 324–335. [CrossRef]
73. Wang, S.; Deng, X.; Wu, Y.; Zhou, S.; Yang, J.; Huang, Y. Understanding the pathogenesis of brain arteriovenous malformation: Genetic variations, epigenetics, signaling pathways, and immune inflammation. *Hum. Genet.* **2023**, *142*, 1633–1649. [CrossRef]
74. Mansur, A.; Radovanovic, I. Vascular malformations: An overview of their molecular pathways, detection of mutational profiles and subsequent targets for drug therapy. *Front. Neurol.* **2023**, *14*, 1099328. [CrossRef] [PubMed]
75. Perez-Alfayate, R.; Grasso, G. State of the Art and Future Direction in Diagnosis, Molecular Biology, Genetics, and Treatment of Brain Arteriovenous Malformations. *World Neurosurg.* **2022**, *159*, 362–372. [CrossRef] [PubMed]
76. Pan, P.; Shaligram, S.S.; Do Prado, L.B.; He, L.; Su, H. The role of mural cells in hemorrhage of brain arteriovenous malformation. *Brain Hemorrhages* **2021**, *2*, 49–56. [CrossRef] [PubMed]
77. Goss, J.A.; Huang, A.Y.; Smith, E.; Konczyk, D.J.; Smits, P.J.; Sudduth, C.L.; Stapleton, C.; Patel, A.; Alexandrescu, S.; Warman, M.L.; et al. Somatic mutations in intracranial arteriovenous malformations. *PLoS ONE* **2019**, *14*, e0226852. [CrossRef]
78. Murphy, P.A.; Lam, M.T.; Wu, X.; Kim, T.N.; Vartanian, S.M.; Bollen, A.W.; Carlson, T.R.; Wang, R.A. Endothelial Notch4 signaling induces hallmarks of brain arteriovenous malformations in mice. *Proc. Natl. Acad. Sci. USA* **2008**, *105*, 10901–10906. [CrossRef]
79. ZhuGe, Q.; Zhong, M.; Zheng, W.; Yang, G.Y.; Mao, X.; Xie, L.; Chen, G.; Chen, Y.; Lawton, M.T.; Young, W.L.; et al. Notch-1 signalling is activated in brain arteriovenous malformations in humans. *Brain* **2009**, *132 Pt 12*, 3231–3241. [CrossRef]
80. Li, S.; Wang, R.; Wang, Y.; Li, H.; Zheng, J.; Duan, R.; Zhao, J. Receptors of the Notch signaling pathway are associated with hemorrhage of brain arteriovenous malformations. *Mol. Med. Rep.* **2014**, *9*, 2233–2238. [CrossRef]
81. Xu, H.; Huo, R.; Li, H.; Jiao, Y.; Weng, J.; Wang, J.; Yan, Z.; Zhang, J.; Zhao, S.; He, Q.; et al. KRAS mutation-induced EndMT of brain arteriovenous malformation is mediated through the TGF-beta/BMP-SMAD4 pathway. *Stroke Vasc. Neurol.* **2023**, *8*, 197–206. [CrossRef]
82. Winkler, E.; Wu, D.; Gil, E.; McCoy, D.; Narsinh, K.; Sun, Z.; Mueller, K.; Ross, J.; Kim, H.; Weinsheimer, S.; et al. Endoluminal Biopsy for Molecular Profiling of Human Brain Vascular Malformations. *Neurology* **2022**, *98*, e1637–e1647. [CrossRef]
83. Adhicary, S.; Fanelli, K.; Nakisli, S.; Ward, B.; Pearce, I.; Nielsen, C.M. Rbpj Deficiency Disrupts Vascular Remodeling via Abnormal Apelin and Cdc42 (Cell Division Cycle 42) Activity in Brain Arteriovenous Malformation. *Stroke* **2023**, *54*, 1593–1605. [CrossRef] [PubMed]
84. Hermanto, Y.; Takagi, Y.; Ishii, A.; Yoshida, K.; Kikuchi, T.; Funaki, T.; Mineharu, Y.; Miyamoto, S. Immunohistochemical Analysis of Sox17 Associated Pathway in Brain Arteriovenous Malformations. *World Neurosurg.* **2016**, *87*, 573–583.e1–e2. [CrossRef] [PubMed]
85. Shabani, Z.; Schuerger, J.; Su, H. Cellular loci involved in the development of brain arteriovenous malformations. *Front. Hum. Neurosci.* **2022**, *16*, 968369. [CrossRef] [PubMed]

86. Tu, T.; Peng, Z.; Zhang, L.; Yang, J.; Guo, K.; Tang, X.; Ye, J.; Zhang, F.; Huang, A.; Yu, J.; et al. Neuroinflammation and hypoxia promote astrocyte phenotypic transformation and propel neurovascular dysfunction in brain arteriovenous malformation. *J. Neuroinflamm.* **2025**, *22*, 124. [CrossRef]
87. Thomas, J.M.; Sasankan, D.; Surendran, S.; Abraham, M.; Rajavelu, A.; Kartha, C.C. Aberrant regulation of retinoic acid signaling genes in cerebral arterio venous malformation nidus and neighboring astrocytes. *J. Neuroinflamm.* **2021**, *18*, 61. [CrossRef]
88. Nakisli, S.; Lagares, A.; Nielsen, C.M.; Cuervo, H. Pericytes and vascular smooth muscle cells in central nervous system arteriovenous malformations. *Front. Physiol.* **2023**, *14*, 1210563. [CrossRef]
89. Dalton, A.; Dobson, G.; Prasad, M.; Mukerji, N. De novo intracerebral arteriovenous malformations and a review of the theories of their formation. *Br. J. Neurosurg.* **2018**, *32*, 305–311. [CrossRef]
90. Andaluz, N.; Myseros, J.S.; Sathi, S.; Crone, K.R.; Tew, J.M., Jr. Recurrence of cerebral arteriovenous malformations in children: Report of two cases and review of the literature. *Surg. Neurol.* **2004**, *62*, 324–330; discussion 30–31. [CrossRef]
91. Hashimoto, N.; Nozaki, K. Do cerebral arteriovenous malformations recur after angiographically confirmed total extirpation? *Crit. Rev. Neurosurg.* **1999**, *9*, 141–146. [CrossRef]
92. Kader, A.; Goodrich, J.T.; Sonstein, W.J.; Stein, B.M.; Carmel, P.W.; Michelsen, W.J. Recurrent cerebral arteriovenous malformations after negative postoperative angiograms. *J. Neurosurg.* **1996**, *85*, 14–18. [CrossRef] [PubMed]
93. Galletti, F.; Costa, C.; Cupini, L.M.; Eusebi, P.; Hamam, M.; Caputo, N.; Siliquini, S.; Conti, C.; Moschini, E.; Lunardi, P.; et al. Brain arteriovenous malformations and seizures: An Italian study. *J. Neurol. Neurosurg. Psychiatry* **2014**, *85*, 284–288. [CrossRef] [PubMed]
94. Cellerini, M.; Mangiafico, S.; Villa, G.; Ammannati, F.; Giordano, G.P. Disappearance of cerebral arteriovenous malformations after partial endovascular embolisation: Four cases with follow-up. *Neuroradiology* **2003**, *45*, 916–920. [CrossRef]
95. Lasjaunias, P. A revised concept of the congenital nature of cerebral arteriovenous malformations. *Interv. Neuroradiol.* **1997**, *3*, 275–281. [CrossRef] [PubMed]
96. Choi, E.J.; Walker, E.J.; Shen, F.; Oh, S.P.; Arthur, H.M.; Young, W.L.; Su, H. Minimal homozygous endothelial deletion of Eng with VEGF stimulation is sufficient to cause cerebrovascular dysplasia in the adult mouse. *Cerebrovasc. Dis.* **2012**, *33*, 540–547. [CrossRef]
97. Chen, W.; Sun, Z.; Han, Z.; Jun, K.; Camus, M.; Wankhede, M.; Mao, L.; Arnold, T.; Young, W.L.; Su, H. De novo cerebrovascular malformation in the adult mouse after endothelial Alk1 deletion and angiogenic stimulation. *Stroke* **2014**, *45*, 900–902. [CrossRef]
98. Walker, E.J.; Su, H.; Shen, F.; Choi, E.J.; Oh, S.P.; Chen, G.; Lawton, M.T.; Kim, H.; Chen, Y.; Chen, W.; et al. Arteriovenous malformation in the adult mouse brain resembling the human disease. *Ann. Neurol.* **2011**, *69*, 954–962. [CrossRef]
99. Shaligram, S.S.; Zhang, R.; Zhu, W.; Ma, L.; Luo, M.; Li, Q.; Weiss, M.; Arnold, T.; Santander, N.; Liang, R.; et al. Bone Marrow-Derived Alk1 Mutant Endothelial Cells and Clonally Expanded Somatic Alk1 Mutant Endothelial Cells Contribute to the Development of Brain Arteriovenous Malformations in Mice. *Transl. Stroke Res.* **2022**, *13*, 494–504. [CrossRef]
100. Hwan Kim, Y.; Vu, P.N.; Choe, S.W.; Jeon, C.J.; Arthur, H.M.; Vary, C.P.H.; Lee, Y.J.; Oh, S.P. Overexpression of Activin Receptor-Like Kinase 1 in Endothelial Cells Suppresses Development of Arteriovenous Malformations in Mouse Models of Hereditary Hemorrhagic Telangiectasia. *Circ. Res.* **2020**, *127*, 1122–1137. [CrossRef]
101. Krebs, L.T.; Starling, C.; Chervonsky, A.V.; Gridley, T. Notch1 activation in mice causes arteriovenous malformations phenocopied by ephrinB2 and EphB4 mutants. *Genesis* **2010**, *48*, 146–150. [CrossRef]
102. Nielsen, C.M.; Cuervo, H.; Ding, V.W.; Kong, Y.; Huang, E.J.; Wang, R.A. Deletion of Rbpj from postnatal endothelium leads to abnormal arteriovenous shunting in mice. *Development* **2014**, *141*, 3782–3792. [CrossRef]
103. Larrivee, B.; Prahst, C.; Gordon, E.; del Toro, R.; Mathivet, T.; Duarte, A.; Simons, M.; Eichmann, A. ALK1 signaling inhibits angiogenesis by cooperating with the Notch pathway. *Dev. Cell* **2012**, *22*, 489–500. [CrossRef] [PubMed]
104. Castonguay, R.; Werner, E.D.; Matthews, R.G.; Presman, E.; Mulivor, A.W.; Solban, N.; Sako, D.; Pearsall, R.S.; Underwood, K.W.; Seehra, J.; et al. Soluble endoglin specifically binds bone morphogenetic proteins 9 and 10 via its orphan domain, inhibits blood vessel formation, and suppresses tumor growth. *J. Biol. Chem.* **2011**, *286*, 30034–30046. [CrossRef] [PubMed]
105. Park, E.S.; Kim, S.; Yao, D.C.; Savarraj, J.P.J.; Choi, H.A.; Chen, P.R.; Kim, E. Soluble Endoglin Stimulates Inflammatory and Angiogenic Responses in Microglia That Are Associated with Endothelial Dysfunction. *Int. J. Mol. Sci.* **2022**, *23*, 1225. [CrossRef] [PubMed]
106. Ruiz, S.; Zhao, H.; Chandakkar, P.; Chatterjee, P.K.; Papoin, J.; Blanc, L.; Metz, C.N.; Campagne, F.; Marambaud, P. A mouse model of hereditary hemorrhagic telangiectasia generated by transmammary-delivered immunoblocking of BMP9 and BMP10. *Sci. Rep.* **2016**, *5*, 37366. [CrossRef]
107. Tillet, E.; Bailly, S. Emerging roles of BMP9 and BMP10 in hereditary hemorrhagic telangiectasia. *Front. Genet.* **2014**, *5*, 456. [CrossRef]
108. Townson, S.A.; Martinez-Hackert, E.; Greppi, C.; Lowden, P.; Sako, D.; Liu, J.; Ucran, J.A.; Liharska, K.; Underwood, K.W.; Seehra, J.; et al. Specificity and structure of a high affinity activin receptor-like kinase 1 (ALK1) signaling complex. *J. Biol. Chem.* **2012**, *287*, 27313–27325. [CrossRef]

109. Saito, T.; Bokhove, M.; Croci, R.; Zamora-Caballero, S.; Han, L.; Letarte, M.; de Sanctis, D.; Jovine, L. Structural Basis of the Human Endoglin-BMP9 Interaction: Insights into BMP Signaling and HHT1. *Cell Rep.* **2017**, *19*, 1917–1928. [CrossRef]
110. Park, E.S.; Kim, S.; Huang, S.; Yoo, J.Y.; Korbelin, J.; Lee, T.J.; Kaur, B.; Dash, P.K.; Chen, P.R.; Kim, E. Selective Endothelial Hyperactivation of Oncogenic KRAS Induces Brain Arteriovenous Malformations in Mice. *Ann. Neurol.* **2021**, *89*, 926–941. [CrossRef]
111. Couto, J.A.; Huang, A.Y.; Konczyk, D.J.; Goss, J.A.; Fishman, S.J.; Mulliken, J.B.; Warman, M.L.; Greene, A.K. Somatic MAP2K1 Mutations Are Associated with Extracranial Arteriovenous Malformation. *Am. J. Hum. Genet.* **2017**, *100*, 546–554. [CrossRef]
112. Chen, W.; Choi, E.J.; McDougall, C.M.; Su, H. Brain arteriovenous malformation modeling, pathogenesis, and novel therapeutic targets. *Transl. Stroke Res.* **2014**, *5*, 316–329. [CrossRef]
113. Darsaut, T.E.; Magro, E.; Bojanowski, M.W.; Chaalala, C.; Nico, L.; Bacchus, E.; Klink, R.; Iancu, D.; Weill, A.; Roy, D.; et al. Surgical treatment of brain arteriovenous malformations: Clinical outcomes of patients included in the registry of a pragmatic randomized trial. *J. Neurosurg.* **2023**, *138*, 891–899. [CrossRef]
114. Huang, P.W.; Peng, S.J.; Pan, D.H.; Yang, H.C.; Tsai, J.T.; Shiau, C.Y.; Su, I.C.; Chen, C.J.; Wu, H.M.; Lin, C.J.; et al. Vascular compactness of unruptured brain arteriovenous malformation predicts risk of hemorrhage after stereotactic radiosurgery. *Sci. Rep.* **2024**, *14*, 4011. [CrossRef]
115. Frenzel, T.; Lee, C.Z.; Kim, H.; Quinnine, N.J.; Hashimoto, T.; Lawton, M.T.; Guglielmo, B.J.; McCulloch, C.E.; Young, W.L. Feasibility of minocycline and doxycycline use as potential vasculostatic therapy for brain vascular malformations: Pilot study of adverse events and tolerance. *Cerebrovasc. Dis.* **2008**, *25*, 157–163. [CrossRef]
116. Muster, R.; Ko, N.; Smith, W.; Su, H.; Dickey, M.A.; Nelson, J.; McCulloch, C.E.; Sneed, P.K.; Clarke, J.L.; Saloner, D.A.; et al. Proof-of-concept single-arm trial of bevacizumab therapy for brain arteriovenous malformation. *BMJ Neurol. Open* **2021**, *3*, e000114. [CrossRef] [PubMed]
117. D'Amato, R.J.; Loughnan, M.S.; Flynn, E.; Folkman, J. Thalidomide is an inhibitor of angiogenesis. *Proc. Natl. Acad. Sci. USA* **1994**, *91*, 4082–4085. [CrossRef] [PubMed]
118. Boon, L.M.; Dekeuleneer, V.; Coulie, J.; Marot, L.; Bataille, A.C.; Hammer, F.; Clapuyt, P.; Jeanjean, A.; Dompmartin, A.; Vikkula, M. Case report study of thalidomide therapy in 18 patients with severe arteriovenous malformations. *Nat. Cardiovasc. Res.* **2022**, *1*, 562–567. [CrossRef] [PubMed]
119. Lekwuttikarn, R.; Lim, Y.H.; Admani, S.; Choate, K.A.; Teng, J.M.C. Genotype-Guided Medical Treatment of an Arteriovenous Malformation in a Child. *JAMA Dermatol.* **2019**, *155*, 256–257. [CrossRef]
120. Edwards, E.A.; Phelps, A.S.; Cooke, D.; Frieden, I.J.; Zapala, M.A.; Fullerton, H.J.; Shimano, K.A. Monitoring Arteriovenous Malformation Response to Genotype-Targeted Therapy. *Pediatrics* **2020**, *146*, e20193206. [CrossRef]
121. Cooke, D.L.; Frieden, I.J.; Shimano, K.A. Angiographic evidence of response to trametinib therapy for a spinal cord arteriovenous malformation. *J. Vasc. Anom.* **2021**, *2*, e018. [CrossRef]
122. Kalailingam, P.; Rannikmae, K.; Hausman-Kedem, M.; Musolino, P.L.; Ruigrok, Y.M. Genetic Insights Into Hemorrhagic Stroke and Vascular Malformations: Pathogenesis and Emerging Therapeutic Strategies. *Stroke* **2025**, *56*, 1298–1311. [CrossRef] [PubMed]
123. Ueki, Y.; Naylor, R.M.; Ghozy, S.A.; Thirupathi, K.; Rinaldo, L.; Kallmes, D.F.; Kadirvel, R. Advances in sporadic brain arteriovenous malformations: Novel genetic insights, innovative animal models and emerging therapeutic approaches. *J. Cereb. Blood Flow. Metab.* **2025**, *45*, 793–799. [CrossRef]
124. Coffman, S.A.; Peterson, K.; Contillo, N.; Fargen, K.M.; Wolfe, S.Q. A comprehensive review on the development of sporadic cerebral arteriovenous malformations: From Padget to next-generation sequencing. *J. Neurosurg.* **2024**, *141*, 323–332. [CrossRef]
125. Scherschinski, L.; Rahmani, R.; Srinivasan, V.M.; Catapano, J.S.; Oh, S.P.; Lawton, M.T. Genetics and Emerging Therapies for Brain Arteriovenous Malformations. *World Neurosurg.* **2022**, *159*, 327–337. [CrossRef]
126. Scimone, C.; Donato, L.; Alibrandi, S.; Conti, A.; Bortolotti, C.; Germano, A.; Alafaci, C.; Vinci, S.L.; D'Angelo, R.; Sidoti, A. Methylome analysis of endothelial cells suggests new insights on sporadic brain arteriovenous malformation. *Heliyon* **2024**, *10*, e35126. [CrossRef]
127. Palmieri, M.; Curro, A.; Tommasi, A.; Di Sarno, L.; Doddato, G.; Baldassarri, M.; Frullanti, E.; Giliberti, A.R.; Fallerini, C.; Spinazzola, A.; et al. Cell-free DNA next-generation sequencing liquid biopsy as a new revolutionary approach for arteriovenous malformation. *JVS Vasc. Sci.* **2020**, *1*, 176–180. [CrossRef]
128. Zenner, K.; Jensen, D.M.; Cook, T.T.; Dmyterko, V.; Bly, R.A.; Ganti, S.; Mirzaa, G.M.; Dobyns, W.B.; Perkins, J.A.; Bennett, J.T. Cell-free DNA as a diagnostic analyte for molecular diagnosis of vascular malformations. *Genet. Med.* **2021**, *23*, 123–130. [CrossRef]
129. Zimmermann, W.H.; Melnychenko, I.; Eschenhagen, T. Engineered heart tissue for regeneration of diseased hearts. *Biomaterials* **2004**, *25*, 1639–1647. [CrossRef]
130. Dye, B.R.; Hill, D.R.; Ferguson, M.A.; Tsai, Y.H.; Nagy, M.S.; Dyal, R.; Wells, J.M.; Mayhew, C.N.; Nattiv, R.; Klein, O.D.; et al. In vitro generation of human pluripotent stem cell derived lung organoids. *eLife* **2015**, *4*, e05098. [CrossRef]

131. Spence, J.R.; Mayhew, C.N.; Rankin, S.A.; Kuhar, M.F.; Vallance, J.E.; Tolle, K.; Hoskins, E.E.; Kalinichenko, V.V.; Wells, S.I.; Zorn, A.M.; et al. Directed differentiation of human pluripotent stem cells into intestinal tissue in vitro. *Nature* **2011**, *470*, 105–109. [CrossRef]
132. Lancaster, M.A.; Knoblich, J.A. Generation of cerebral organoids from human pluripotent stem cells. *Nat. Protoc.* **2014**, *9*, 2329–2340. [CrossRef] [PubMed]
133. Oh, E.J.; Kim, H.M.; Kwak, S.; Huh, C.; Chung, H.Y. The Formation of Human Arteriovenous Malformation Organoids and Their Characteristics. *Cells* **2024**, *13*, 1955. [CrossRef] [PubMed]
134. Nikolova, M.T.; He, Z.; Wimmer, R.A.; Seimiya, M.; Nikoloff, J.M.; Penninger, J.M.; Gray Camp, J.; Treutlein, B. Fate and state transitions during human blood vessel organoid development. *bioRxiv* **2022**. [CrossRef] [PubMed]
135. Salewskij, K.; Penninger, J.M. Blood Vessel Organoids for Development and Disease. *Circ. Res.* **2023**, *132*, 498–510. [CrossRef]
136. Cai, H.; Tian, C.; Chen, L.; Yang, Y.; Sun, A.X.; McCracken, K.; Tchieu, J.; Gu, M.; Mackie, K.; Guo, F. Vascular network-inspired diffusible scaffolds for engineering functional midbrain organoids. *Cell Stem Cell* **2025**, *32*, 824–837.e5. [CrossRef]
137. Kistemaker, L.; van Bodegraven, E.J.; de Vries, H.E.; Hol, E.M. Vascularized human brain organoids: Current possibilities and prospects. *Trends Biotechnol.* **2025**, *43*, 1275–1285. [CrossRef]

brain sciences

MDPI

Brief Report

The Value of Non-Invasive Optimal Vessel Analysis Quantitative Magnetic Resonance Angiography for Studying Flow and Collateral Patterns in Patients with Bilateral Carotid Steno-Occlusive Disease

Fiona Helg [1], Elisa Colombo [1,2], Corinne Inauen [3], Lara Maria Höbner [1], Martina Sebök [1,2], Tilman Schubert [4], Jorn Fierstra [1,2], Antonio Spinello [1], Susanne Wegener [2,3], Andreas R. Luft [2,3,5], Zsolt Kulcsar [4], Luca Regli [1,2] and Giuseppe Esposito [1,2,*]

[1] Department of Neurosurgery, Clinical Neuroscience Center, University Hospital Zurich, 8091 Zurich, Switzerland; fiona.helg@uzh.ch (F.H.); elisa.colombo@usz.ch (E.C.); lara.hoebner@usz.ch (L.M.H.); martina.seboek@usz.ch (M.S.); jorn.fierstra@usz.ch (J.F.); antonio.spinello@usz.ch (A.S.); luca.regli@usz.ch (L.R.)

[2] Faculty of Medicine, University of Zurich, 8006 Zurich, Switzerland; susanne.wegener@usz.ch (S.W.); andreas.luft@usz.ch (A.R.L.)

[3] Department of Neurology, Clinical Neuroscience Center, University Hospital Zurich, 8091 Zurich, Switzerland; corinne.inauen@usz.ch

[4] Department of Neuroradiology, Clinical Neuroscience Center, University Hospital Zurich, 8091 Zurich, Switzerland; tilman.schubert@usz.ch (T.S.); zsolt.kulcsar@usz.ch (Z.K.)

[5] Cereneo Center for Neurology and Rehabilitation, 6354 Vitznau, Switzerland

* Correspondence: giuseppe.esposito@usz.ch

Abstract: Background/Objectives: Bilateral steno-occlusive disease of the internal carotid artery (ICA) carries an increased stroke risk with associated high morbidity and mortality. Management of these patients is often complex. In this study, we evaluate the value of non-invasive optimal vessel analysis quantitative magnetic resonance angiography (NOVA-qMRA) for studying flow and collateral patterns in patients with bilateral carotid steno-occlusive disease. **Methods**: Patients with bilateral ICA-stenosis $\geq 50\%$ who received NOVA-qMRA were included in this study. The volume flow rates (VFRs) of the A2-segment of the anterior cerebral artery (A2-ACA), M1-segment of the middle cerebral artery (M1-MCA), and P2-segment of the posterior cerebral artery (P2-PCA) were analyzed. Demographic, clinical, and treatment data were collected. **Results**: Twenty-two patients (mean age $\pm$ SD: 68 $\pm$ 10 years) were included. Nineteen patients (86%) were symptomatic. Thirteen patients (59%) were revascularized; among them, M1-VFR was significantly lower (p-value = 0.01) on the side selected for revascularization (88 mL/min $\pm$ 53) compared to the contralateral one (130 mL/min $\pm$ 56). P2-VFR was significantly higher (p-value = 0.04) in the treated subgroup (108 mL/min $\pm$ 41) than in the non-treated one (83 mL/min $\pm$ 34). **Conclusions**: The present study supports the use of NOVA-qMRA to study flow and collateral patterns in patients with bilateral steno-occlusive carotid disease, especially M1- and P2-VFR. This information may be helpful for decision-making and to tailor revascularization treatment.

Keywords: stroke; steno-occlusive disease; NOVA-qMRA

1. Introduction

Stroke represents a major burden to the healthcare system with it being the second leading cause of death globally and a relevant cause of morbidity [1]. Bilateral ICA-stenosis and/or -occlusion is bearing a poor prognosis with an increased risk of stroke and consecutive disability, coma, and death [2].

Therapeutic management for this condition varies and is debated [3]. Given the variable symptomatology of bilateral steno-occlusive carotid disease, clinical presentation must be supported by further parameters to tailor the therapeutic strategy [4–6].

Magnetic resonance angiography (MRA) represents a well-established tool to study stroke patients and large cerebral artery stenosis or occlusion by using time-of-flight (TOF) sequences [7–10]. Unlike traditional methods that often rely on invasive procedures, contrast agents, or ionizing radiation, non-invasive optimal vessel analysis (NOVA)-qMRA uses TOF and phase contrast (PC) sequences. The synergy between TOF and PC sequences not only provides detailed anatomical localization but also highly accurate flow quantification of the major cerebral vessels (in mL/min), making it a superior method for assessing intracranial arterial VFRs (Figure 1). This way, NOVA enables us to study cerebral collateral pathways and quantify their activation [11–13]. The duration of the MRI procedure typically takes about 30 to 60 min depending on the number of intracranial vessels being assessed. After the acquisition of the imaging sequences, NOVA-qMRA requires the use of dedicated post-processing software installed on an external workstation used by a trained physician to compute the VFRs on patient-specific relevant vessels.

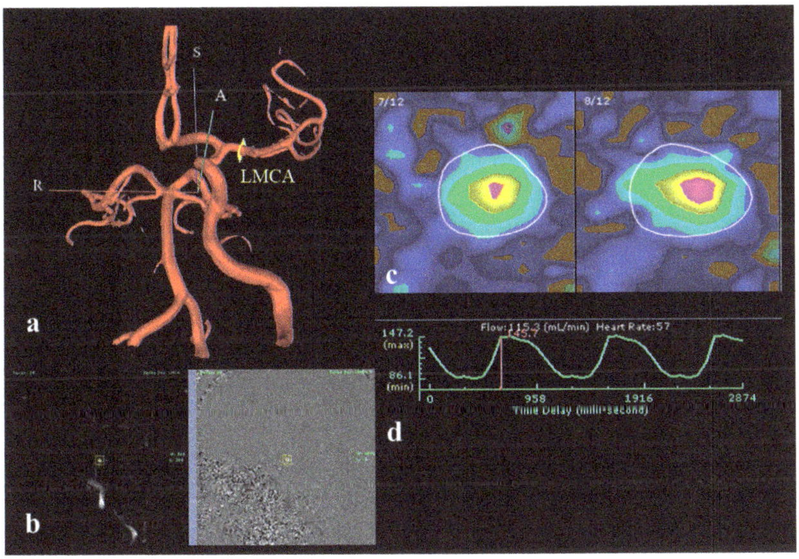

Figure 1. Workflow of the imaging post-processing in the NOVA software (VasSol, Chicago, IL, USA) The post-processing starts with the surface rendering of the cerebral vasculature from the 3D TOF MRA. A region of interest (ROI) is then placed perpendicular to the axis of the vessel of interest; in this exemplifying case, it is the left MCA. In this Figure R (red line) means Right, S (blue line) means Superior and A (green) means anterior: the axes are given for three-dimensional clarity (**a**). The cut is then adjusted according to the gated 2D phase contrast sequences (**b**) and proofed with the velocity contouring of the vessels, where the greatest intravascular velocity is portrayed in purple and the concentric slower velocity and progressively identified by yellow, green and light blue (**c**). The corresponding waveform, including the volume flow rate of the specific vessel, is automatically obtained (**d**).

Due to the complexity and interindividual variability in the angioanatomy of patients with bilateral ICA-stenosis and/or -occlusion, a tailored treatment strategy is required [14]. Besides clinical presentation, flow analysis might be useful as an additional parameter to aid the therapeutic decision-making. In this study, we report on a series of patients with bilateral steno-occlusive carotid disease where flow and collateral patterns were studied via NOVA-qMRA.

2. Materials and Methods

Kantonale Ethikkommission (Kanton Zürich, Switzerland) approval was obtained (KEK-Nr: PB_2023_01011) and all patients signed an informed consent form for the sharing and scientific diffusion of their clinical and radiological data.

2.1. Patient Cohort

Patients with bilateral ICA-stenosis ≥50% who received NOVA-qMRA between January 2019 and January 2022 were included in this study. The severity of ICA steno-occlusive disease was classified according to the North American Symptomatic Carotid Endarterectomy Trial (NASCET) criteria, a widely used classification system based on measuring the degree of arterial narrowing caused by atherosclerotic plaques, with the aim of guiding clinical decisions regarding medical or surgical treatment [15]. According to the NASCET criteria, the degree of stenosis is calculated as a percentage reduction in the lumen diameter of the ICA by comparing the residual lumen diameter at the site of maximal stenosis to the normal lumen diameter of the distal ICA, which serves as the reference point. Patients were divided into two groups, i.e., treated and non-treated, depending on whether they were revascularized or not. Demographic, clinical, radiological, and therapeutic data of the included patients during the hospital stay were collected. The National Institutes of Health Stroke Scale (NIHSS) and modified Rankin scale (mRS) at the time of hospital admission and discharge were collected to document functional status and outcome. The Trial of Org 10172 in the acute stroke treatment (TOAST) system was used to identify the likely etiology of the stroke of the included patients. This system does not specify nor quantify the severity of the intracranial atherosclerosis, but it does categorize ischemic strokes into 5 subtypes based on the underlying mechanism of injury [16].

2.2. Imaging Data

The volume flow rates (VFRs) of the following arterial segments were collected: A2-segment of the anterior cerebral artery (A2-ACA), M1-segment of the middle cerebral artery (M1-MCA), and P2-segment of the posterior cerebral artery (P2-PCA). The hemispheric VFR (hVFR) was calculated as the summation of the ipsilateral A2-, M1-, and P2-VFRs [16]. The choice of the arterial segments provided a comprehensive assessment of the functionality of both the anterior (via ACoA) and posterior (via PCoA) collateral pathways. These segments were specifically targeted because they serve as critical "bridges" in redistributing blood flow in the presence of steno-occlusive disease, offering insights into collateral circulation. The VFRs were compared between the treated- and non-treated subgroups. Within the treated group, the VFRs of the revascularized vs. non-revascularized hemisphere were also compared (Figure 2).

In symptomatic patients, the timing at which the NOVA-qMRA was performed was defined in the acute phase (0–7 days), subacute phase (8 days to 6 weeks), and chronic phase (>6 weeks) from symptoms' onset [17].

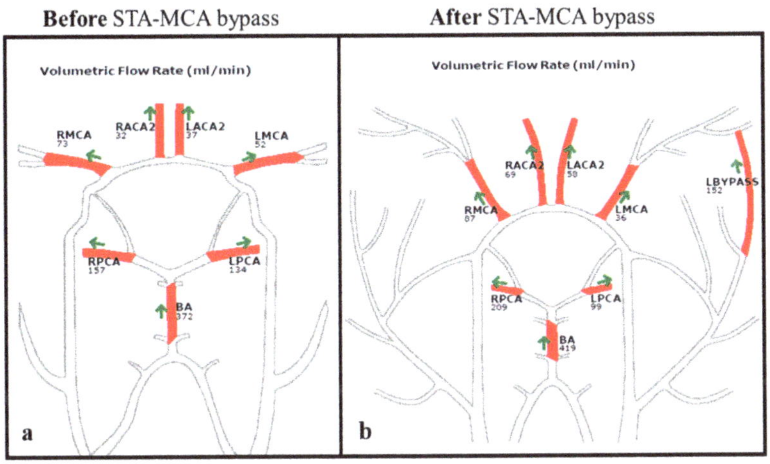

Figure 2. NOVA-maps of a 67-year-old patient who presented with an acute left ICA-occlusion and contralateral chronic ICA-occlusion. On the **left**, the preoperative NOVA-map shows a reduced left MCA-M1-VFR of 52 mL/min (the normal range for LMCA VFR in subjects above 61 years of age is between 81 mL/min and 201 mL/min) and an increased left PCA-P2-VFR of 134 mL/min (the normal range for LPCA VFR in subjects above 61 years of age is between 34 mL/min and 88 mL/min) (**a**); on the **right** is the NOVA-map 2 days after an acute left flow augmentation STA-MCA bypass showing adequate VFR of the bypass and a reduction in the LPCA VFR, demonstrating less need for collateral pathways (**b**).

2.3. Statistical Analysis

Statistical analysis was performed using R Studio (2023.06.2). After assessing the normal distribution of the data using the Shapiro–Wilk test, VFRs of the segments A2, M1, and P2 were analyzed and compared, either in an intra- or intergroupal manner. For intragroupal comparisons, one-tailed, paired *t*-tests were conducted, and for intergroupal comparisons, one-tailed, unpaired *t*-tests were performed. A p-value < 0.05 was considered to represent statistical significance.

3. Results

3.1. Demographic and Clinical Data

In total, 22 patients (1 woman and 21 men, mean age ± SD: 68 ± 10 years) with bilateral ICA-stenosis and/or -occlusion were included from our prospective register. Twenty patients presented severe atherosclerosis defined as Grade 1 according to the TOAST classification and two presented with TOAST Grade 2 [18]. Further clinical and demographic data are summarized in Table 1.

At the time of hospital admission, only one patient (4.5%) presented with an NIHSS > 7, and two patients (9%) had an mRS > 2. At discharge, two patients (9%) showed an NIHSS > 7 and one patient (4.5%) presented an mRS > 2. Twelve patients (55%) received surgical treatment, of which four (33%) underwent carotid endarterectomy (CEA), seven (58%) underwent flow augmentation superficial temporal artery to middle cerebral artery (STA-MCA) bypass, and one patient (8%) underwent a combined approach consisting of CEA of the left external carotid artery (ECA) followed by ipsilateral STA-MCA bypass. One patient (5%) received carotid artery stenting. Nine patients (41%) were managed conservatively. The therapeutic strategies are summarized in Table 2.

Table 1. Clinical data of included patients with bilateral ICA-stenosis and/or -occlusion (all patients n = 22).

	n (%)
Male gender	21 (95)
Symptomatic disease	19 (86)
Unilateral ICA-occlusion + contralateral stenosis ≥ 70%	7 (32)
Bilateral ICA-stenosis ≥ 70%	2 (9)
Bilateral ICA-occlusion	3 (14)
Unilateral occlusion and contralateral stenosis ≥ 50%, <70%	10 (45)
TOAST 1	20 (91)
TOAST 2	2 (9)
Additional Basilar artery stenosis	2 (9)
Additional unilateral vertebral artery stenosis or occlusion	4 (18)
Additional bilateral vertebral artery stenosis or occlusion	1 (5)

ICA = internal carotid artery; TOAST = trial of ORG 10172 in acute stroke treatment.

Table 2. Therapeutic strategies and localization.

Therapy	*n* (%)		Bilateral	Left Side Only	Right Side Only
Conservative	9 (41)		NA	NA	NA
Endovascular	1 (5) *		0	1	0
Surgery	12 (55)		1	8	3
	4	CEA			
	7	STA-MCA bypass			
	1	Combined approach [1]			

CEA = carotid endarterectomy, STA-MCA bypass = superficial temporal artery-middle cerebral artery bypass, [1] Combined approach = CEA of the left ECA (external carotid artery), and ipsilateral STA-MCA bypass *: carotid artery stenting (CAS), NA = Not applicable.

3.2. Hemodynamic Assessment

Nineteen patients (86%) presented with symptoms. The timing of the NOVA-qMRA after the cerebrovascular insult (CVI) is shown in Table 3. In three patients (14%), bilateral ICA-stenosis was discovered incidentally.

Table 3. Timing of NOVA-qMRA after CVI for the 19 symptomatic patients.

	Acute (0–7 Days)	Subacute (8 Days–6 Weeks)	Chronic (>6 Weeks)
Timing of NOVA-qMRA after CVI	9 (47%)	5 (26%)	5 (26%)

NOVA-qMRA = non-invasive optimal vessel analysis quantitative magnetic resonance angiography; CVI = cerebrovascular insult.

3.3. Treated Group

Thirteen patients received a cerebral revascularization procedure based on the NOVA-qMRA VFRs co-adjuvate by the clinical presentation. In the treated group, two patients (15%) presented with bilateral ICA-stenosis ≥ 70%, three (23%) with bilateral ICA-occlusion, five (38%) had unilateral ICA-occlusion and contralateral stenosis ≥ 70%, and three had unilateral ICA-occlusion and contralateral ICA-stenosis ≥ 50% and <70%. Out of the treated patients, 11 (84%) exhibited symptoms. Before treatment, the mean VFR of the hemisphere selected for revascularization was 253 mL/min, whereas the mean value of the contralateral hemisphere was 304 mL/min. The mean M1-VFR on the side selected for revascularization was significantly lower than that of the contralateral side (88 mL/min vs. 130 mL/min, *p*-value of 0.01). Please refer to Table 2 for an overview of the therapeutic strategy and the chosen revascularized side in this subgroup of patients, and to Table 4 for a visual summary of the segmental VFRs in the treated group.

Table 4. Comparison between segmental VFRs (A2, M1, P2) on the hemisphere selected for revascularization and segmental VFRs of the contralateral side.

VFR (mL/min)	Side Chosen for Revascularization (Mean ± SD)	Contralateral Side (Mean ± SD)	*p*-Values
A2	63 ± 33	68 ± 30	0.22
M1	88 ± 53	130 ± 56	0.01
P2	108 ± 41	105 ± 66	0.45

3.4. Non-Treated Group

Nine patients were treated conservatively. Among these, two patients (22%) presented with unilateral ICA-occlusion and contralateral stenosis $\geq$ 70%, while the remaining seven patients (78%) had unilateral ICA-occlusion and contralateral ICA-stenosis $\geq$ 50% and <70%. In the non-treated group, eight patients (89%) were symptomatic. In this subgroup, no significant differences were observed after comparing the segmental VFRs of the right and left sides (see Table 5). The mean hemispheric VFR of the left side was 292 mL/min, whereas the mean VFR of the contralateral side was 305 mL/min.

Table 5. Segmental (A2, M1, P2) VFRs of the non-treated subgroup.

VFR (mL/min)	Left Side (Mean ± SD)	Right Side (Mean ± SD)
A2	78 ± 11	82 ± 27
M1	127 ± 35	150 ± 48
P2	84 ± 44	83 ± 34

3.5. Comparison Between Treated and Non-Treated Groups

When comparing the segmental VFRs between the treated and non-treated groups, the M1-VFR was found to be significantly higher (*p*-value = 0.05) in the non-treated subgroup. Furthermore, the P2- and A2-VFRs were found to be significantly higher (*p*-values of 0.04 and 0.03, respectively) in the treated subgroup.

4. Discussion

This study highlights the potential value of NOVA-qMRA in evaluating blood flow and collateral circulation in patients with bilateral steno-occlusive carotid disease. Managing these patients is particularly challenging, as their clinical presentation can vary widely and is often nonspecific [19–21]. Incorporating flow data derived from NOVA-qMRA into clinical assessments could enhance therapeutic decision-making, especially in cases where the laterality of symptoms is ambiguous. This information may prove invaluable in guiding the choice of the hemisphere to revascularize [8,17–24].

We analyzed NOVA measurements from 22 patients with bilateral internal carotid artery (ICA) stenosis and/or occlusion, 19 of whom presented with neurological symptoms. Among these patients, 13 underwent revascularization. Flow velocity and volume flow rates (VFRs) were measured in key arterial segments, defined as A2, M1, and

P2. In the treated group, the segmental VFR analysis revealed a significantly lower M1-VFR on the revascularized side compared to the contralateral side (88 ± 53 mL/min vs. 130 ± 56 mL/min, $p = 0.01$). Conversely, in the non-treated subgroup, there were no significant differences in M1- or P2-VFRs between the two hemispheres.

Interestingly, the P2-VFRs were significantly higher in the treated group compared to the non-treated group. This finding could reflect the increased activation of the collateral leptomeningeal pathways through the posterior cerebral artery [16,25,26]. Such collateral flow activation may serve as a compensatory mechanism in response to diminished anterior circulation flow, further underlining the utility of NOVA-qMRA in identifying critical hemodynamic patterns.

The clinical outcomes in our cohort were encouraging. At the time of hospital discharge, among the patients included in the analyzed cohort, only one presented a neurological worsening, while the rest of the cohort did not show any relevant neurological exacerbation [25,27,28]. Furthermore, our findings suggest that higher M1-VFRs and lower P2-VFRs are associated with better-preserved cerebral hemodynamics and flows [16,18,27–29]. These observations align with the growing understanding of the importance of collateral circulation in maintaining adequate cerebral perfusion in the context of ICA disease. However, there are some limitations to this study that should be acknowledged. First, the small sample size limits the statistical power and generalizability of our findings. Larger studies are needed to validate and extend these results. Second, the study cohort was recruited from a single tertiary referral center, which introduces an inherent selection bias and may not reflect the broader patient population. Furthermore, this study represents a retrospective analysis that aimed to provide initial data on the implementation of NOVA-qMRA in the study of anterior cerebral circulation, and it did not provide a thorough comparison of NOVA-qMRA with other imaging techniques in this cohort of patients; thus, the power of the analysis is reduced. Despite these limitations, this pilot study provides important preliminary evidence supporting the integration of NOVA-qMRA into the diagnostic workup of patients with bilateral steno-occlusive carotid disease.

5. Conclusions

This study endorses the added value of NOVA-qMRA to the diagnostic workup process of patients with bilateral steno-occlusive carotid disease. The analysis of segmental VFRs, especially of M1- and P2-VFR, might be helpful to select and tailor revascularization treatment.

Author Contributions: Conceptualization, G.E., E.C., S.W. and A.R.L.; methodology, G.E.; formal analysis, F.H. and E.C.; investigation, F.H.; data curation, F.H., E.C., L.M.H. and A.S.; writing—original draft preparation, F.H. and E.C.; writing—review and editing F.H., E.C., G.E., M.S., T.S., J.F. and L.R.; supervision, G.E., L.R., Z.K. and C.I. All authors have read and agreed to the published version of the manuscript.

Funding: This research received no external funding.

Institutional Review Board Statement: Kantonale Ethikkommission (Kanton Zürich) approval was obtained (KEK-Nr: PB_2023_01011, 26 March 2024).

Informed Consent Statement: All patients signed an informed consent form for the sharing and scientific diffusion of their clinical and radiological data.

Data Availability Statement: Data are available upon request to the corresponding author for scientific purposes only. The data are not publicly available due to data protection and privacy.

Conflicts of Interest: The authors declare no conflicts of interest.

Abbreviations

The following abbreviations are used in this manuscript:

ICA	Internal Carotid Artery
NOVA-qMRA	Non-invasive optimal vessel analysis quantitative magnetic resonance angiography
VFR	Volume flow rate
ACA	Anterior cerebral artery
MCA	Middle cerebral artery
PCA	Posterior cerebral artery
TOF	Time-of-flight
PC	Phase contrast
NIHSS	National Institutes of Health Stroke Scale
mRS	Modified Rankin scale
STA	Superior temporal artery
NASCET	North American Symptomatic Carotid Endarterectomy Trial
CVI	Cerebrovascular insult
TOAST	Trial of ORG 10172 in acute stroke treatment
ECA	External carotid artery
CAS	Carotid artery stenting

References

1. Donkor, E.S. Stroke in the 21st Century: A Snapshot of the Burden, Epidemiology, and Quality of Life. *Stroke Res. Treat.* **2018**, *2018*, 3238165. [CrossRef] [PubMed]
2. Persoon, S.; Klijn, C.J.; Algra, A.; Kappelle, L.J. Bilateral carotid artery occlusion with transient or moderately disabling ischaemic stroke: Clinical features and long-term outcome. *J. Neurol.* **2009**, *256*, 1728–1735. [CrossRef] [PubMed]
3. Beutler, B.D.; Rangaswamy, R.; Bruno, A.J.; Tabaac, B.J. Acute bilateral internal carotid artery occlusion: A novel approach to management of a catastrophic clinical entity. *Clin. Imaging* **2021**, *76*, 166–174. [CrossRef]
4. Reinhard, M.; Müller, T.; Roth, M.; Guschlbauer, B.; Timmer, J.; Hetzel, A. Bilateral severe carotid artery stenosis or occlusion-cerebral autoregulation dynamics and collateral flow patterns. *Acta Neurochir.* **2003**, *145*, 1053–1060. [CrossRef]
5. Chaves, C.; Hreib, K.; Allam, G.; Liberman, R.F.; Lee, G.; Caplan, L.R. Patterns of cerebral perfusion in patients with asymptomatic internal carotid artery disease. *Cerebrovasc. Dis.* **2006**, *22*, 396–401. [CrossRef] [PubMed]
6. Huang, J.; Liu, H.; Chen, H.; Yuan, L.; Fang, L.; Yang, Z. Acute Bilateral Internal Carotid Artery Occlusion Presenting with Symmetric Cortical Infarctions Exhibits Dramatic Improvement After Mechanical Thrombectomy. *World Neurosurg.* **2020**, *141*, 149–152. [CrossRef] [PubMed]
7. Amin-Hanjani, S.; Du, X.; Zhao, M.; Walsh, K.; Malisch, T.W.; Charbel, F.T. Use of quantitative magnetic resonance angiography to stratify stroke risk in symptomatic vertebrobasilar disease. *Stroke* **2005**, *36*, 1140–1145. [CrossRef] [PubMed]
8. Barlinn, K.; Alexandrov, A.V. Vascular imaging in stroke: Comparative analysis. *Neurotherapeutics* **2011**, *8*, 340–348. [CrossRef]
9. Korogi, Y.; Takahashi, M.; Mabuchi, N.; Miki, H.; Shiga, H.; Watabe, T.; O'Uchi, T.; Nakagawa, T.; Horikawa, Y.; Fujiwara, S. Intracranial vascular stenosis and occlusion: Diagnostic accuracy of three-dimensional, Fourier transform, time-of-flight MR angiography. *Radiology* **1994**, *193*, 187–193. [CrossRef]
10. Heiserman, J.E.; Drayer, B.P.; Keller, P.J.; Fram, E.K. Intracranial vascular stenosis and occlusion: Evaluation with three-dimensional time-of-flight MR angiography. *Radiology* **1992**, *185*, 667–673. [CrossRef] [PubMed]
11. Zhao, M.; Charbel, F.T.; Alperin, N.; Loth, F.; Clark, M.E. Improved phase-contrast flow quantification by three-dimensional vessel localization. *Magn. Reson. Imaging* **2000**, *18*, 697–706. [CrossRef]
12. Calderon-Arnulphi, M.; Amin-Hanjani, S.; Alaraj, A.; Zhao, M.; Du, X.; Ruland, S.; Zhou, X.; Thulborn, K.; Charbel, F. In vivo evaluation of quantitative MR angiography in a canine carotid artery stenosis model. *AJNR Am. J. Neuroradiol.* **2011**, *32*, 1552–1559. [CrossRef] [PubMed]
13. Brisman, J.L. Wingspan stenting of symptomatic extracranial vertebral artery stenosis and perioperative evaluation using quantitative magnetic resonance angiography: Report of two cases. *Neurosurg. Focus* **2008**, *24*, E14. [CrossRef]
14. Fatic, N.; Jaffer, U.; Ivana, S.; Gordana, G.-V.; Markovic, D.; Kostic, D.; Davidovic, L. Bilateral Internal Carotid Artery Occlusion, External Carotid Artery Stenosis, and Vertebral Artery Kinking: May It Be Asymptomatic? *Ann. Vasc. Surg.* **2017**, *44*, 416.e5–416.e8. [CrossRef] [PubMed]

15. Arning, C.; Widder, B.; von Reutern, G.M.; Stiegler, H.; Görtler, M. Ultraschallkriterien zur Graduierung von Stenosen der A. carotis interna-Revision der DEGUM-Kriterien und Transfer in NASCET-Stenosierungsgrade. *Ultraschall Med.* **2010**, *31*, 251–257. [CrossRef]
16. Adams, H.P., Jr.; Bendixen, B.H.; Kappelle, L.J.; Biller, J.; Love, B.B.; Gordon, D.L.; Marsh, E.E., 3rd. Classification of subtype of acute ischemic stroke. Definitions for use in a multicenter clinical trial. TOAST. Trial of Org 10172 in Acute Stroke Treatment. *Stroke* **1993**, *24*, 35–41. [CrossRef] [PubMed]
17. Sebök, M.; Höbner, L.M.; Fierstra, J.; Schubert, T.; Wegener, S.; Kulcsár, Z.; Luft, A.R.; Regli, L.; Esposito, G. Flow-augmentation STA MCA bypass for acute and subacute ischemic stroke due to internal carotid artery occlusion and the role of advanced neuroim aging with hemodynamic and flow-measurement in the decision-making: Preliminary data. *Quant. Imaging Med. Surg.* **2024**, *14*, 777–788. [CrossRef] [PubMed]
18. Velz, J.; Esposito, G.; Wegener, S.; Kulcsar, Z.; Luft, A.; Regli, L. Diagnostisches und therapeutisches Handeln bei Karotisstenose [Diagnostic and Therapeutic Management of Carotid Artery Disease]. *Praxis* **2020**, *109*, 705–723. [CrossRef] [PubMed]
19. Karki, M.; Devarakonda, P.K.; Dhulipalla, L.; Pattipati, M.; Ayala-Rodriguez, C. Bilateral Internal Carotid Artery Occlusion, an Unusual Clinical Entity in a Young Adult. *Cureus* **2021**, *13*, e15971. [CrossRef]
20. van Niftrik, C.H.B.; Sebök, M.; Germans, M.R.; Halter, M.; Pokorny, T.; Stumpo, V.; Bellomo, J.; Piccirelli, M.; Pangalu, A.; Katan, M.; et al. Increased Risk of Recurrent Stroke in Symptomatic Large Vessel Disease with Impaired BOLD Cerebrovascular Reactivity. *Stroke* **2024**, *55*, 613–621. [CrossRef]
21. Qiao, X.; Duan, J.; Zhang, N.; Duan, Y.; Wang, X.; Pei, Y.; Xu, Z.; Yang, B.; Qi, M.; Li, J. Risk Factors of Impaired Perfusion in Patients With Symptomatic Internal Carotid Artery Steno-Occlusive Disease. *Front. Neurol.* **2022**, *13*, 801413. [CrossRef]
22. Amin-Hanjani, S.; Du, X.; Pandey, D.K.; Thulborn, K.R.; Charbel, F.T. Effect of age and vascular anatomy on blood flow in major cerebral vessels. *J. Cereb. Blood Flow Metab.* **2015**, *35*, 312–318. [CrossRef]
23. Amin-Hanjani, S.; Rose-Finnell, L.; Richardson, D.; Ruland, S.; Pandey, D.; Thulborn, K.R.; Liebeskind, D.S.; Zipfel, G.J.; Elkind, M.S.V.; Kramer, J.; et al. Vertebrobasilar Flow Evaluation and Risk of Transient Ischaemic Attack and Stroke study (VERiTAS): Rationale and design. *Int. J. Stroke* **2010**, *5*, 499–505. [CrossRef]
24. Starke, R.M.; Chwajol, M.; Lefton, D.; Sen, C.; Berenstein, A.; Langer, D.J. Occipital artery-to-posterior inferior cerebellar artery bypass for treatment of bilateral vertebral artery occlusion: The role of quantitative magnetic resonance angiography noninvasive optimal vessel analysis: Technical case report. *Neurosurgery* **2009**, *64*, E779–E781. [CrossRef] [PubMed]
25. van Niftrik, C.H.B.; Sebök, M.; Wegener, S.; Esposito, G.; Halter, M.; Hiller, A.; Stippich, C.; Luft, A.R.; Regli, L.; Fierstra, J. Increased Ipsilateral Posterior Cerebral Artery P2-Segment Flow Velocity Predicts Hemodynamic Impairment. *Stroke* **2021**, *52*, 1469–1472. [CrossRef] [PubMed]
26. Jud, S.; Klövekorn, R.; van Niftrik, C.H.B.; Herzog, L.; Sebök, M.; Schweizer, J.; Luft, A.R.; Fierstra, J.; Wegener, S. High posterior cerebral artery flow predicts ischemia recurrence in patients with internal carotid artery occlusion. *Front. Neurol.* **2023**, *14*, 1193640. [CrossRef] [PubMed]
27. Sebök, M.; Niftrik, C.H.B.V.; Lohaus, N.; Esposito, G.; El Amki, M.; Winklhofer, S.; Wegener, S.; Regli, L.; Fierstra, J. Leptomeningeal collateral activation indicates severely impaired cerebrovascular reserve capacity in patients with symptomatic unilateral carotid artery occlusion. *Cereb. Blood Flow Metab.* **2021**, *41*, 3039–3051. [CrossRef] [PubMed]
28. Connolly, F.; Röhl, J.E.; Lopez-Prieto, J.; Danyel, L.A.; Schreiber, S.J.; Valdueza, J.M. Pattern of Activated Pathways and Quality of Collateral Status in Patients with Symptomatic Internal Carotid Artery Occlusion. *Cerebrovasc. Dis.* **2019**, *48*, 244–250. [CrossRef] [PubMed]
29. Sebök, M.; Esposito, G.; Niftrik, C.H.B.V.; Fierstra, J.; Schubert, T.; Wegener, S.; Held, J.; Kulcsár, Z.; Luft, A.R.; Regli, L. Flow augmentation STA-MCA bypass evaluation for patients with acute stroke and unilateral large vessel occlusion: A proposal for an urgent bypass flowchart. *J. Neurosurg.* **2022**, *137*, 1047–1055. [CrossRef] [PubMed]

brain sciences

MDPI

Systematic Review

Neurosurgical Microvascular Anastomosis: Systematic Review of the Existing Simulators and Proposal of a New Training Classification System

Lelio Guida [1], Martina Sebök [2], Marcelo Magaldi Oliveira [3], Christiaan Hendrik Bas van Niftrik [2], Fady T. Charbel [4], Marco Cenzato [5], Luca Regli [2] and Giuseppe Esposito [2,*]

[1] Department of Pediatric Neurosurgery, Assistance Pubilque Hôpitaux de Paris, Hôpital Necker Enfants Malades, Université de Paris Cité, 75015 Paris, France; lelio.guida@aphp.fr
[2] Departement of Neurosurgery, Clinical Neuroscience Center, University Hospital of Zurich, University of Zurich, 8091 Zurich, Switzerland; martina.seboek@usz.ch (M.S.); bas.vanniftrik@usz.ch (C.H.B.v.N.); luca.regli@usz.ch (L.R.)
[3] Department of Surgery, School of Medicine, Federal University of Minas Gerais, Belo Horizonte 31270-901, MG, Brazil; mmagaldi@hotmail.com
[4] Department of Neurosurgery, University of Illinois at Chicago, Chicago, IL 60612, USA; fcharbel@uic.edu
[5] Department of Neurosurgery, Niguarda Great Metropolitan Hospital of Milan, 20162 Milan, Italy; marco.cenzato@ospedaleniguarda.it
* Correspondence: giuseppe.esposito@usz.ch; Tel.: +41-44-255-2660

Abstract: Background: The literature lacks a combined analysis of neurosurgical microvascular anastomosis training models. We performed a systematic literature search to provide an overview of the existing models and proposed a classification system based on the level of simulation and reproducibility of the microvascular anastomosis. Methods: The systematic literature search followed the PRISMA guidelines. We consulted MEDLINE, Web of Knowledge, and EMBASE independently for papers about bypass training models. Every training model was analyzed according to six tasks supposed to esteem their fidelity to the real operative setting by using a scoring system from zero to two. Finally, authors classified the models into five classes, from A to E, by summing the individual scores. Results: This study included 109 papers for analysis. Training models were grouped into synthetic tubes, ex vivo models (animal vessels, fresh human cadavers, human placentas) and in vivo simulators (live animals—rats, rabbits, pigs). By applying the proposed classification system, live animals and placentas obtained the highest scores, falling into class A (excellent simulators). Human cadavers and animal vessels (ex vivo) were categorized in class B (good simulators), followed by synthetic tubes (class C, reasonable simulators). Conclusions: The proposed classification system helps the neurosurgeon to analyze the available training models for microvascular anastomosis critically, and to choose the most appropriate one according to the skills they need to improve

Keywords: neurosurgical bypass; micro-anastomosis; microsurgical training; microvascular surgery

1. Introduction

Cerebral bypass surgery has become a niche procedure that has to be performed in high-volume cerebrovascular reference centers by experienced and dedicated microvascular surgeons [1–3]. Maintaining sufficient know-how and improving technical skills represents one of the significant challenges for cerebrovascular training centers [4].

Adequate training in microsuturing and microvascular anastomosis is essential to develop the appropriate dexterity [5,6]. Ideally, training models should offer an adequate setting to train each step of this delicate procedure. Several training models have been proposed in the literature, which are traditionally grouped into ex vivo or in vivo models.

This paper analyzes, discusses, and classifies the main existing models used to practice microvascular anastomosis, based on the level of simulation and anastomosis reproducibility. To the authors' knowledge, there is no such attempt in the literature so far.

2. Materials and Methods

2.1. Research Strategy

A comprehensive literature search was performed, following the PRISMA statement. MEDLINE, EMBASE and Web of Science were consulted between January 2019 and July 2023, using combinations of keywords and lexical variant about "training in microsurgical vascular anastomosis" ((education OR training OR simulator OR simulation) AND (anastomosis AND (microvascular) OR (microsurgical AND vascular) OR (microsurgery AND vascular)) OR ((micro-anastomosis AND vascular) OR (micro-anastomosis and vascular))). Since this review does not have a clear link to human health, it was not eligible for registration in PROSPERO.

All the original papers for training purposes on microvascular anastomoses written in English were included. Microsurgical anastomosis or micro-anastomosis refers to any vascular suture performed under an operative microscope, without a strict designation of minimum vessel size. Supermicrosurgical anastomosis is an anastomosis performed at 30–50× magnification on 0.3 to 0.8 mm vessels [7].

Exclusion criteria were papers about basic microsuture models (e.g., gazes), papers about microsurgical anastomosis of nerves, and micro-anastomosis papers not intended for training. Two independent reviewers (LG and MS) screened titles to find eligible papers; they read abstracts for primary evaluation of the studies and found additional studies in reference lists of relevant articles. No articles were retrieved from secondary sources.

2.2. Technical Classification of Brain Bypass Simulators: Six Tasks

The international board of experts in micro-neurovascular surgery defined 6 tasks during the international Bypass 2020 symposium in Zurich, Switzerland:

1. Vessel dissection: training with the dissection and the removal of adventitia.
2. Subarachnoidal dissection: training with the dissection of subarachnoidal spaces (cisterns).
3. Anastomosis variety: performing the standard micro-anastomoses within the same simulator (end-to-end, end-to-side, side-to-side).
4. Number of anastomoses/vessels/diameters of vessel: performing many microvascular anastomoses in the same simulator thanks to the availability of vessels of different diameters.
5. Stenosis-leaks: developing problem-solving strategies in case of anastomosis stenosis or anastomotic leaks (it requires perfusion and/or pressurization tests).
6. Thrombosis: developing problem-solving strategies in case of thrombosis of the micro-anastomosis.

By attributing the scores, authors considered all the simulators as perfused.

2.3. Scoring System

The authors applied to each simulator a scoring system ranging from zero to two:

- 0 points: the surgeon cannot execute the task by the simulator;
- 1 point: the task is described to be accomplished in an acceptable way;
- 2 points: the task is reported to be optimally doable by the simulator.

Agreement between the authors was ascertained by using Cohen's K. Therefore, according to the total score, models were classified into five classes, from class A (excellent simulator) to class E (not suitable as a simulator) (Table 1).

Table 1. Features of the classification system.

	Tasks	Score	Sum	Grade
1	Vessel dissection	2 task optimally doable	10–12	A (excellent simulator)
2	Subarachnoidal dissection		7–9	B (good simulator)
3	Variety of the anastomosis	1 task doable but not in a proper way	4–6	C (reasonable simulator)
4	Number anastomosis/vessel/diameter			
5	Stenosis leaks	0 task not doable	1–3	D (poor simulator)
6	Thrombosis		0	E (not a simulator)

3. Results

The literature search identified 327 non-duplicate records, of which 218 were excluded, and 109 articles were included in the analysis (Figure 1).

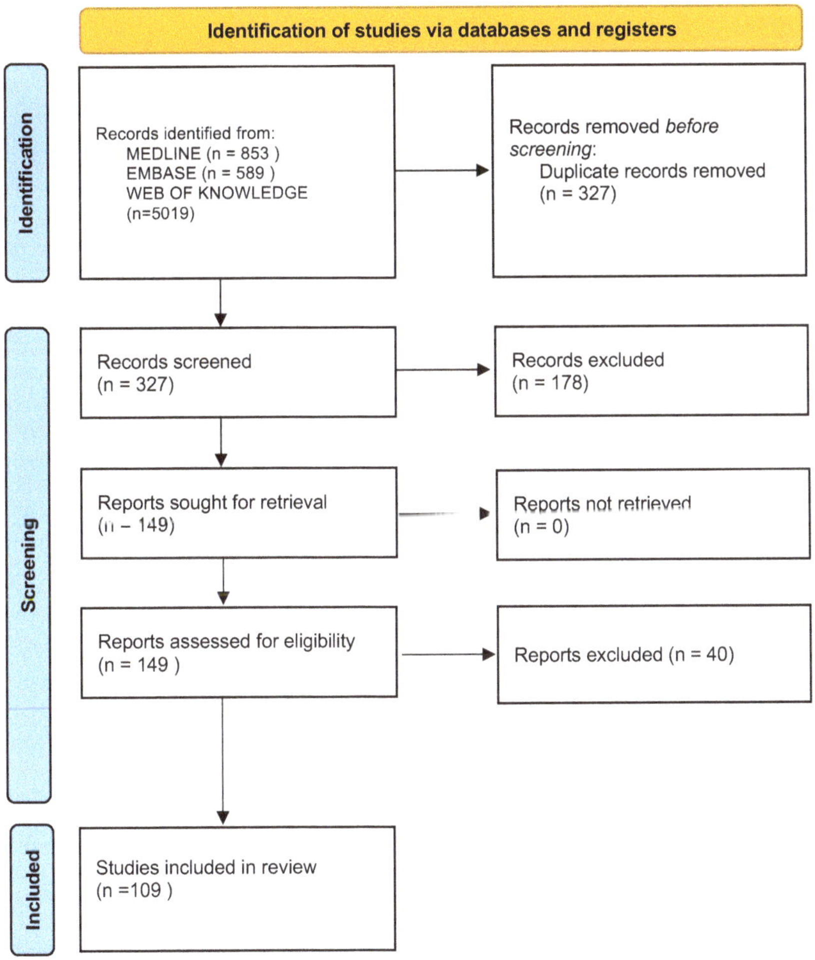

Figure 1. The PRISMA flowchart of the research strategy [8].

The models identified for analysis are described in the following sections.

3.1. Synthetic Tubes

Synthetic tubes have gained increasing success over the years because of their availability and low costs. Originally, manufacturers produced tubes in silicon [9], but current research proposes several alternative materials to better simulate the consistency of real arterial vessels (Gore-Tex, polyurethane, PVC, and PVA gelatin tubes).

In a recent blind randomized comparative survey between silicone and PVA tubes, the latter was demonstrated to better simulate rat vessels [10]. A three-layered synthetic vessel model has also been proposed [11].

Surgeons can train with single tubes, use practice cards composed of parallel tubes affixed to a pocketbook-sized card [12], or use commercialized supports [13]. Synthetic tubes offer the possibility to simulate standard types of vascular micro-anastomosis (task 3). The patency and strength of the anastomosis may be tested through the infusion of fluids [14] (task 5).

Disadvantages of these models include the impossibility to train with vessel and subarachnoid dissection (tasks 1 and 2) and to simulate thrombosis (task 6).

More complex and expensive models have been developed to overcome these limitations. Inoue proposed a model of an A3-A3 side-to-side bypass by putting two parallel prosthetic tubes on the bottom of a 6.5 cm deep paper box [15]. Takeuci presented an anatomic model using a mannequin head and small balloons filled with water, simulating the consistency of brain and Silastic tubes [16]. Ishikawa and Belykh developed skulls and brain models with craniotomies to simulate trans-Sylvian, subtemporal, suboccipital, and interhemispheric approaches [17,18]. Mori created an artificial skull and brain model to simulate posterior circulation revascularization [19]. In 2018, Cikla developed a skull and brain model with perfused artificial vessels to simulate both intra- and extracranial circulation and anastomoses [20]. Finally, the recently introduced virtual/augmented reality neurosurgical simulator boxes using synthetic perfused vessels in an anatomic accurate brain (e.g., Mycro model, Upsurgeon) represent an affordable and useful tool as an alternative to animal models [21].

3.2. Ex Vivo Training Models

3.2.1. Animal Vessels (In Vitro)

Microvascular trainees can perform anastomoses on vessels harvested from animals sacrificed for other purposes. These materials are ideal because of their similarity to macroscopic and microscopic human vessels [22]. Arteries can be isolated and explanted or anastomosed in situ. Once the trainee completes the anastomosis, vessels can be perfused and pressurized [23] to assess the presence of leakages or stenosis (task 6). Chicken wings represent the most commonly used model, since they are widely available and affordable [24,25]. The chicken brachial artery is generally dissected from the surrounding connective tissues (task 1), cut, and sutured under a microscope. The harvesting of both brachial and radial arteries and their reimplantation has been suggested to simulate a superficial temporal artery–middle cerebral artery (STA-MCA) bypass [26]. Explanted animal vessels have been put deep into a grapefruit, between two slices [27], to simulate side-to-side distal anterior cerebral artery bypass. Other biological materials include the following:

- Cryogenically preserved rat [28] or human vessels (from tissues in lymph node dissection) [29,30];
- Porcine coronary arteries perfused through a pulsatile pump [31];
- Sections of turkey neck with both carotid arteries perfused [32];
- Turkey wings [33];
- Fresh chicken legs [34];
- Chicken feet [35];
- Oxen tongues [36];
- Pig spleen after splenectomy [37];
- Perfused porcine thighs [38];
- Bovine heart model [39];
- Rat cadavers with an extracorporeal perfusion device [40].

Turkey brachial arteries have been revealed to better approximate the real dimensions of human STA and MCA, and they were more appreciated than chicken wings in a survey among anastomosis course participants [41].

These models have several advantages: good reproducibility of a human artery's physical characteristics (i.e., elasticity and consistency), accessibility [42], and conservation (most of the materials can be cheaply bought at supermarkets and stored over the long term in a freezer). A very recent comparative trial comparing non-living and living animal models found that trainees working with non-living chicken thigh models had better results than students training with living rats [43].

3.2.2. Fresh Human Cadavers

As shown by Sindhu et al. in a randomized controlled trial, the higher the model fidelity to real-life experience in the operating room, the faster the acquisition of the required skill [44].

Several different cadaveric models have been developed. Entirely pressurized fresh cadavers are useful to simulate high-flow conventional carotid-to-middle cerebral artery bypass with interposition of a previously harvested radial artery graft [45]. Cadaveric heads, whose arteries and veins have been cannulated and connected to a closed pumping circuit with subarachnoid cisternal tubes, can simulate the cisternal circulation of blood and CSF [46,47]. Latex-injected non-pressurized cadaveric heads are used to perform the main types of cerebral anastomoses after the removal of superficial intravascular latex [48]. Perfused and fixed human cadaveric brain [49] has been enclosed with white silk clothing (simulating the dura) and inserted into human skulls [50].

Despite the high anatomical fidelity, these models are expensive; they are not easily accessible and do not offer a large number of anastomoses to perform. These disadvantages restrict their use to specific purposes for advanced training or research (for instance, assessing the intracranial feasibility of new intracranial bypass techniques).

3.2.3. Placenta

Human and bovine placentas represent effective models for microsurgical training [51–53]. According to the histological composition of its vessels, the human placenta may be considered an appropriate model for STA-MCA anastomosis. In contrast, the thicker and larger diameter of bovine placenta is a good model for internal carotid artery–radial artery–middle cerebral artery (ICA-RA-MCA) bypass [54].

Recently, Magaldi Oliveira systematically defined the nomenclature of placenta vessels and correlated them with major intracranial arteries [51]. When perfused and pressurized, placental arteries simulate intracranial vessels, and the trainee can perform a great variety of simulation scenarios in a single model, allowing for many repetitive exercises and surgical error exploration. With a single placenta model, the trainee can perform a lot of micro-anastomoses and other procedures such vessel graft reimplantation/transplantation. A recently introduced pulsatile flow system can further improve the surgical fidelity of these models [55] (tasks 4). A placenta can be inserted into a skull model [54] to increase the anatomical fidelity. Trainees can check bypass vessel patency with indocyanine green light microscopic vision (task 5) or analyze it with the application of the anastomosis lapse index (ALI), based on the number of average errors per anastomosis performed [56]. Human [57] and bovine [54] placentas are usually affordable and obtainable, being a waste product of birth and calving. Placenta models are among the most promising tools available for training in microvascular anastomoses, due to their similarity to cerebral vessels, accessibility, and affordability.

3.3. In Vivo Training Models (Live Animals)

Microsurgical training based on live animals has been the paradigm of microsurgical training for years, and it currently remains a very accurate, practical, and appreciated method to simulate microvascular anastomoses [58]. In vivo models offer the unique advantage of reproducing physiologic heart pulsation and coagulation. These models allow one to simulate and manage acute intraprocedural complications such as intraluminal thrombosis (task 6). Rats are most commonly used because of their availability, uncomplicated perioperative care, and limited costs (about USD 120/animal [59]). Several experimental models have been proposed over the years:

- Side-to-side anastomosis involving a bilateral common carotid artery [60], portal vein and vena cava [61], femoral vein and artery [62], bilateral common iliac arteries [58], and internal and external carotid artery [60];
- End-to-end anastomosis involving the common carotid [58], abdominal aorta [63], femoral artery [64], and external jugular vein [65];
- End-to-side anastomosis involving the bilateral common carotid artery ("half-ring model") [66], common carotid artery and external jugular vein [66], superficial caudal epigastric artery and contralateral femoral artery [66], iliolumbar vein and inferior vena cava [67], left and right common iliac arteries [58,68], middle sacral artery and common iliac artery [68].

Most animals are euthanized after the surgery: in these cases, the quality of anastomosis is assessed by harvesting the artery from the living animal or during the autopsy.

Contrarily, some authors have reported on the long-term patency and onset of late complications after training, for example, in the side-to-side internal and external carotid artery bypass models and in the side-to-side femoral artery and vein anastomosis model [69] (task 6).

Two further proposed models involve rats. The multiple lymphatic–venous anastomosis (MVLA) model consists of the anastomosis of lymphatic vessels into the lumbar vein [70]; the rat tail revascularization model offers the advantage of assessing the functionality of the anastomosis by evaluating its vitality [71].

Even if in vivo models cannot reproduce surgical anatomy, they have unique advantages in terms of high-fidelity simulation of almost all surgical steps, including the occurrence and management of intra-operative (anastomosis leak, acute thrombosis, vasospasm, or vascular stenosis) and postoperative complications (delayed thrombosis of the anastomosis, and formation of pseudoaneurysms) (tasks 5–6) [72]. These are the reasons why living rats are still among the commonly used and appreciated training models worldwide [73].

However, the availability of these models progressively reduces because of ethical reasons and the high costs of managing an animal laboratory. A recently published systematic review highlighted the lack of evidence regarding the need to teach microsurgical or microvascular skills [74].

3.4. Classification

There was a strong agreement between authors (92%), with a Cohen K of 0.9. Based on the proposed scoring system (Table 1), the simulation devices are classified as follows (Table 2):

Table 2. By using this scoring system, models have been classified into 5 classes, from class A (excellent simulator) to class E (not suitable as simulator): see Table 1.

Task	Synthetic Tubes	Animal Vessels (Ex Vivo)	Human Cadavers	Placenta	Live Animals (In Vivo)
Vessel dissection	0	1	1	2	2
Subarachnoid dissection	0	0	2	2	1
Variety of the anastomosis	2	2	2	2	2
Number anastomosis/vessel/diameter	2	2	1	2	1
Stenosis leaks	2	2	2	2	2
Thrombosis	0	0	0	0	2
TOTAL OF POINTS (class of the simulator)	6 (C)	7 (B)	8 (B)	10 (A)	10 (A)

1—Synthetic tubes—Grade C—reasonable simulators: They allow one to perform all the types of micro-anastomoses (task 3) and to perform several anastomoses (task 4). More sophisticated models using synthetic tubes allow for the evaluation of the immediate patency and strength of the anastomosis (task 5) [14]. Conversely, tubes are not suitable for training surgeons in vessel or subarachnoid microdissection (task 1 and 2), or to simulate the onset of thrombosis (tasks 7).

2.1—Animal vessels (ex vivo)—Grade B—good simulators: They allow one to train with all the micro-anastomoses (task 3) several times thanks to their availability (task 4), with the advantage of improving some abilities in vessel microdissection (adventitia removal) (task 1), even if the experience of dissecting a vessel from muscles and fat does not perfectly fit subarachnoid dissection. When perfused/pressurized, they mimic human vessel pulsation, allowing the surgeon to assess the presence of stenosis and leaks [23,75] (task 5). However, these models are not suitable to simulate thrombosis (task 6).

2.2—Fresh human cadavers—Grade B—good simulators: Fresh human cadavers allow one to train some abilities with vessel microdissection (task 1) and to perform all the standard micro-anastomoses (task 3). This model optimally allows one to train in arachnoid dissection (task 2). Perfusion and pressurization of the model allow for the evaluation of stenosis or leaks of the micro-anastomosis (task 5). Trainees can perform micro-anastomosis with vessels of different diameters and depths (task 4). Cadavers models are limited by the impossibility to reproduce thrombosis (task 6).

2.3—Placenta—Grade A—excellent simulator: Placenta models allow the optimal achievement of all the tasks, with the exception of simulating thrombosis scenarios (task 6). The big advantage is that it is possible to perform the tasks many times as needed, in vessels of different sizes (task 4) [51]. Dissecting placenta vessels simulates arachnoidal dissection.

3—Live animals (in vivo)—Grade A—excellent simulators: Given the presence of an active coagulation system, these are the only simulators that develop thrombotic complications (task 6). These models offer a unique surgical experience when facing challenging complications such as bleeding, micro-anastomotic leaks, and thrombosis. However, live animals are not optimal to repeat the exercise as many times as needed and allow limited training in subarachnoid dissection. In selected protocols, a post-anastomotic follow-up period can be applied to evaluate the delayed bypass patency [67]. Moreover, ethical concerns exist regarding the use of live animals.

4. Discussion

The proposed classification system provides a valuable resource to the microvascular surgeon to critically analyze the multiplicity of available devices and choose the most appropriate model for cerebral bypass surgery according to the skills they need to improve (Figure 2). To the authors' knowledge, this is the first paper to propose a classification system of the training models.

A limitation of this classification is that it only takes into account the technical aspects of performing a micro-anastomosis and considers neither costs nor availability nor the ethical issues of the models. This is mostly true for class A and B models that allow for achieving the highest number of skills. Placenta has strong overall availability and cheaper direct and indirect costs in comparison to human cadavers and in vivo models. In this sense, placenta models represent valid simulators for every trainee (mostly intermediate and advanced), especially in reduced-budget educational programs. Placenta also represent a very good model for experienced surgeons who want to regularly exercise their skills or try/master new techniques.

A significant advantage of this classification is its dynamic nature. It can be continually updated if researchers develop new educational models ameliorate existing models.

Importantly, the highest scored models (grades A and B) do not represent the best simulators for all trainees. Mokhtari highlighted that entry-level surgeons who had previously undergone training with Silastic tubes performed significantly better in terms of anastomotic quality and average time when working with live animals [63].

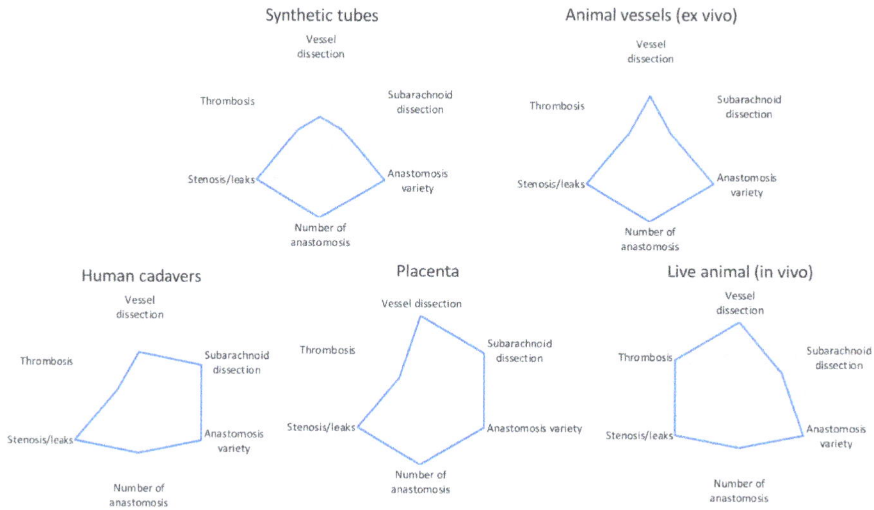

Figure 2. Spider graphs presenting the features of the training models. In clockwise sense: basic microsuture models, synthetic tubes, animal vessels (in vitro), human cadavers, placenta, and live animals (in vivo).

In 2016, the analysis of the 10-year training results in an Okayama research center revealed that initially performing microsurgery on silicon tubes and chicken wings enabled a reduction in the number of animals required later in the training program [76].

An analysis by Pafitanis, involving novices training with coupler-assisted microvascular anastomoses of a three-layer silicon vessel, objectively assessed the learning curve of the trainees. This analysis proposed objective thresholds for ethical animal model training and safe, supervised clinical sessions in the operating theater. These studies support the idea that the educational process of the cerebral bypass surgeon requires stepwise training.

Based on this classification, we suggest that entry-level trainees first master the micro-anastomosis techniques on class C simulators. Thereafter, intermediate and advanced trainees could use placenta to master microdissection and micro-anastomoses techniques. If needed, advanced trainees may consider the use of fresh cadavers with high fidelity of the brain and angioanatomy, which offer the unique advantage of simulating EC-IC or IC-IC bypasses with or without interposition of a graft, or live animals, for working with real rheological properties.

In this sense, this scoring system can support the development of educational programs in neurovascular micro-neurosurgery, helping to select the most adapted training models according to trainee level.

Finally, despite the notable impact of training on the learning curve of cerebrovascular microsurgeons, it is mandatory to emphasize the importance of working alongside expert cerebral bypass surgeons [1,77].

5. Conclusions

The proposed classification considers the most relevant skills required by a neurosurgeon to perform a microvascular anastomosis. This system helps trainees to critically analyze the available models and to choose the most appropriate according to their level (entry-level vs. intermediate vs. advanced) and the skills to be improved. This way, it may also further reduce the use of live animals as training models.

Funding: This research received no external funding.

Conflicts of Interest: The authors declare no conflicts of interest.

References

1. Esposito, G.; Regli, L. Intraoperative tools for cerebral bypass surgery. *Acta Neurochir.* **2018**, *160*, 775–778. [CrossRef]
2. Sebök, M.; Esposito, G.; van Niftrik, C.H.B.; Fierstra, J.; Schubert, T.; Wegener, S.; Held, J.; Kulcsár, Z.; Luft, A.R.; Regli, L. Flow augmentation STA-MCA bypass evaluation for patients with acute stroke and unilateral large vessel occlusion: A proposal for an urgent bypass flowchart. *J. Neurosurg.* **2022**, *137*, 1047–1055. [CrossRef]
3. Sebök, M.; Höbner, L.M.; Fierstra, J.; Schubert, T.; Wegener, S.; Kulcsár, Z.; Luft, A.R.; Regli, L.; Esposito, G. Flow-augmentation STA-MCA bypass for acute and subacute ischemic stroke due to internal carotid artery occlusion and the role of advanced neuroimaging with hemodynamic and flow-measurement in the decision-making: Preliminary data. *Quant. Imaging Med. Surg.* **2024**, *14*, 777–788. [CrossRef]
4. Esposito, G.; Amin-Hanjani, S.; Regli, L. Role of and Indications for Bypass Surgery after Carotid Occlusion Surgery Study (COSS)? *Stroke* **2016**, *47*, 282–290. [CrossRef]
5. Streefkerk, H.J.N.; Van der Zwan, A.; Verdaasdonk, R.M.; Beck, H.J.M.; Tulleken, C.A.F. Cerebral revascularization. *Adv. Tech. Stand. Neurosurg.* **2003**, *28*, 145–225.
6. Santyr, B.; Abbass, M.; Chalil, A.; Vivekanandan, A.; Krivosheya, D.; Denning, L.M.; Mattingly, T.K.; Haji, F.A.; Lownie, S.P. High-fidelity, simulation-based microsurgical training for neurosurgical residents. *Neurosurg. Focus.* **2022**, *53*, E3. [CrossRef]
7. Masia, J.; Olivares, L.; Koshima, I.; Teo, T.C.; Suominen, S.; Van Landuyt, K.; Demirtas, Y.; Becker, C.; Pons, G.; Garusi, C.; et al. Barcelona Consensus on Supermicrosurgery. *J. Reconstr. Microsurg.* **2013**, *30*, 53–58. [CrossRef]
8. Page, M.J.; McKenzie, J.E.; Bossuyt, P.M.; Boutron, I.; Hoffmann, T.C.; Mulrow, C.D.; Shamseer, L.; Tetzlaff, J.M.; Akl, E.A.; Brennan, S.E.; et al. The PRISMA 2020 statement: An updated guideline for reporting systematic reviews. *BMJ* **2021**, *372*, n71. [CrossRef]
9. Peled, I.J.; Kaplan, H.Y.; Wexler, M.R. Microsilicone anastomoses. *Ann. Plast. Surg.* **1983**, *10*, 331–332. [CrossRef]
10. Atlan, M.; Lellouch, A.G.; Legagneux, J.; Chaouat, M.; Masquelet, A.C.; Letourneur, D. A New Synthetic Model for Microvascular Anastomosis Training? A Randomized Comparative Study between Silicone and Polyvinyl Alcohol Gelatin Tubes. *J. Surg. Educ.* **2018**, *75*, 182–187. [CrossRef]
11. Cooper, L.; Sindali, K.; Srinivasan, K.; Jones, M.; Nugent, N. Developing a Three-Layered Synthetic Microsurgical Simulation Vessel. *J. Reconstr. Microsurg.* **2019**, *35*, 15–21. [CrossRef]
12. Matsumura, N.; Hayashi, N.; Hamada, H.; Shibata, T.; Horie, Y.; Endo, S. A newly designed training tool for microvascular anastomosis techniques: Microvascular Practice Card. *Surg. Neurol.* **2009**, *71*, 616–620. [CrossRef] [PubMed]
13. Galmiche, C.; Hidalgo Diaz, J.J.; Vernet, P.; Facca, S.; Menu, G.; Liverneaux, P. Learning of supermicrosurgical vascular anastomosis: MicroChirSim® procedural simulator versus Anastomosis Training Kit® procedural simulator. *Hand Surg. Rehabil.* **2018**, *37*, 20–23. [CrossRef] [PubMed]
14. Meier, S.A.; Lang, A.; Beer, G.M. Polyurethane vessels for microvascular surgical training to reduce animal use. *ALTEX* **2004**, *21*, 135–138. [PubMed]
15. Inoue, T.; Tsutsumi, K.; Saito, K.; Adachi, S.; Tanaka, S.; Kunii, N. Training of A3-A3 side-to-side anastomosis in a deep corridor using a box with 6.5-cm depth: Technical note. *Surg. Neurol.* **2006**, *66*, 638–641. [CrossRef]
16. Takeuchi, M.; Hayashi, N.; Hamada, H.; Matsumura, N.; Nishijo, H.; Endo, S. A new training method to improve deep microsurgical skills using a mannequin head. *Microsurgery* **2008**, *28*, 168–170. [CrossRef]
17. Ishikawa, T.; Yasui, N.; Ono, H. Novel brain model for training of deep microvascular anastomosis. *Neurol. Med. Chir.* **2010**, *50*, 627–629. [CrossRef]
18. Belykh, E.; Abramov, I.; Bardonova, L.; Patel, R.; McBryan, S.; Bouza, L.E.; Majmundar, N.; Zhao, X.; Byvaltsev, V.A.; Johnson, S.A.; et al. Seven bypasses simulation set: Description and validity assessment of novel models for microneurosurgical training. *J. Neurosurg.* **2023**, *138*, 732–739. [CrossRef]
19. Mori, K.; Yamamoto, T.; Nakao, Y.; Esaki, T. Surgical simulation of cerebral revascularization via skull base approaches in the posterior circulation using three-dimensional skull model with artificial brain and blood vessels. *Neurol. Med. Chir.* **2011**, *51*, 93–96. [CrossRef]
20. Cikla, U.; Sahin, B.; Hanalioglu, S.; Ahmed, A.S.; Niemann, D.; Baskaya, M.K. A novel, low-cost, reusable, high-fidelity neurosurgical training simulator for cerebrovascular bypass surgery. *J. Neurosurg.* **2018**, *130*, 1663–1671. [CrossRef]
21. Petrone, S.; Cofano, F.; Nicolosi, F.; Spena, G.; Moschino, M.; Di Perna, G.; Lavorato, A.; Lanotte, M.M.; Garbossa, D. Virtual-Augmented Reality and Life-Like Neurosurgical Simulator for Training: First Evaluation of a Hands-On Experience for Residents. *Front. Surg.* **2022**, *9*, 862948. [CrossRef] [PubMed]
22. Kang, B.Y.; Jeon, B.J.; Lee, K.T.; Mun, G.H. Comprehensive Analysis of Chicken Vessels as Microvascular Anastomosis Training Model. *Arch. Plast. Surg.* **2017**, *44*, 12–18. [CrossRef] [PubMed]
23. Krishnan, K.G.; Dramm, P.; Schackert, G. Simple and viable in vitro perfusion model for training microvascular anastomoses. *Microsurgery* **2004**, *24*, 335–338. [CrossRef] [PubMed]

24. Hino, A. Training in microvascular surgery using a chicken wing artery. *Neurosurgery* **2003**, *52*, 1495–1497; discussion 1497–1498. [CrossRef]
25. Dave, A.; Singhal, M.; Tiwari, R.; Chauhan, S.; De, M. Effectiveness of a microsurgery training program using a chicken wing model. *J. Plast. Surg. Hand Surg.* **2022**, *56*, 191–197. [CrossRef]
26. Kim, B.J.; Kim, S.T.; Jeong, Y.G.; Lee, W.H.; Lee, K.S.; Paeng, S.H. An efficient microvascular anastomosis training model based on chicken wings and simple instruments. *J. Cerebrovasc. Endovasc. Neurosurg.* **2013**, *15*, 20–25. [CrossRef]
27. Cikla, U.; Rowley, P.; Simoes, E.L.J.; Ozaydin, B.; Goodman, S.L.; Avci, E.; Baskaya, M.K.; Patel, N.J. Grapefruit Training Model for Distal Anterior Cerebral Artery Side-to-Side Bypass. *World Neurosurg.* **2020**, *138*, 39–51. [CrossRef]
28. Lausada, N.R.; Escudero, E.; Lamonega, R.; Dreizzen, E.; Raimondi, J.C. Use of cryopreserved rat arteries for microsurgical training. *Microsurgery* **2005**, *25*, 500–501. [CrossRef]
29. Ishii, N.; Kiuchi, T.; Oji, T.; Kishi, K. Microsurgical Training using Reusable Human Vessels from Discarded Tissues in Lymph Node Dissection. *Arch. Plast. Surg.* **2016**, *43*, 595–598. [CrossRef]
30. Joy, M.T.; Applebaum, M.A.; Anderson, W.M.; Serletti, J.M.; Capito, A.E. Impact of High-Fidelity Microvascular Surgery Simulation on Resident Training. *J. Reconstr. Microsurg.* **2024**, *40*, 211–216. [CrossRef]
31. Schoffl, H.; Hager, D.; Hinterdorfer, C.; Dunst, K.M.; Froschauer, S.; Steiner, W.; Kwasny, O.; Huemer, G.M. Pulsatile perfused porcine coronary arteries for microvascular training. *Ann. Plast. Surg.* **2006**, *57*, 213–216. [CrossRef] [PubMed]
32. Colpan, M.E.; Slavin, K.V.; Amin-Hanjani, S.; Calderon-Arnuphi, M.; Charbel, F.T. Microvascular anastomosis training model based on a Turkey neck with perfused arteries. *Neurosurgery* **2008**, *62* (Suppl. S2), ONS407–ONS410; discussion ONS410–ONS411. [CrossRef] [PubMed]
33. Bates, B.J.; Wimalawansa, S.M.; Monson, B.; Rymer, M.C.; Shapiro, R.; Johnson, R.M. A simple cost-effective method of microsurgical simulation training: The turkey wing model. *J. Reconstr. Microsurg.* **2013**, *29*, 615–618. [CrossRef] [PubMed]
34. Cifuentes, I.J.; Rodriguez, J.R.; Yañez, R.A.; Salisbury, M.C.; Cuadra, Á.J.; Varas, J.E.; Dagnino, B.L. A Novel Ex Vivo Training Model for Acquiring Supermicrosurgical Skills Using a Chicken Leg. *J. Reconstr. Microsurg.* **2016**, *32*, 699–705. [CrossRef] [PubMed]
35. Satterwhite, T.; Son, J.; Echo, A.; Lee, G. The chicken foot dorsal vessel as a high-fidelity microsurgery practice model. *Plast. Reconstr. Surg.* **2013**, *131*, 311e–312e. [CrossRef]
36. Camargo, C.P.; Silva, D.I.d.S.B.d.C.E.; Maluf, F.C.; Morais-Besteiro, J.; Gemperli, R. A non-living, effective model for microvascular training. *Acta Cir. Bras.* **2017**, *32*, 1087–1092. [CrossRef]
37. Maluf, I.; Silva, A.B.D.D.; Groth, A.K.; Lopes, M.A.C.; Kurogi, A.S.; Freitas, R.D.S.; Tomasich, F.D.S. An alternative experimental model for training in microsurgery. *Rev. Col. Bras. Cir.* **2014**, *41*, 72–74. [CrossRef]
38. Nam, S.M.; Shin, H.S.; Kim, Y.B.; Park, E.S.; Choi, C.Y. Microsurgical training with porcine thigh infusion model. *J. Reconstr. Microsurg.* **2013**, *29*, 303–306. [CrossRef]
39. Olijnyk, L.D.; Carvalho, R.F.D.; Severino, A.G.; Patel, K.; Jotz, G.P.; Silva, C.E.D.; Stefani, M.A. Ex vivo model with bovine heart: A proposal for training microscopic dissection and vascularmicroanastomoses. *Rev. Col. Bras. Cir.* **2019**, *45*, e1992. [CrossRef]
40. Zucal, I.; Feder, A.L.; Kyaw, T.; Khin, S.; Heidekrueger, P.I.; Prantl, L.; Haerteis, S.; Aung, T. An Innovative Simulation Model for Microvascular Training. *Plast. Reconstr. Surg.* **2022**, *150*, 189e–193e. [CrossRef]
41. Abla, A.A.; Uschold, T.; Preul, M.C.; Zabramski, J.M. Comparative use of turkey and chicken wing brachial artery models for microvascular anastomosis training. *J. Neurosurg.* **2011**, *115*, 1231–1235. [CrossRef] [PubMed]
42. Tamrakar, K. Learning Microvascular Anastomosis in Low Socioeconomic Vascular Models during Residency. *Cureus* **2017**, *9*, e1199. [CrossRef]
43. Le Hanneur, M.; BouchÉ, P.A.; Vignes, J.L.; Poitevin, N.; Legagneux, J.; Fitoussi, F. Non-living vs. living animal models for microvascular surgery training: A randomized comparative study. *Plast. Reconstr. Surg.* **2024**, *153*, 853–860. [CrossRef]
44. Sidhu, R.S.; Park, J.; Brydges, R.; MacRae, H.M.; Dubrowski, A. Laboratory-based vascular anastomosis training: A randomized controlled trial evaluating the effects of bench model fidelity and level of training on skill acquisition. *J. Vasc. Surg.* **2007**, *45*, 343–349. [CrossRef] [PubMed]
45. Russin, J.J.; Mack, W.J.; Carey, J.N.; Minneti, M.; Giannotta, S.L. Simulation of a high-flow extracranial-intracranial bypass using a radial artery graft in a novel fresh tissue model. *Neurosurgery* **2012**, *71*, ons315–ons319; discussion ons319–ons320. [CrossRef]
46. Aboud, E.; Al-Mefty, O.; Yaşargil, M.G. New laboratory model for neurosurgical training that simulates live surgery. *J. Neurosurg.* **2002**, *97*, 1367–1372. [CrossRef] [PubMed]
47. Carrizales-Rodriguez, J.; Borrayo-Dorado, S.; Méndez-Guerrero, I.; Sanchez, J.; Rios-Ramirez, F.; Cardenas-Garcia, Y.; Abdala-Vargas, N.; Höllig, A.; Méndez-Rosito, D. The Hibiscus Model: A Feasible Cadaveric Model Using Continuous Arterial Circulation for Intracranial Bypass Training and Its Validation. *World Neurosurg.* **2023**, *174*, e17–e25. [CrossRef]
48. Steinberg, J.A.; Rennert, R.C.; Levy, M.; Khalessi, A.A. A Practical Cadaveric Model for Intracranial Bypass Training. *World Neurosurg.* **2019**, *121*, e576–e583. [CrossRef]
49. Olabe, J.; Olabe, J.; Sancho, V. Human cadaver brain infusion model for neurosurgical training. *Surg. Neurol.* **2009**, *72*, 700–702. [CrossRef]
50. Olabe, J.; Olabe, J.; Roda, J.M.; Sancho, V. Human cadaver brain infusion skull model for neurosurgical training. *Surg. Neurol. Int.* **2011**, *2*, 54. [CrossRef]

51. Oliveira, M.M.; Wendling, L.; Malheiros, J.A.; Nicolato, A.; Prosdocimi, A.; Guerra, L.; Costa, P.H.; Ferrarez, C.E.; Ferreira, M.T.; Sauvageau, E.; et al. Human Placenta Simulator for Intracranial-Intracranial Bypass: Vascular Anatomy and 5 Bypass Techniques. *World Neurosurg.* **2018**, *119*, e694–e702. [CrossRef] [PubMed]
52. De Oliveira, M.M.R.; Ferrarez, C.E.; Ramos, T.M.; Malheiros, J.A.; Nicolato, A.; Machado, C.J.; Ferreira, M.T.; De Oliveira, F.B.; De Sousa, C.F.P.M.; Costa, P.H.V.; et al. Learning brain aneurysm microsurgical skills in a human placenta model: Predictive validity. *J. Neurosurg.* **2018**, *128*, 846–852. [CrossRef]
53. Belykh, E.G.; Lei, T.; Oliveira, M.M.; Almefty, R.O.; Yagmurlu, K.; Elhadi, A.M.; Sun, G.; Bichard, W.D.; Spetzler, R.F.; Preul, M.C.; et al. Carotid Endarterectomy Surgical Simulation Model Using a Bovine Placenta Vessel. *Neurosurgery* **2015**, *77*, 825–829; discussion 829–830. [CrossRef] [PubMed]
54. Belykh, E.; Lei, T.; Safavi-Abbasi, S.; Yagmurlu, K.; Almefty, R.O.; Sun, H.; Almefty, K.K.; Belykh, O.; Byvaltsev, V.A.; Spetzler, R.F.; et al. Low-flow and high-flow neurosurgical bypass and anastomosis training models using human and bovine placental vessels: A histological analysis and validation study. *J. Neurosurg.* **2016**, *125*, 915–928. [CrossRef] [PubMed]
55. Gallardo, F.C.; Bustamante, J.L.; Martin, C.; Orellana, C.M.; Caviglia, M.R.; Oriola, G.G.; Diaz, A.I.; Rubino, P.A.; Quesada, V.Q. Novel Simulation Model with Pulsatile Flow System for Microvascular Training, Research, and Improving Patient Surgical Outcomes. *World Neurosurg.* **2020**, *143*, 11–16. [CrossRef] [PubMed]
56. Ghanem, A.M.; Al Omran, Y.; Shatta, B.; Kim, E.; Myers, S. Anastomosis Lapse Index (ALI): A Validated End Product Assessment Tool for Simulation Microsurgery Training. *J. Reconstr. Microsurg.* **2016**, *32*, 233–241. [CrossRef]
57. Magaldi, M.O.; Nicolato, A.; Godinho, J.V.; Santos, M.; Prosdocimi, A.; Malheiros, J.A.; Lei, T.; Belykh, E.; Almefty, R.O.; Almefty, K.K.; et al. Human Placenta Aneurysm Model for Training Neurosurgeons in Vascular Microsurgery. *Oper. Neurosurg.* **2014**, *10*, 592–601. [CrossRef]
58. Tayebi Meybodi, A.; Lawton, M.T.; Yousef, S.; Mokhtari, P.; Gandhi, S.; Benet, A. Microsurgical Bypass Training Rat Model: Part 2-Anastomosis Configurations. *World Neurosurg.* **2017**, *107*, 935–943. [CrossRef]
59. Byvaltsev, V.A.; Akshulakov, S.K.; Polkin, R.A.; Ochkal, S.V.; Stepanov, I.A.; Makhambetov, Y.T.; Kerimbayev, T.T.; Staren, M.; Belykh, E.; Preul, M.C. Microvascular Anastomosis Training in Neurosurgery: A Review. *Minim. Invasive Surg.* **2018**, *2018*, 6130286. [CrossRef]
60. Matsumura, N.; Hamada, H.; Yamatani, K.; Hayashi, N.; Hirashima, Y.; Endo, S. Side-to-side arterial anastomosis model in the rat internal and external carotid arteries. *J. Reconstr. Microsurg.* **2001**, *17*, 263–266. [CrossRef]
61. Lee, S.H.; Fisher, B. Portacaval shunt in the rat. *Surgery* **1961**, *50*, 668–672.
62. Matsumura, N.; Endo, S.; Hamada, H.; Kurimoto, M.; Hirashima, Y.; Takaku, A. An experimental model for side-to-side microvascular anastomosis. *J. Reconstr. Microsurg.* **1999**, *15*, 581–583. [CrossRef] [PubMed]
63. Mokhtari, P.; Meybodi, A.T.; Lawton, M.T.; Payman, A.; Benet, A. Transfer of Learning from Practicing Microvascular Anastomosis on Silastic Tubes to Rat Abdominal Aorta. *World Neurosurg.* **2017**, *108*, 230–235. [CrossRef] [PubMed]
64. Liu, H.L. Microvascular anastomosis of submillimeter vessels-a training model in rats. *J. Hand Microsurg.* **2013**, *5*, 14–17. [CrossRef] [PubMed]
65. Nasir, S.; Aydin, M.A.; Karahan, N.; Demiryürek, D.; Sargon, M. New microvenous anastomosis model for microsurgical training: External jugular vein. *J. Reconstr. Microsurg.* **2006**, *22*, 625–630. [CrossRef]
66. Mikami, T.; Suzuki, H.; Ukai, R.; Komatsu, K.; Kimura, Y.; Akiyama, Y.; Wanibuchi, M.; Mikuni, N. Surgical Anatomy of Rats for the Training of Microvascular Anastomosis. *World Neurosurg.* **2018**, *120*, e1310–e1318. [CrossRef]
67. Onoda, S.; Kimata, Y.; Matsumoto, K. Iliolumbar Vein as a Training Model for Microsurgical End-to-Side Anastomosis. *J. Craniofac Surg.* **2016**, *27*, 767–768. [CrossRef]
68. Yin, X.; Ye, G.; Lu, J.; Wang, L.; Qi, P.; Wang, H.; Wang, J.; Hu, S.; Yang, X.; Chen, K.; et al. A Novel Rat Model for Comprehensive Microvascular Training of End-to-End, End-to-Side, and Side-to-Side Anastomoses. *J. Reconstr. Microsurg.* **2019**, *35*, 499–504. [CrossRef]
69. Pruthi, N.; Sarma, P.; Pandey, P. Training in Micro-Vascular Anastomosis Using Rat Femoral Vessels: Comparison of Immediate and Delayed Patency Rates. *Turk. Neurosurg.* **2018**, *28*, 56–61. [CrossRef]
70. Yamamoto, T.; Yamamoto, N.; Yamashita, M.; Furuya, M.; Hayashi, A.; Koshima, I. Establishment of supermicrosurgical lymphaticovenular anastomosis model in rat. *Microsurgery* **2017**, *37*, 57–60. [CrossRef]
71. Sakrak, T.; Köse, A.A.; Karabağli, Y.; Koçman, A.E.; Ozbayoğlu, A.C.; Cetin, C. Rat tail revascularization model for advanced microsurgery training and research. *J. Reconstr. Microsurg.* **2011**, *27*, 391–396. [CrossRef] [PubMed]
72. Esposito, G.; Rossi, F.; Matteini, P.; Scerrati, A.; Puca, A.; Albanese, A.; Rossi, G.; Ratto, F.; Maira, G.; Pini, R. In vivo laser assisted microvascular repair and end-to-end anastomosis by means of indocyanine green-infused chitosan patches: A pilot study. *Lasers Surg. Med.* **2013**, *45*, 318–325. [CrossRef] [PubMed]
73. Shurey, S.; Akelina, Y.; Legagneux, J.; Malzone, G.; Jiga, L.; Ghanem, A.M. The rat model in microsurgery education: Classical exercises and new horizons. *Arch. Plast. Surg.* **2014**, *41*, 201–208. [CrossRef] [PubMed]
74. Brown, J.S.; Rapaport, B.H.J. Role of live animals in the training of microvascular surgery: A systematic review. *Br. J. Oral. Maxillofac. Surg.* **2019**, *57*, 616–619. [CrossRef] [PubMed]
75. Pafitanis, G.; Cooper, L.; Vijayan, R.; Ghanem, A.; Myers, S. Putting the heart into microvascular training: The micropump, a practical "heart-like" device to enhance vascular anastomosis non-living simulation. *J. Plast. Reconstr. Aesthetic Surg. JPRAS* **2017**, *70*, 1787–1788. [CrossRef]

76. Onoda, S.; Kimata, Y.; Sugiyama, N.; Tokuyama, E.; Matsumoto, K.; Ota, T.; Thuzar, M. Analysis of 10-Year Training Results of Medical Students Using the Microvascular Research Center Training Program. *J. Reconstr. Microsurg.* **2016**, *32*, 336–341. [CrossRef]
77. Esposito, G.; Fierstra, J.; Regli, L. Distal outflow occlusion with bypass revascularization: Last resort measure in managing complex MCA and PICA aneurysms. *Acta Neurochir.* **2016**, *158*, 1523–1531. [CrossRef]

brain sciences

Article

Coincidence of Concentric Vessel-Wall Contrast Enhancement in Moyamoya Disease and Acute Postoperative Ischemic Stroke During Revascularization Procedures

Patrick Haas [1,*], Till-Karsten Hauser [2], Lucas Moritz Wiggenhauser [1], Leonie Zerweck [2], Marcos Tatagiba [1], Nadia Khan [1,3] and Constantin Roder [1]

1 Department of Neurosurgery and Moyamoya Center, University of Tübingen, Hoppe-Seyler-Straße 3, 72076 Tübingen, Germany; lucas.moritz.wiggenhauser@med.uni-tuebingen.de (L.M.W.); marcos.tatagiba@med.uni-tuebingen.de (M.T.); nadia.khan@kispi.uzh.ch (N.K.); constantin.roder@med.uni-tuebingen.de (C.R.)
2 Department of Neuroradiology, University of Tübingen, Hoppe-Seyler-Straße 3, 72076 Tübingen, Germany; till-karsten.hauser@med.uni-tuebingen.de (T.-K.H.); leonie.zerweck@med.uni-tuebingen.de (L.Z.)
3 Moyamoya Center, University Children's Hospital Zurich, University of Zurich, Steinwiesstrasse 75, 8032 Zurich, Switzerland
* Correspondence: patrick.haas@med.uni-tuebingen.de; Tel./Fax: +49-7071-29-80325

Abstract: Background: Concentric vessel-wall contrast enhancement (VW-CE) of the terminal carotid artery and its proximal branches may be linked to ischemic strokes, disease activity and progression in Moyamoya disease (MMD). The objective of this retrospective cohort study is to analyze the association between VW-CE and perioperative acute ischemic stroke (PAIS) occurring within 24 h after revascularization. Methods: All previously untreated MMD patients who required revascularization and who had undergone preoperative MRI with VW-CE-sequences were included. PAIS was detected by CT and/or diffusion-weighted MRI sequences within 24 h postoperatively. Results: Of the 110 patients included (female-to-male ratio: 2.7:1, median age: 45.1 (16.6–69.2); n = 247 revascularizations), a priori VW-CE was present in 67.3% (mean time from MRI to first surgery: 86 days ± 82 days). PAIS occurred in five patients undergoing primary revascularization (PAIS rate per revascularization: 2.1%), all of whom had a preoperative pathological VW-CE in the vascular segment corresponding to the stroke area. Two (40%) incidents of PAIS occurred in revascularized territory, while three (60%) occurred in non-revascularized vascular territory. In each case, the supplying artery exhibited VW-CE, indicating disease activity. No additional PAIS occurred during subsequent revascularizations in cases of multistage procedures (n = 38), such as ACA or PCA revascularization as a second step. Conclusions: Preoperative VW-CE in one or more vascular segments may be a marker for postoperative stroke in the respective vascular territory at the time of revascularization. VW-CE imaging should be routinely performed when planning revascularization in MMD. If VW-CE is found, strict perioperative monitoring of these high-risk patients should be performed to achieve the best results possible.

Keywords: cerebral revascularization; Moyamoya disease; postoperative ischemic stroke; contrast-enhanced vessel wall imaging

1. Introduction

Moyamoya disease (MMD) can cause ischemic stroke due to alterations in the vascular architecture of the terminal segments of the internal carotid arteries (ICAs), proximal anterior cerebral artery (ACA) or middle cerebral artery (MCA), as perfusion deficits can no longer be compensated for by an insufficient rete mirabile. If indicated, revascularization with extra-/intracranial (EC-IC) bypasses is regarded as the gold standard of therapy, as it has been demonstrated to reduce the recurrence rate of stroke in hemodynamically insufficient patients [1]. However, ischemic strokes may also occur perioperatively, although the precise pathomechanism is not yet fully understood. Several studies have investigated the risk and protective factors for perioperative acute ischemic stroke (PAIS) after revascularization procedures in patients with MMD, mainly focusing on comorbidities [2–7]. The potential pathomechanisms underlying this phenomenon have been subject to considerable debate: among those discussed are hemodynamic effects due to a vascular steal or watershed shift after direct revascularization on the one hand, as well as altered cerebral blood flow caused by anesthetics and changes of arterial blood pressure on the other [8–10]. A potential correlation between the vascular territory affected by PAIS and MMD remains uncertain, as postoperative strokes may also occur in the hemisphere contralateral to the operated side [11,12]. As PAIS is potentially one of the most serious complications in the surgical treatment of MMD, a deeper understanding is crucial for improving patient outcomes.

Vessel-wall imaging in MMD has recently received increased scientific attention [13,14]. Contrast enhancement in the affected vessel walls (VW-CE) may be an indicator of disease activity in the vessel wall [15]. Vessel-wall alterations in MMD have been previously identified through autopsy studies, and they are characterized by proliferating smooth muscle cells and macrophage infiltration [16]. Although the significance of VW-CE is not yet fully understood, studies have indicated that contrast uptake in affected vessel walls may predict disease progression and increase the risk of poor patient outcomes [15,17–19]. Consequently, MRI screening for VW-CE is routinely performed in all MMD patients at our center. This study retrospectively investigates the occurrence of PAIS during EC-IC revascularization in MMD and its correlation with preoperative VW-CE imaging findings.

2. Methods

2.1. Inclusion and Exclusion Criteria

MMD was defined according to the Japanese Guidelines for the Management of Moyamoya disease [20]. Diagnosis and therapy were based on the consensus recommendations of the European Stroke Organization [21]. The study included adult MMD patients who had not previously undergone revascularization and who were treated with EC-IC bypass for the first time at our center between 12/2013 and 12/2023. Only patients who had received preoperative high-resolution MRI with contrast-enhanced fat-saturated vessel-wall imaging were included in this study. Patient files were scanned for clinical signs of ischemic stroke and imaging was used to confirm PAIS (MRI and/or CT) with an onset < 24 h after surgery. In general, all patients underwent routine postoperative imaging by CT or MRI within 24 h after revascularization.

2.2. VW-CE MR Imaging Protocol

VW-CE MRI was performed on a 3Tesla scanner (Magnetom Vida Fit, Siemens Healthineers, Forchheim, Germany) with a 64 Channel Head/Neck Coil. The sequence parameters were: 3D T1 SPACE (Sampling Perfection with Application optimized Contrasts using different flip-angle evolution) with a time of repetition (TR) of 600 ms, time of echo (TE) of 23 ms, flip angle of 120°, slice thickness of 0.8, field of view (FOV) of 185 × 220 mm, a time of acquisition (TA) of 3:45 and a 384 × 324 matrix, resulting in a voxel size of 0.29 × 0.29 × 0.80 mm. A contrast agent (dosage: 0.1 mmol Gadobutrol/kg) was administered during the measurement of a perfusion sequence (TA 2:29). The VW-CE sequence was started after a whole-brain T1 sequence (TA 1:46); so, the VW-CE imaging was started at around 4:25 min after the contrast administration. Blood suppression was achieved by inversion recovery, and no pulse gating was used.

2.3. Data Processing, Workflow and Statistics

All the data were stored in a custom database (REDCap) and statistically analyzed (JMP, SAS Institute, Cary, NC, USA). Levene's test for homogeneity of variance was applied and pooled/unpooled t-tests were performed accordingly. p-values < 0.05 were considered significant. Contingency tables were analyzed with Fisher's exact test. Nominal logistic regression models were used for multivariate analysis. A stepwise regression approach was used to select all the effects. Odds ratios (ORs) with 95% confidence intervals were calculated as a measure of the strength of association.

2.4. Severity of PAIS

The Clavien–Dindo classification (CDC) was used to assess the severity of the PAIS, which is standard for all complications in our clinic [22]. The modified Rankin Scale (mRS) and the National Institute of Health Stroke Scale (NIHSS) were recorded preoperatively and postoperatively to assess the clinical condition of the patient.

2.5. Standardized Diagnostic Protocol

As part of a standardized diagnostic protocol, patients suspected of having MMD undergo conventional angiography and CO_2-evoked blood-oxygenation-level dependent (BOLD) MRI to determine vasoreactivity as a correlate of cerebral perfusion reserve, as previously described [23–28]. In cases of borderline findings, PET imaging with acetazolamide challenge is also performed. The indication for EC-IC revascularization is then determined on the basis of all the findings. For multi-territorial findings, revascularization of bilaterally affected MCA territories is performed in a single-stage procedure. Any additional affected ACA or PCA territories are then revascularized in secondary or tertiary procedures as part of a multi-stage tailored procedure, as described previously [25]. In the event of an initial ischemic stroke, a period of 6 to 12 weeks is typically allowed to elapse between its occurrence and the first revascularization in order to permit stabilization of the patient's blood flow and clinical condition. This period of time is in accordance with the European consensus recommendations [21]. All patients are hydrated by intravenous administration of balanced full-electrolyte solutions for a minimum duration of 12 h prior to surgery. Antihypertensive medication, with the exception of beta-blockers, are discontinued during anesthesia. Perioperative blood pressure monitoring begins with an invasive arterial blood pressure measurement while the patient is still conscious to avoid blood pressure fluctuations due to the induction of anesthesia.

2.6. Standard Protocol Approvals, Registrations, and Patient Consent

All procedures performed in studies involving human participants were in accordance with the ethical standards of the institutional research committee and with the 1964 Helsinki Declaration and its later amendments or comparable ethics standards. Approval from the local ethics committee was obtained (105/2024BO2). Due to the retrospective character of this analysis, no specific formal consent from the participating patients was obtained.

3. Results

Inclusion criteria were met by n = 110 patients. The female-to-male sex ratio was 2.7:1, and the median age was 45.1 years (16.6–69.2) (Table 1). A total of n = 247 vascular territories were revascularized, of which n = 157 were direct or combined (direct and indirect) bypasses (63.6%). The majority of patients underwent single-stage revascularization surgery (65.5%; unilateral or bilateral revascularization), while 31.8% of patients underwent two-stage revascularization and three patients underwent up to four stages of revascularization (all of them with secondary disease progression in a not-yet revascularized territory). The most common target regions for the first revascularizing procedure were the MCA territory on the right, with a total of n = 84, and on the left, with n = 82, followed by the ACA territory (right n = 36, left = 32). The mean time between preoperative VW-CE MRI and first revascularization procedure was 86 ± 82 d. The overall prevalence of contrast uptake in the arterial wall (VW-CE) was 67.3%. The distal C7 segment of the ICA (right 29.9%; left 32.2%) and the proximal branches A1 (right 13.8%; left 12.6%) and M1 (right 39.1%; left 36.8%) of the ACA and MCA were most frequently affected by VW-CE (Figure 1).

Table 1. Basic patient characteristics.

Patient Characteristics	n (%)
Sex	
- female	80 (72.7%)
- male	30 (27.2%)
Age (at first surgery)	median 45.1 y (16.6–69.2)
Ethnicity	
- Caucasian	99 (90.0%)
- Asian	10 (9.1%)
- Arabic	1 (0.9%)
Initial MMD onset	
- hemorrhagic stroke	7 (6.4%)
- ischemic stroke or TIA/PRIND	77 (70.0%)
- minor (e.g., headache) or incidental	26 (23.6%)
Moyamoya disease	
- unilateral left	21 (19.1%)
- unilateral right	16 (14.5%)
- bilateral	73 (66.4%)
Suzuki classification (Right/Left)	
- grade 1	5/4
- grade 2	11/9
- grade 3	27/34
- grade 4	22/22
- grade 5	16/16
- grade 6	8/9
vessel-wall imaging	110 (100%)
- VW-CE	74 (67.3%)
Time interval between VW-CE imaging and the first surgery	mean 86 d ± 82 d

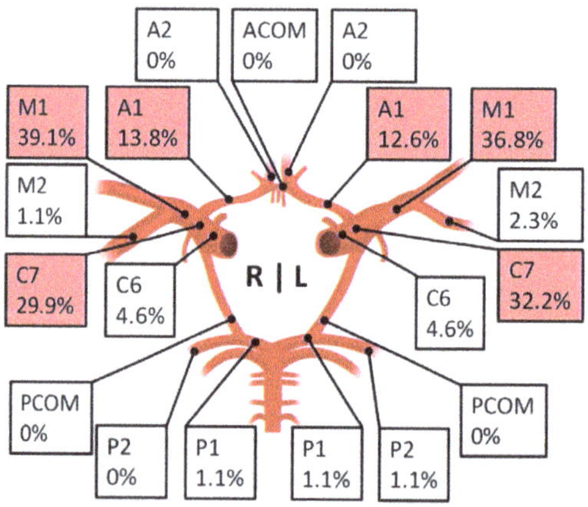

Figure 1. A total of 67.3% of all MMD patients with VW-CE imaging showed contrast enhancement of the vessel wall (VW-CE). The percentage prevalence of these VW-CEs in the different vessel segments of the arterial circle of Willis is shown (right hemisphere (R); left hemisphere (L)). (ICA: C6 and C7; MCA: M1 and M2; ACA: A1, ACOM and A2; PCA: P1, PCOM and P2). Note: Very rarely, VW-CE were also seen in the C5 section of the ICA; these are not shown for reasons of clarity.

Unless otherwise specified, the value indicates the number of patients and the corresponding percentage.

Perioperative Acute Ischemic Stroke After Revascularization

The overall incidence rate of PAIS (n = 5) per bypass (n = 247) was 2.1%, 3.3% per revascularizing operation (n = 152) and 4.5% at the first surgery (n = 110). When only looking at patients with VW-CE, the PAIS rate at the first surgery was 6.8%. Figure 2 depicts the preoperative angiograms of patients with PAIS. All five cases of PAIS occurred in vascular territory supplied by a vessel affected by VW-CE: PAIS in the ACA or MCA territory (n = 4) occurred in the ipsilateral C7, A1 or M1 segment affected by CE-VW. One PAIS occurred in the PCA territory, which corresponded to a VW-CE in the ipsilateral P1 and P2 segments (Figure 3). Only three of the five cases of PAIS (60%) occurred in the revascularized territory itself. The severity of PAIS according to the Clavien–Dindo Classification (CDC) was $\leq$grade 2 in n = 4 cases and grade 5 in n = 1 case. This case showed a poor outcome due to bilateral infarction in the ACA territory (Figure 3B). The remaining cases exhibited only a modest decline in the NIHSS and mRS, accompanied by stable, or even improved, progression at the 6-month follow-up (Table 2). After univariate analysis of the comorbidities of smoking, diabetes mellitus (DM), alcohol consumption, body mass index (BMI) and patient characteristics (age, sex, ethnicity, initial disease manifestation asymptomatic vs. TIA vs. ischemic vs. hemorrhagic stroke), only increased BMI showed a significant association with PAIS (BMI (non-PAIS) 27.2 $\pm$ 5.4 vs. BMI (PAIS) 32.8 $\pm$ 6.5; p = 0.0273; OR = 1.2 95%CI 1.0–1.4). In a multivariate analysis of these variables, again, only BMI could be identified as a risk factor for PAIS. The occurrence of VW-CE was not significantly associated with PAIS.

Table 2. PAIS patient characteristics.

Case	Age [Years]	Sex	Suzuki (Left/ Right)	VW-CE	Revascularization	Ethnicity	BMI	Smoking	HTN	DM	Initial MMD Onset	NIHSS Preop/ Postop/ 6mFU	mRS Preop/ Postop/ 6mFU
A	63	female	3/3	C7 right A1 right	STA-MCA right combined	Caucasian	26.6	no	yes	no	ischemic	0/5/3	2/3/3
B	46	female	2/4	C7 left	STA-MCA right combined	Caucasian	37.3	no	yes	yes	ischemic	0/3/3	1/1/1
C	22	female	5/3	C7 right M1 right C7 left	STA-MCA bilaterally combined	Caucasian	41.9	no	yes	no	ischemic	3/4/3	2/3/2
D	46	female	4/6	C7 left M1 left A1 left	STA-MCA bilaterally direct	Caucasian	29.1	no	no	no	ischemic	2/32/ #	3/5/ #
E	59	male	4/4	P1 left P2 left	STA-MCA bilaterally direct	Caucasian	29.1	yes	yes	no	ischemic	0/4/ *	1/2 *

arterial hypertension (HTN), diabetes mellitus (DM), National Institute of Health Stroke Scale (NIHSS), modified Rankin Scale (mRS). Follow-up conducted 6 months after revascularization (6mFU); #—lost to follow-up; *—6mFU still pending.

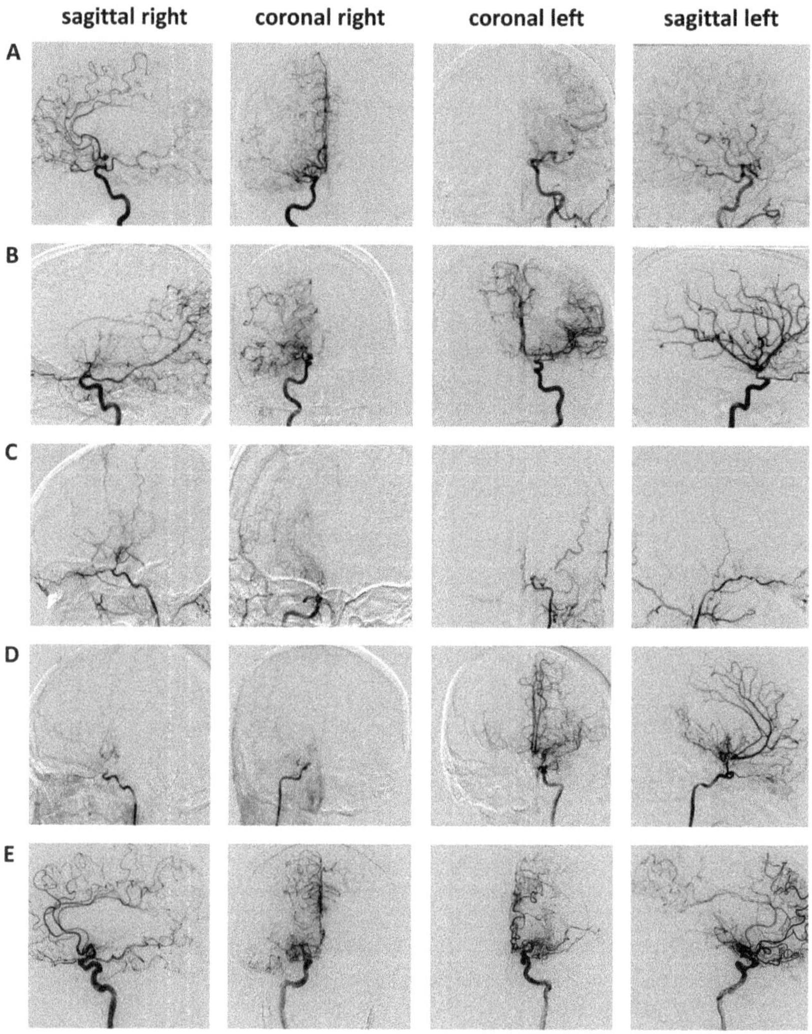

Figure 2. Preoperative angiograms of the five patients (**A–E**) with PAIS. (**A**) ACA supply on both sides via the right ICA. (**B**) Bilateral ACA supply via the left ICA. See the corresponding infarct pattern in Figure 3B. (**C**) Advanced ICA stenoses on both sides. (**D**) Right ICA occlusion, left hemispheric A1 stenosis and M1 occlusion. A matching PAIS pattern was also seen bilaterally in the ACA territory, with VW-CE of the left ICA. Secondary findings: two supraophthalmic ICA aneurysms on the left side. (**E**) Left ICA with collateralization to parietooccipital, consistent with PAIS (Figure 3E). Note: Angiograms of the basilar artery are not shown for reasons of clarity.

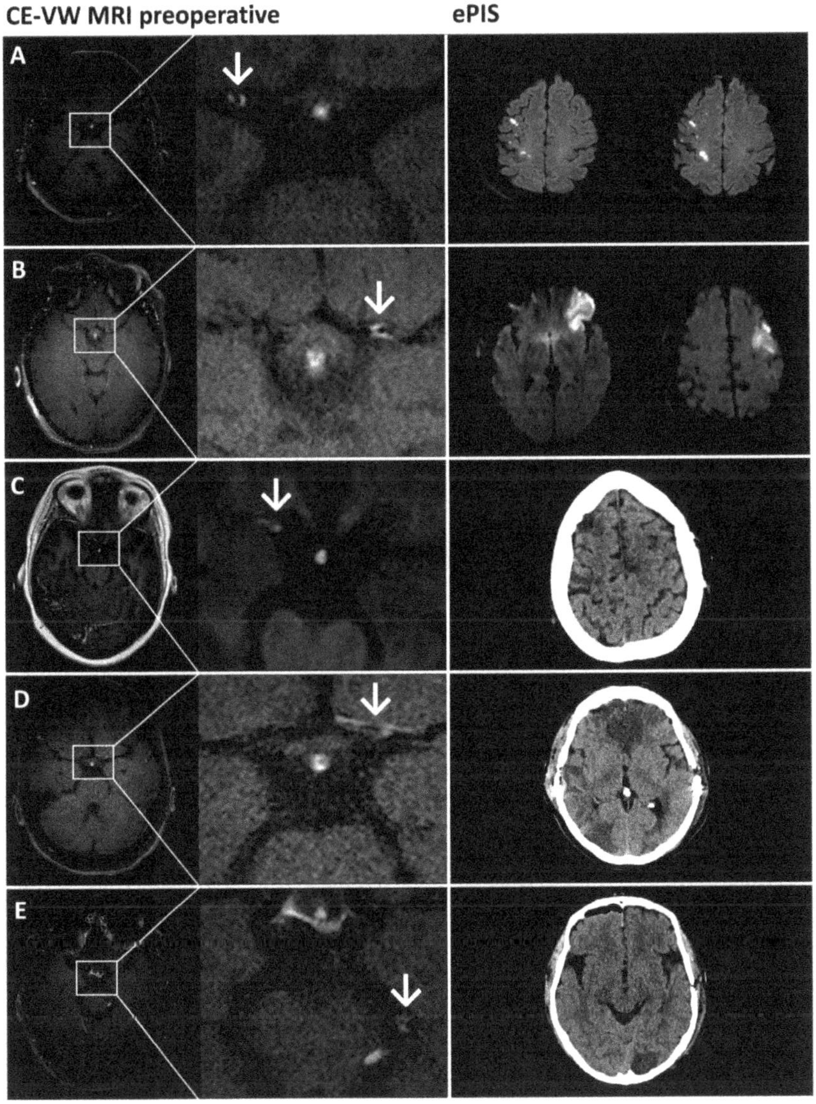

Figure 3. Imaging of five patients (**A–E**) who had a PAIS. Left column: preoperative VW-CE imaging (MRI). White arrows mark a VW-CE (exemplary slices). Right column: postoperative imaging to visualize a PAIS. The first two cases (**A**,**B**) received diffusion-weighted MRI sequences, while the other (**C–E**) received CT imaging. (**A**) Ischemia in the MCA and ACA/MCA watershed area with bilateral ACA supply via the right ICA (Figure 2A), which is possibly hemodynamically induced. (**B**) The initial situation is analogous to that of case (**A**), with bilateral ACA supply via the left ICA. However, in this instance, the infarcts are wedge-shaped, which may be indicative of a thromboembolic process. (**C**) Right frontal ischemia in preoperatively advanced ICA stenosis on both sides. (**D**) Territorial infarcts of the ACA on both sides and parietooccipital with ACA supply on both sides via the left ICA, corresponding to VW-CE, which is most likely hemodynamically caused by intraoperative blood pressure fluctuations. (**E**) Occipital ischemia on the left and collaterals (Figure 2E) via the left ICA with VW-CE at the P1/P2 transition.

4. Discussion

This study is the first to investigate perioperative acute ischemic stroke (PAIS) in MMD patients following revascularization, employing a novel imaging perspective. This perspective is based on the clinical observation of a potential correlation between the contrast enhancement of vessels proximal to the stroke area upon preoperative baseline MRI. All patients with PAIS exhibited preoperative concentric contrast enhancement of the arterial walls of the terminal segments of the ICA and/or proximal branches of the ACA, MCA, or PCA supplying the territory affected by PAIS. This anatomical association has not previously been observed and requires further investigation. The occurrence of VW-CE was not significantly associated with PAIS in the studied cohort, which may be attributed to the generally low incidence of PAIS itself. Postoperative acute stroke rates vary in the literature, partly due to differences in the time intervals studied or because calculations were made per bypass rather than per operation in the case of multi-territorial revascularization in single-stage procedures. While some authors report PAIS within 24 h after surgery, as we do, others have identified PAIS with a latency of up to 7 days [5,29,30]. Our PAIS rate of 3.3% per revascularizing surgery and 2.1% per bypass seems plausible given the rates described in the literature, which range from 2.1% to 6.9% [2,3,5,29,31].

Although PAISs were generally quite rare in the relatively large sample analyzed, which limits stochastic analysis, this observation merits further attention. It is possible that a pathological VW-CE may correspond to a disease activity that may result in the deterioration and instability of perfusion distal to the affected vessel segment. A correlation between disease progression in MMD and VW-CE has already been previously demonstrated [15,19]. This finding is consistent with other studies that have demonstrated a correlation between postoperative stroke and the imaging progression of steno-occlusive changes or clinically unstable disease [2,19,32]. Several studies have provided support for this hypothesis, identifying preoperative ischemic events as a risk factor for PAIS [3,5,6,33,34]. All identified patients with PAIS initially presented with symptoms of an ischemic stroke. However, this was not demonstrated to be a significant risk factor for PAIS. It is noteworthy that no spatial correlation with the occurrence of PAIS has yet been established, as several authors have correctly described the occurrence of ischemic stroke in locations contralateral to the operated hemisphere or clearly distant from the surgical site [3,7,11,12]. Therefore, not all occurrences of PAIS can be explained by a watershed shift phenomenon, which could be seen as a paradoxical decrease in cerebral blood flow in the adjacent cortex near the site of local hyperperfusion, or a steal phenomenon with increased retrograde flow versus decreased antegrade flow [8,9]. The data presented here suggest such a spatial correlation between the VW-CE and the area affected by PAIS. This may be a potential factor influencing the sequence of multi-stage procedures and the urgency of planning patient-specific revascularization procedures. The time interval between VW-CE imaging and surgical treatment in this study should not diminish the significance of the results given the presumed long-lasting and durable nature of the VW-CE in MMD, which approximates to at least 24 months [17,19]. During this period, a slow intensity increase of VW-CE can be observed for approximately 12 months, followed by a decrease in intensity for another 12 months.

In our cohort, no further PAISs were observed in multi-stage procedures. This may be attributed to the protective effect of enhanced blood flow resulting from the initial revascularization or a stabilization of hemodynamics in segments with disease progression, as a decreasing rate of PAIS in secondary interventions has also been reported in other studies [3]. However, this may also be biased by the fact that the hemisphere or vascular territory with an assignable VW-CE is often the hemisphere with the most pronounced symptoms and a limited perfusion reserve, and it is therefore treated first in the primary intervention. In view of our study results, the question arises as to whether revascularization should be postponed due to an increased PAIS rate until the VW-CE has subsided. Studies specifically addressing this issue are not known. However, based on the current state of the evidence, the risk–benefit ratio should be clearly in favor of prompt revascularization as VW-CE indicates increased disease activity and, consequently, an elevated risk of stroke [15,17,19].

With regard to comorbidities, this study identified obesity as a risk factor for PAIS, while other studies have also identified diabetes mellitus as an independent vascular risk factor [3,4,35]. These findings are conclusive in that both conditions may be interdependent and have been shown to have an overall negative impact on the cerebral vasoarchitecture through microvascular dysfunction [36]. In addition, patients diagnosed with PAIS exhibited a higher incidence of significantly reduced high-density lipoprotein (HDL) levels [37]. There was no evidence in this study that ethnicity had an impact on VW-CE or PAIS. However, the low proportion of non-Caucasian patients in the cohort analyzed is a limiting factor. Whether the observations from this study are also present in Asian patients with MMD would certainly be an interesting question for future studies.

The findings of this study indicate a possible direct relationship between VW-CE and PAIS. Nevertheless, it is not feasible to ascertain a causal relationship and the origin of these ischemic strokes. It seems reasonable to suggest that a VW-CE vessel segment may act as an indicator of an actively progressing stenosis, with hemodynamic restriction occurring distal to it. This is corroborated by the increased susceptibility of MMD patients to perioperative fluctuations in blood pressure levels. Conversely, it is also possible that VW-CE segments could be the origin of thromboembolic infarcts, which has already been demonstrated to be a factor in MMD [38,39]. This is also supported by the effect of antiplatelet therapy (APT), as a reduction in the risk of PAIS with APT was found in at least some, but not all, studies [1,40,41]. Overall, APT is most likely to result in improved overall survival in MMD, while the risk of hemorrhage appears to be reduced [1,42]. However, the present study cannot make a conclusion about the effect of APT on PAIS, as all patients included received APT as standard. Thus, MMD may be a mixed picture of hemodynamic and thromboembolic ischemia.

This study did not specifically address intraoperative risk factors. However, as previously stated, the distinctive features of surgical procedures may be a pivotal factor in the development of PAIS in a territory at risk due to VW-CE. Hemodynamic variations due to anesthetic management with vasoreactive drugs and a hematocrit shift due to volume management have been identified as risk factors for PAIS [10]. Therefore, patient-specific blood pressure management both intraoperatively and postoperatively may reduce the risk of PAIS [31]. In addition, the carbon dioxide sensitivity of the cerebral vasculature must be taken into account, as an increased incidence of PAIS has been described, at least in ventilation-associated hypocapnia and hypercapnia [5,43]. This emphasizes the necessity for close coordination between the surgeon and anesthesiologist regarding, e.g., perioperative blood pressure levels and ventilation parameters.

Limitations

This is a retrospective analysis, which always has the risk of a certain bias. Due to the rarity of perioperative stroke, the cohort examined is rather small in comparison to the entire cohort treated. Nevertheless, the risk of an underpowered analysis seems low given the large study population in total. Still, further investigations of larger populations should certainly be considered. We therefore expect to see higher data densities in the future as we continue our imaging protocol and aim to analyze the pathophysiological impact of vessel-wall contrast enhancement in a translational clinical trial. Moreover, the analysis of individual dynamics of contrast enhancement before surgery was not possible, as only one preoperative VW-CE imaging was performed for each of the patients. Furthermore, this study concentrated on the diagnosis of VW-CE and PAIS. However, it is not possible to draw conclusions regarding the causal relationships between these factors alone, and further research is required to ascertain the significance of VW-CE in MMD.

5. Conclusions

Acute perioperative ischemic stroke represents a rare but serious adverse event of revascularization procedures in MMD. The findings of our study indicate a potential correlation between PAIS and the preoperative observation of concentric contrast enhancement of the affected vessel walls. In several studies this vessel-wall contrast enhancement was found to be associated with disease progression in the respective vessel segment. Patients with VW-CE may be at an elevated risk for acute perioperative ischemic strokes and should be monitored meticulously. Further research is required to gain a deeper insight into the relationship between VW-CE and the progression of MMD. This could potentially lead to improved patient outcomes by determining the appropriate treatment, including the timing of surgery and the sequence of territories to be revascularized in cases of multi-territorial involvement. Additionally, a more comprehensive understanding of the underlying pathophysiological processes leading to Moyamoya disease could be achieved.

Author Contributions: Clinical data acquisition was conducted by authors P.H., N.K. and C.R. Imaging and radiological evaluation was performed by T.-K.H. Manuscript writing and corrections were made by P.H., C.R., L.Z., N.K., L.M.W., T.-K.H. and M.T. All authors have read and agreed to the published version of the manuscript.

Funding: L.Z. is supported by the Medical Faculty Tübingen (TÜFF program, 2723-0-0).

Institutional Review Board Statement: All procedures performed in studies involving human participants were in accordance with the ethical standards of the institutional research committee and with the 1964 Helsinki Declaration and its later amendments or comparable ethics standards. Approval of the local ethics committee was obtained on 5 June 2024 (105/2024BO2).

Informed Consent Statement: Due to the retrospective character of this analysis, no specific formal consent from the participating patients was obtained.

Data Availability Statement: The original contributions presented in the study are included in the article, further inquiries can be directed to the corresponding author.

Conflicts of Interest: The authors declare no conflicts of interest.

Abbreviations

ACA	anterior cerebral artery
APT	antiplatelet therapy
BMI	body mass index
BOLD	blood-oxygenation-level dependent
CDC	Clavien–Dindo Classification
CT	computed tomography scan
DM	diabetes mellitus
EC-IC	extracranial–intracranial
PAIS	perioperative acute ischemic stroke
HDL	high-density lipoprotein
HTN	(arterial) hypertension
ICA	internal carotid artery
MCA	middle cerebral artery
MMD	Moyamoya disease
MRI	magnetic resonance imaging
OR	odds ratio
VW-CE	contrast-enhancing vessel wall
TIA	transitory ischemic attack

References

1. Yamada, S.; Oki, K.; Itoh, Y.; Kuroda, S.; Houkin, K.; Tominaga, T.; Miyamoto, S.; Hashimoto, N.; Suzuki, N. Effects of Surgery and Antiplatelet Therapy in Ten-Year Follow-Up from the Registry Study of Research Committee on Moyamoya Disease in Japan. *J. Stroke Cerebrovasc. Dis.* **2016**, *25*, 340–349. [CrossRef] [PubMed]

2. Kazumata, K.; Ito, M.; Tokairin, K.; Ito, Y.; Houkin, K.; Nakayama, N.; Kuroda, S.; Ishikawa, T.; Kamiyama, H. The frequency of postoperative stroke in moyamoya disease following combined revascularization: A single-university series and systematic review. *J. Neurosurg.* **2014**, *121*, 432–440. [CrossRef] [PubMed]
3. Wang, J.; Jiang, H.; Tang, J.; Lin, C.; Ni, W.; Gu, Y. Postoperative cerebral infarction after revascularization in patients with moyamoya disease: Incidence and risk factors. *Front. Neurol.* **2022**, *13*, 1053193. [CrossRef] [PubMed]
4. Wei, W.; Chen, X.; Yu, J.; Li, X.-Q. Risk factors for postoperative stroke in adults patients with moyamoya disease: A systematic review with meta-analysis. *BMC Neurol.* **2019**, *19*, 98. [CrossRef]
5. Hyun, S.-J.; Kim, J.-S.; Hong, S.-C. Prognostic factors associated with perioperative ischemic complications in adult-onset moyamoya disease. *Acta Neurochir.* **2010**, *152*, 1181–1188. [CrossRef]
6. Antonucci, M.; Burns, T.; Pulling, T.; Rosenberg, J.; Marks, M.; Steinberg, G.; Zaharchuk, G. Acute Preoperative Infarcts and Poor Cerebrovascular Reserve Are Independent Risk Factors for Severe Ischemic Complications following Direct Extracranial-Intracranial Bypass for Moyamoya Disease. *Am. J. Neuroradiol.* **2016**, *37*, 228–235. [CrossRef]
7. Jung, Y.J.; Ahn, J.S.; Kwon, D.H.; Kwun, B.D. Ischemic complications occurring in the contralateral hemisphere after surgical treatment of adults with moyamoya disease. *J. Korean Neurosurg. Soc.* **2011**, *50*, 492–496. [CrossRef]
8. Tashiro, R.; Fujimura, M.; Kameyama, M.; Mugikura, S.; Endo, H.; Takeuchi, Y.; Tomata, Y.; Niizuma, K.; Tominaga, T. Incidence and Risk Factors of the Watershed Shift Phenomenon after Superficial Temporal Artery-Middle Cerebral Artery Anastomosis for Adult Moyamoya Disease. *Cerebrovasc. Dis.* **2019**, *47*, 178–187. [CrossRef]
9. Oshima, H.; Katayama, Y.; Hirayama, T. Intracerebral steal phenomenon associated with global hyperemia in moyamoya disease during revascularization surgery. *J. Neurosurg.* **2000**, *92*, 949–954. [CrossRef]
10. Li, J.; Zhao, Y.; Zhao, M.; Cao, P.; Liu, X.; Ren, H.; Zhang, D.; Zhang, Y.; Wang, R.; Zhao, J. High variance of intraoperative blood pressure predicts early cerebral infarction after revascularization surgery in patients with Moyamoya disease. *Neurosurg. Rev.* **2020**, *43*, 759–769. [CrossRef]
11. Hara, S.; Nariai, T.; Inaji, M.; Tanaka, Y.; Maehara, T. Imaging Pattern and the Mechanisms of Postoperative Infarction After Indirect Revascularization in Patients with Moyamoya Disease. *World Neurosurg.* **2021**, *155*, e510–e521. [CrossRef] [PubMed]
12. Guzman, R.; Lee, M.; Achrol, A.; Bell-Stephens, T.; Kelly, M.; Do, H.M.; Marks, M.P.; Steinberg, G.K. Clinical outcome after 450 revascularization procedures for moyamoya disease. *J. Neurosurg.* **2009**, *111*, 927–935. [CrossRef] [PubMed]
13. Lu, M.; Zhang, H.; Liu, D.; Liu, X.; Zhang, L.; Peng, P.; Yuan, F.; Liu, S.; Sheng, F.; Liu, Y.; et al. Association of intracranial vessel wall enhancement and cerebral hemorrhage in moyamoya disease: A high-resolution magnetic resonance imaging study. *J. Neurol.* **2021**, *268*, 4768–4777. [CrossRef] [PubMed]
14. Brinjikji, W.; Mossa-Basha, M.; Huston, J.; Rabinstein, A.A.; Lanzino, G.; Lehman, V.T. Intracranial vessel wall imaging for evaluation of steno-occlusive diseases and intracranial aneurysms. *J. Neuroradiol.* **2017**, *44*, 123–134. [CrossRef] [PubMed]
15. Wang, S.S.-Y.; Hauser, T.-K.; Haas, P.; Tellermann, J.; Hurth, H.; Ernemann, U.; Tatagiba, M.; Bender, B.; Khan, N.; Roder, C. Intensity Score of Vessel Wall Contrast Enhancement in MRI Allows Prediction of Disease Progression in Moyamoya Angiopathy. *Neurosurgery* **2024**, *95*, 1000–1009. [CrossRef]
16. Masuda, J.; Ogata, J.; Yutani, C. Smooth muscle cell proliferation and localization of macrophages and T cells in the occlusive intracranial major arteries in moyamoya disease. *Stroke* **1993**, *24*, 1960–1967. [CrossRef]
17. Lu, M.; Zhang, H.; Liu, D.; Hao, F.; Zhang, L.; Peng, P.; Yuan, F.; Liu, S.; Sheng, F.; Liu, Y.; et al. Vessel wall enhancement as a predictor of arterial stenosis progression and poor outcomes in moyamoya disease. *Eur. Radiol.* **2023**, *33*, 2489–2499. [CrossRef]
18. Wang, M.; Yang, Y.; Zhou, F.; Li, M.; Liu, R.; Guan, M.; Li, R.; He, L.; Xu, Y.; Zhang, B.; et al. The Contrast Enhancement of Intracranial Arterial Wall on High-resolution MRI and Its Clinical Relevance in Patients with Moyamoya Vasculopathy. *Sci. Rep.* **2017**, *7*, 44264. [CrossRef]
19. Roder, C.; Hauser, T.-K.; Ernemann, U.; Tatagiba, M.; Khan, N.; Bender, B. Arterial wall contrast enhancement in progressive moyamoya disease. *J. Neurosurg.* **2019**, *132*, 1845–1853. [CrossRef]
20. Fujimura, M.; Tominaga, T.; Kuroda, S.; Takahashi, J.C.; Endo, H.; Ogasawara, K.; Miyamoto, S.; Labor Welfare Research Committee on Moyamoya Disease (Spontaneous Occlusion of Circle of Willis) of the Ministry of Health; the Guideline Committee 2021 of the Japan Stroke Society. 2021 Japanese Guidelines for the Management of Moyamoya Disease: Guidelines from the Research Committee on Moyamoya Disease and Japan Stroke Society. *Neurol. Med.-Chir.* **2022**, *62*, 165–170. [CrossRef]
21. Bersano, A.; Khan, N.; Fuentes, B.; Acerbi, F.; Canavero, I.; Tournier-Lasserve, E.; Vajcoczy, P.; Zedde, M.L.; Hussain, S.; Lémeret, S.; et al. European Stroke Organisation (ESO) Guidelines on Moyamoya angiopathy Endorsed by Vascular European Reference Network (VASCERN). *Eur. Stroke J.* **2023**, *8*, 55–84. [CrossRef] [PubMed]
22. Clavien, P.A.; Barkun, J.; de Oliveira, M.L.; Vauthey, J.N.; Dindo, D.; Schulick, R.D.; de Santibañes, E.; Pekolj, J.; Slankamenac, K.; Bassi, C.; et al. The clavien-dindo classification of surgical complications: Five-year experience. *Ann. Surg.* **2009**, *250*, 187–196. [CrossRef] [PubMed]
23. Hauser, T.-K.; Seeger, A.; Bender, B.; Klose, U.; Thurow, J.; Ernemann, U.; Tatagiba, M.; Meyer, P.T.; Khan, N.; Roder, C. Hypercapnic BOLD MRI compared to H215O PET/CT for the hemodynamic evaluation of patients with Moyamoya Disease. *NeuroImage Clin.* **2019**, *22*, 101713. [CrossRef] [PubMed]
24. Roder, C.; Klose, U.; Hurth, H.; Brendle, C.; Tatagiba, M.; Ernemann, U.; Khan, N.; Hauser, T.-K. Longitudinal Reproducibility of CO_2-Triggered BOLD MRI for the Hemodynamic Evaluation of Adult Patients with Moyamoya Angiopathy. *Cerebrovasc. Dis.* **2021**, *50*, 332–338. [CrossRef]

25. Roder, C.; Bürkle, E.; Ebner, F.H.; Tatagiba, M.; Ernemann, U.; Buck, A.; Meyer, P.T.; Khan, N. Estimation of Severity of Moyamoya Disease with [15O]Water-Positron Emission Tomography Compared with Magnetic Resonance Imaging and Angiography. *World Neurosurg.* **2018**, *117*, e75–e81. [CrossRef]
26. Zerweck, L.; Roder, C.; Hauser, T.-K.; Thurow, J.; Mengel, A.; Tatagiba, M.; Khan, N.; Meyer, P.T.; Ernemann, U.; Klose, U. Hemodynamic evaluation of patients with Moyamoya Angiopathy: Comparison of resting-state fMRI to breath-hold fMRI and [15O]water PET. *Neuroradiology* **2022**, *64*, 553–563. [CrossRef]
27. Zerweck, L.; Pohmann, R.; Klose, U.; Martirosian, P.; Haas, P.; Ernemann, U.; Khan, N.; Roder, C.; Hauser, T.-K.; Hennersdorf, F. Evaluation of the contribution of individual arteries to the cerebral blood supply in patients with Moyamoya angiopathy: Comparison of vessel-encoded arterial spin labeling and digital subtraction angiography. *Neuroradiology* **2024**, *66*, 1131–1140. [CrossRef]
28. Zerweck, L.; Hauser, T.-K.; Roder, C.; Blazhenets, G.; Khan, N.; Ernemann, U.; Meyer, P.T.; Klose, U. Evaluation of the cerebrovascular reactivity in patients with Moyamoya Angiopathy by use of breath-hold fMRI: Investigation of voxel-wise hemodynamic delay correction in comparison to [15O]water PET. *Neuroradiology* **2023**, *65*, 539–550. [CrossRef]
29. Schubert, G.A.; Biermann, P.; Weiss, C.; Seiz, M.; Vajkoczy, P.; Schmiedek, P.; Thomé, C. Risk Profile In Extracranial/Intracranial Bypass Surgery—The Role of Antiplatelet Agents, Disease Pathology, and Surgical Technique In 168 Direct Revascularization Procedures. *World Neurosurg.* **2014**, *82*, 672–677. [CrossRef]
30. Kuroda, S.; Houkin, K.; Nunomura, M.; Abe, H. Frontal lobe infarction due to hemodynamic change after surgical revascularization in moyamoya disease. two case reports. *Neurol. Med.-Chir.* **2000**, *40*, 315–320. [CrossRef]
31. Li, C.; Zhang, N.; Yu, S.; Xu, Y.; Yao, Y.; Zeng, M.; Li, D.; Xia, C. Individualized Perioperative Blood Pressure Management for Adult Moyamoya Disease: Experience from 186 Consecutive Procedures. *J. Stroke Cerebrovasc. Dis.* **2021**, *30*, 105413. [CrossRef] [PubMed]
32. Funaki, T.; Takahashi, J.C.; Takagi, Y.; Kikuchi, T.; Yoshida, K.; Mitsuhara, T.; Kataoka, H.; Okada, T.; Fushimi, Y.; Miyamoto, S. Unstable moyamoya disease: Clinical features and impact on perioperative ischemic complications. *J. Neurosurg.* **2015**, *122*, 400–407. [CrossRef] [PubMed]
33. Kim, S.-H.; Choi, J.-U.; Yang, K.-H.; Kim, T.-G.; Kim, D.-S. Risk factors for postoperative ischemic complications in patients with moyamoya disease. *J. Neurosurg. Pediatr.* **2005**, *103*, 433–438. [CrossRef] [PubMed]
34. Zhao, M.; Deng, X.; Zhang, D.; Wang, S.; Zhang, Y.; Wang, R.; Zhao, J. Risk factors for and outcomes of postoperative complications in adult patients with moyamoya disease. *J. Neurosurg.* **2019**, *130*, 531–542. [CrossRef]
35. Pettersson, S.D.; Olofsson, H.K.; Ali, S.; Szarek, D.; Miękisiak, G.; Ogilvy, C.S. Risk Factors for Ischemic Stroke After Revascularization Surgery in Patients with Moyamoya Disease: An Age-Stratified Comparative Meta-Analysis. *World Neurosurg.* **2023**, *173*, 146–157.e14. [CrossRef]
36. van Sloten, T.T.; Sedaghat, S.; Carnethon, M.R.; Launer, L.J.; Stehouwer, C.D. Cerebral microvascular complications of type 2 diabetes: Stroke, cognitive dysfunction, and depression. *Lancet Diabetes Endocrinol.* **2020**, *8*, 325–336. [CrossRef]
37. Yu, X.; Ge, P.; Zhai, Y.; Wang, R.; Zhang, Y.; Zhang, D. Hypo-high density lipoproteinemia is a predictor for recurrent stroke during the long-term follow-up after revascularization in adult moyamoya disease. *Front. Neurol.* **2022**, *13*, 891622. [CrossRef]
38. Kim, D.Y.; Son, J.P.; Yeon, J.Y.; Kim, G.M.; Kim, J.S.; Hong, S.C.; Bang, O.Y. Infarct Pattern and Collateral Status in Adult Moyamoya Disease: A Multimodal Magnetic Resonance Imaging Study. *Stroke* **2017**, *48*, 111–116. [CrossRef]
39. Pompsch, M.; Veltkamp, R.; Diehl, R.R.; Kraemer, M. Microembolic signals and antiplatelet therapy in Moyamoya angiopathy. *J. Neurol.* **2022**, *269*, 6605–6612. [CrossRef]
40. Liu, T.; Qin, M.; Xiong, X.; Feng, L.; Lai, X.; Gao, Y. Benefits and risks of antiplatelet therapy for moyamoya disease: A systematic review and meta-analysis. *Front. Neurol.* **2023**, *14*, 1132339. [CrossRef]
41. Luo, Y.; Cao, Z.; Ye, H.; Wu, S.; Sun, X. Antiplatelet therapy may improve the prognosis of patients with moyamoya disease: A 12-year retrospective study. *J. Neurol.* **2023**, *270*, 3876–3884. [CrossRef] [PubMed]
42. Seo, W.; Kim, J.; Choi, E.; Kim, Y.; Chung, J.; Saver, J.L.; Bang, O.Y.; Kim, G. Association of Antiplatelet Therapy, Including Cilostazol, With Improved Survival in Patients With Moyamoya Disease in a Nationwide Study. *J. Am. Hear. Assoc.* **2021**, *10*, e017701. [CrossRef] [PubMed]
43. Kuwabara, Y.; Ichiya, Y.; Sasaki, M.; Yoshida, T.; Masuda, K.; Matsushima, T.; Fukui, M. Response to hypercapnia in moyamoya disease. Cerebrovascular response to hypercapnia in pediatric and adult patients with moyamoya disease. *Stroke* **1997**, *28*, 701–707. [CrossRef] [PubMed]

brain sciences

MDPI

Article

BOLD Cerebrovascular Reactivity and NOVA Quantitative MR Angiography in Adult Patients with Moyamoya Vasculopathy Undergoing Cerebral Bypass Surgery

Loris Garbani Nerini [1,2,3], Jacopo Bellomo [1,2], Lara Maria Höbner [1,2], Vittorio Stumpo [1,2], Elisa Colombo [1,2], Christiaan Hendrik Bas van Niftrik [1,2], Tilman Schubert [2,4], Zsolt Kulcsár [2,4], Susanne Wegener [2,5], Andreas Luft [2,5], Luca Regli [1,2], Jorn Fierstra [1,2], Martina Sebök [1,2,*,†] and Giuseppe Esposito [1,2,†]

1 Department of Neurosurgery, University Hospital Zurich, Frauenklinikstrasse 10, 8091 Zurich, Switzerland; loris.garbaninerini@uzh.ch (L.G.N.); jacopo.bellomo@usz.ch (J.B.); lara.hoebner@usz.ch (L.M.H.); vittorio.stumpo@usz.ch (V.S.); elisa.colombo@usz.ch (E.C.); bas.vanniftrik@usz.ch (C.H.B.v.N.); luca.regli@usz.ch (L.R.); jorn.fierstra@usz.ch (J.F.); giuseppe.esposito@usz.ch (G.E.)
2 Clinical Neuroscience Center, University Hospital Zurich, Frauenklinikstrasse 10, 8091 Zurich, Switzerland; tilman.schubert@usz.ch (T.S.); zsolt.kulcsar@usz.ch (Z.K.); susanne.wegener@usz.ch (S.W.); andreas.luft@usz.ch (A.L.)
3 University of Zürich (UZH), Raemistrasse 100, CH-8091 Zurich, Switzerland
4 Department of Neuroradiology, University Hospital Zurich, Frauenklinikstrasse 10, 8091 Zurich, Switzerland
5 Department of Neurology, University Hospital Zurich, Frauenklinikstrasse 26, 8091 Zurich, Switzerland
* Correspondence: martina.seboek@usz.ch; Tel.:+41-44-2551111
† Shared last authorship.

Abstract: Revascularization surgery for the symptomatic hemisphere with hemodynamic impairment is effective for Moyamoya vasculopathy patients. However, careful patient selection is crucial and ideally supported by advanced quantitative hemodynamic imaging. Recently, blood oxygenation level-dependent cerebrovascular reactivity (BOLD-CVR) and quantitative magnetic resonance angiography with non-invasive optimal vessel analysis (qMRA-NOVA) have gained prominence in assessing these patients. This study aims to present the results of BOLD-CVR and qMRA-NOVA imaging along with the changes in cerebral hemodynamics and flow status following flow augmentation with superficial temporal artery–middle cerebral artery (STA-MCA) bypass in our Moyamoya vasculopathy patient cohort. Symptomatic patients with Moyamoya vasculopathy treated at the Clinical Neuroscience Center of the University Hospital Zurich who underwent hemodynamic and flow imaging (BOLD-CVR and qMRA-NOVA) before and after bypass were included in the analysis. Reduced hemispheric volume flow rates, as well as impaired BOLD-CVR, were measured in all 12 patients with Moyamoya vasculopathy before STA-MCA bypass surgery. Following the surgical procedure, post-operative BOLD-CVR demonstrated a non-significant increase in BOLD-CVR values within the revascularized, symptomatic middle cerebral artery territory and cerebral hemisphere. The results of the statistical tests should be viewed as indicative due to the small sample size. Additionally, post-operative qMRA-NOVA revealed a significant improvement in the hemispheric volume flow rate of the affected hemisphere due to the additional bypass flow rate. Our findings affirm the presence of hemodynamic and flow impairments in the symptomatic hemisphere of the Moyamoya vasculopathy patients. Bypass surgery proves effective in improving both BOLD-CVR impairment and the hemispheric volume flow rate in our patient cohort.

Keywords: moyamoya; BOLD-CVR; NOVA; STA-MCA bypass; hemodynamics; quantitative flow

1. Introduction

Moyamoya disease is a rare idiopathic vasculopathy characterized by the progressive stenosis or occlusion of the distal internal carotid arteries (ICAs), as well as the proximal anterior (ACAs) and middle cerebral arteries (MCAs), followed by the development of a collateral network of arteries [1,2]. The term "Moyamoya", derived from Japanese, translates to "puff of smoke", capturing the extensive cerebral collateral network associated with the disease. The formation of collaterals serves as a compensatory mechanism in response to the decreased cerebral flow caused by the stenosis or occlusion of intracranial arteries. However, this compensatory attempt is often insufficient, resulting in clinical manifestations such as ischemic strokes and transient ischemic attacks (TIAs). Additionally, the dense collateral network tends to cause bleeding, leading to hemorrhagic strokes [1,3].

The treatment objective of symptomatic Moyamoya patients is to enhance cerebral perfusion, thereby reducing the risk for future ischemic and hemorrhagic events [4–6]; revascularization surgery via direct, indirect, and combined bypass procedures stands as the sole proven and effective treatment based on clinical trials [7–9]. The most recent guidelines on Moyamoya Angiopathy from the European Stroke Organisation (ESO) recommend revascularization surgery using either a direct or a combined bypass procedure [10].

In the historical context, various imaging techniques [11] have been used to assess the vessel status of patients with Moyamoya vasculopathy, with digital subtraction angiography (DSA) remaining a gold-standard technique [12]. However, when analyzing the cerebral perfusion status, techniques such as single-photon emission computed tomography (SPECT) and positron emission tomography (PET) have been utilized. It is noteworthy that these latter methods necessitate exposure to ionizing radiation and have limited availability in routine clinical practice [8,12,13]. Arterial spin labeling is an effective method for detecting the cerebral blood flow in patients with Moyamoya vasculopathy [14].

Recently, two innovative magnetic resonance imaging techniques for the quantitative assessment of the cerebrovascular reserve capacity and blood flow in cerebral vessels have emerged and are increasingly applied in the evaluation of patients with cerebrovascular steno-occlusive disease:

(1) Blood oxygenation level-dependent (BOLD) magnetic resonance imaging (MRI), to evaluate the cerebrovascular reactivity (CVR) at the brain parenchyma level, utilizing the physiological vasodilatory response to CO_2 [15–17];
(2) Quantitative magnetic resonance angiography (qMRA) with non-invasive optimal vessel analysis (NOVA), which measures the volume flow rate (VFR) of large intracranial arteries in mL/min [15,18,19].

The objective of this study is to present the results of BOLD-CVR hemodynamic investigation and qMRA-NOVA flow imaging in our cohort of patients with Moyamoya vasculopathy, along with the changes in cerebral hemodynamics and flow status following revascularization surgery.

2. Methods

2.1. Patient Selection

This retrospective cohort study with prospectively collected data includes all adult (>18 years old) patients with symptomatic Moyamoya vasculopathy who underwent a bypass surgery at the Clinical Neuroscience Center of the University Hospital Zurich between May 2019 and May 2023 and who received advanced MR imaging studies (BOLD-CVR and qMRA-NOVA). Following cerebral revascularization, qMRA-NOVA was performed before discharge, and BOLD-CVR was performed 3 months after bypass. All 12 included patients received a combined bypass procedure (direct STA-MCA bypass with indirect synangiosis). The indirect revascularization techniques varied, with 9 patients undergoing encephalo-duro-synangiosis (EDS), 2 patients encephalo-duro-myo-synangiosis (EDMS), and 1 patient encephalo-duro-periosteo-synangiosis (EDPS).

Ethical approval for this study was obtained from the Ethics Committee of the Canton of Zurich under the reference number KEK 2020-02314. All participants provided their consent by signing a general informed consent form.

2.2. Quantitative Advanced MRI Techniques

MRI data were obtained using a 3 Tesla Skyra VD13 system with a 32-channel head matrix following a protocol previously published [20,21]. A (3D) T1-weighted, magnetization-prepared rapid acquisition gradient echo (MP RAGE) image, oriented similarly to the BOLD fMRI scans, was conducted for the purpose of overlay to capture structural information of the entire brain. Additionally, a 3D time-of-flight (TOF) angiography and 2D phase-contrast imaging, utilizing the 3D coordinates determined from the NOVA, were performed to enable VFR analysis [15].

2.2.1. BOLD-CVR Measurement and Analysis

To quantitatively analyze cerebrovascular reactivity at the brain parenchymal level, the BOLD signal was integrated with a standardized vasodilatory CO_2 stimulus that was achieved through a computer-controlled gas blender employing prospective gas-targeting algorithms (RespirAct^{TM}), as per established protocols [22,23]. Following the examination of raw CVR data, this approach yielded quantitative BOLD-CVR values (%BOLD signal change/mmHg CO_2) assessed for the entire brain, both grey and white matter, and for both hemispheres. Furthermore, employing a vascular atlas on the normalized CVR maps allowed for the calculation of quantitative BOLD-CVR values specific to the vascular territories of both hemispheres, in accordance with previously published methods [15,16].

For this patient cohort, BOLD-CVR values were assessed for the whole brain, as well as for symptomatic and non-symptomatic brain hemispheres, and for symptomatic and non-symptomatic vascular territories (anterior cerebral artery (ACA), middle cerebral artery (MCA), and posterior cerebral artery (PCA) territories).

2.2.2. qMRA NOVA

Volume flow measurements were conducted using the commercially available NOVA (non-invasive optimal vessel analysis) software from VasSol, Inc. Chicago, IL, USA [19]. For the analysis, we focused on the volume flow rates (VFRs) of specific arterial segments: the second segment of the anterior cerebral artery (ACA-A2), the first segment of the middle cerebral artery (MCA-M1), and the second segment of the posterior cerebral artery (PCA-P2). The hemispheric volume flow rate (hVFR) was computed by summing the VFR values for ACA-A2, MCA-M1, and PCA-P2. In the post-bypass qMRA-NOVA analysis, the affected hVFR is calculated as the sum of the VFRs of ACA-A2, MCA-M1, PCA-P2, and the bypass VFR [15,24].

2.3. Direct STA-MCA Bypass and Indirect Revascularization

There is no consensus on the optimal type of revascularization surgery. At our institution, we use the STA-MCA bypass as a direct revascularization procedure, connecting the STA to a cortical M4 branch in an end-to-side fashion using microsurgical techniques. Notably, the distal part of the donor STA branch is cut in a fish-mouth fashion to increase its opening diameter, and a linear arteriotomy is performed on the cortical recipient M4 branch, which should be at least 2.5 times the diameter of the recipient. A detailed description of the flow-augmentation bypass procedure is available elsewhere (4). Several indirect techniques have been proposed, evolving over time. We use a combination of vascularized tissue based on patient characteristics and tissue availability, including EDS, EDMS, and EDPS. Combining direct and indirect revascularization procedures leverages the advantages of both techniques [8,25,26].

2.4. Statistical Analysis

The statistical analysis was conducted using R. Dichotomous variables are expressed as the frequency (%), while continuous variables are presented as the mean ± standard deviation, and are compared with a paired Student's t-test. A p value less than 0.05 was considered statistically significant.

3. Results

3.1. Study Population Characteristics

Out of the twelve patients included, one individual underwent two bypass operations, initially in one symptomatic hemisphere and, subsequently, after 7 months, in the other meanwhile-symptomatic cerebral hemisphere. For the BOLD-CVR and qMRA-NOVA analyses, each of the two operations was treated separately, resulting in 13 imaging samples. Among the 12 patients who underwent surgery, 9 underwent postoperative qMRA-NOVA analysis, and 11 underwent postoperative BOLD-CVR analysis. In the case of the patient who underwent bypass in both hemispheres, BOLD and NOVA analyses were performed after each operation, leading to 10 qMRA-NOVA and 12 BOLD-CVR imaging samples for the postoperative analysis.

Table 1 presents the baseline characteristics and clinical neurological scores of the included cohort of patients with Moyamoya vasculopathy. Among the included patients, six had unilateral vasculopathy, while the remaining six had bilateral vasculopathy. Three patients (25%) presented with hemorrhagic stroke, four patients (33.3%) with ischemic stroke, and five patients (41.7%) with transient ischemic attacks. Figure 1 illustrates a representative case of a patient with Moyamoya vasculopathy who underwent a surgical revascularization via STA-MCA bypass.

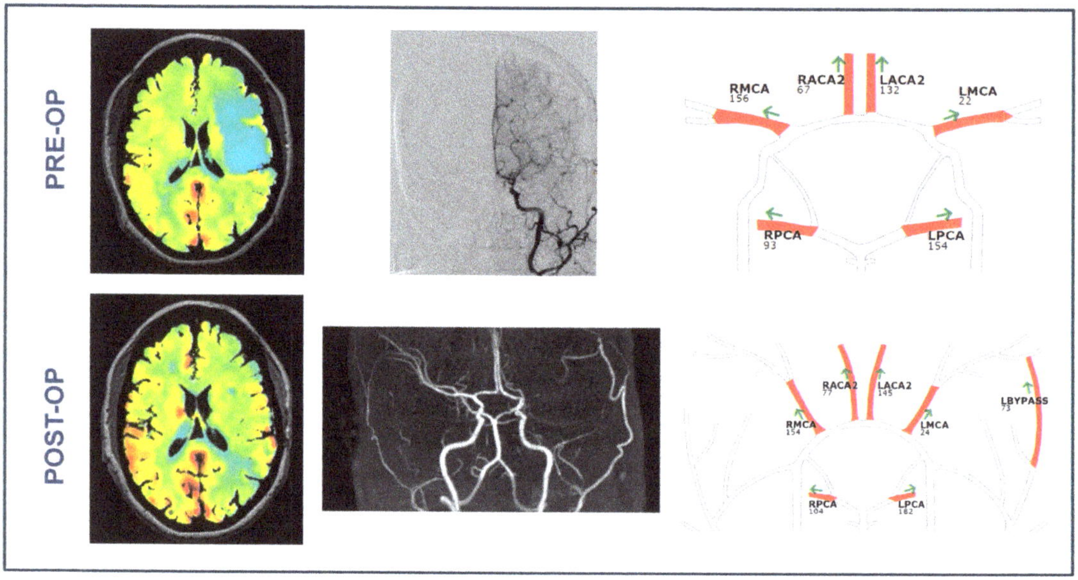

Figure 1. Illustrative case. A 49-year-old patient with Moyamoya vasculopathy presented with bilateral stenosis of the supraclinoid ICA and M1 occlusion on the left side. The patient already experienced two episodes of transitory ischemic attacks in her history, with transient weakness of the right arm and leg, with the last episode occurring two months preoperatively. At the admission, the patient did not have any neurological symptoms. The angiography confirmed the diagnosis and showed a significant presence of collaterals in the left MCA territory. The patient therefore underwent STA-MCA flow-augmentation bypass surgery with encephalo-duro-synangiosis on the left hemisphere. Pre-bypass qMRA NOVA showed an increased flow in the left ACA and PCA, as well as a marked flow reduction in the left MCA. BOLD-CVR showed a steal phenomenon with impaired CVR (hemodynamic failure grade II) for the left MCA territory. After the bypass in the left hemisphere, the qMRA-NOVA showed a patent bypass with a flow of 73 mL/min. The BOLD-CVR showed cortical improvement in the left MCA territory after the bypass operation.

Table 1. Baseline characteristics of included patient cohort.

	Total Patient Cohort (n = 12)
Age (mean ± SD)	50.25 ± 13.34
Gender: male, n (%)	7 (58.3)
Smoking, n (%)	5 (41.7)
Arterial hypertension, n (%)	3 (25.0)
Dyslipidemia, n (%)	2 (16.7)
Diabetes mellitus, n (%)	4 (33.3)
mRS (median (IQR))	
Before surgery	1 (2)
After surgery	0 (1)
NIHSS (median (IQR))	
Before surgery	0 (2)
After surgery	0 (0)

IQR = interquartile range; mRS = modified Rankin scale; n = number; NIHSS = National Institutes of Health Stroke Scale; SD = standard deviation.

In the case of the patient who underwent bypass in both hemispheres, BOLD and NOVA analyses were performed after each operation, leading to 10 qMRA-NOVA and 12 BOLD-CVR imaging samples for postoperative analysis (Supplementary Table S1).

3.2. BOLD-CVR and qMRA-NOVA Imaging Data before Bypass Surgery

Table 2 shows the quantitative hemodynamic BOLD-CVR values, while Table 3 presents the qMRA-NOVA flow values before bypass. When comparing the BOLD-CVR values between the symptomatic and non-symptomatic hemispheres, the symptomatic MCA territory exhibited lower BOLD-CVR values (BOLD-CVR symptomatic MCA territory vs. non-symptomatic MCA territory (%BOLD/mmHgCO_2): 0.03 ± 0.07 vs. 0.10 ± 0.11; $p = 0.09$), though the difference did not reach statistical significance. The results of the statistical tests should be viewed as indicative due to the small sample size. Similarly, for the ACA territory, the symptomatic territory showed lower absolute values compared to the non-symptomatic one, without a statistically significant difference. A similar trend was noted when comparing the symptomatic and the non-symptomatic hemispheres (BOLD-CVR symptomatic vs. non-symptomatic hemisphere (%BOLD/mmHgCO_2): 0.09 ± 0.07 vs. 0.12 ± 0.08) (Table 2).

Table 2. BOLD-CVR values before the bypass surgery in 12 patients (13 imaging samples).

BOLD-CVR (%BOLD/mmHgCO_2)	**Mean ± SD**
CVR whole brain	0.11 ± 0.07
CVR symptomatic hemisphere	0.09 ± 0.07
CVR non-symptomatic hemisphere	0.12 ± 0.08
CVR symptomatic ACA territory	0.08 ± 0.08
CVR non-symptomatic ACA territory	0.11 ± 0.08
CVR symptomatic MCA territory	0.03 ± 0.07
CVR non-symptomatic MCA territory	0.10 ± 0.11
CVR symptomatic PCA territory	0.23 ± 0.06
CVR non-symptomatic PCA territory	0.25 ± 0.06

ACA = anterior cerebral artery; BOLD = blood oxygenation-level dependent; CO_2 = carbon dioxide; CVR = cerebrovascular reactivity; MCA = middle cerebral artery; PCA = posterior cerebral artery; SD = standard deviation.

In the comparison of qMRA-NOVA-derived volume flow rates, a statistically significant difference was observed between the symptomatic and non-symptomatic M1-VFR (symptomatic vs. non-symptomatic (mL/min): 16.15 ± 18.45 vs. 101.38 ± 86.97; $p < 0.004$). Regarding P2-VFR, although no statistically significant difference was found, the symptomatic P2 exhibited a higher flow compared to the non-symptomatic P2 (P2-VFR symptomatic vs. non-symptomatic (mL/min): 164.69 ± 63.20 vs. 123.54 ± 61.59; $p = 0.10$). No difference was observed between symptomatic and non-symptomatic A2-

VFRs. The cumulative flow of the symptomatic hemisphere was lower than the flow in the non-symptomatic hemisphere (VFR of symptomatic hemisphere vs. VFR of non-symptomatic hemisphere (mL/min): 282.77 ± 89.70 vs. 322.15 ± 109.05), though this difference did not reach statistical significance (Table 3).

Table 3. qMRA-NOVA flow values before bypass surgery in 12 patients (13 imaging samples).

qMRA-NOVA (mL/min):	Mean ± SD
VFR symptomatic A2-ACA vessel	96.69 ± 53.94
VFR non-symptomatic A2-ACA vessel	97.23 ± 70.46
VFR symptomatic M1-MCA vessel	16.15 ± 18.45
VFR non-symptomatic M1-MCA vessel	101.38 ± 86.97
VFR symptomatic P2-PCA vessel	164.69 ± 63.20
VFR non-symptomatic P2-PCA vessel	123.54 ± 61.59
VFR symptomatic hemisphere	282.77 ± 89.70
VFR non-symptomatic hemisphere	322.15 ± 109.05

A2 = second segment of the anterior cerebral artery; M1 = first segment of the middle cerebral artery; P2 = second segment of the posterior cerebral artery; VFR = volume flow rate.

3.3. *BOLD Cerebrovascular Reactivity after Bypass*

Following cerebrovascular revascularization with STA-MCA bypass, every vascular territory in both the affected and unaffected hemispheres exhibited an improvement in BOLD-CVR, although no statistically significant differences were observed for any (Table 4). The symptomatic MCA territory demonstrated the most significant improvement in BOLD-CVR after bypass surgery (Δ 0.04%BOLD/mmHgCO_2), followed by the BOLD-CVR improvement of the affected hemisphere (Δ 0.03%BOLD/mmHgCO_2). Figure 2 illustrates the difference in the BOLD-CVR values of the symptomatic (affected) hemisphere and of the MCA territory before and after bypass revascularization for each patient. Looking at the individual data, we can see that three patients out of twelve showed a decrease in the CVR values of the affected hemisphere following the bypass surgery. All three patients presented with ischemic symptoms, and the bypass was patent following the surgery.

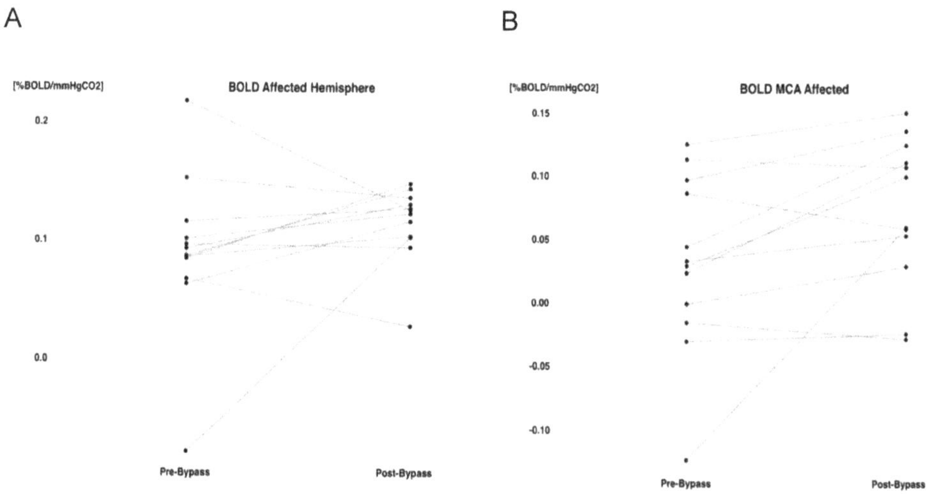

Figure 2. Graphical representation of BOLD-CVR values of the symptomatic (affected); (**A**) hemisphere and MCA. (**B**) territory before and after STA-MCA bypass.

Table 4. Comparison of pre- and post-bypass BOLD-CVR values in 11 Moyamoya patients (12 imaging series).

BOLD-CVR (%BOLD/mmHgCO_2)			
(Mean ± SD)	**Pre-Bypass (n = 12)**	**Post-Bypass (n = 12)**	***p*-Value**
CVR whole brain	0.11 ± 0.07	0.12 ± 0.04	0.52
CVR symptomatic hemisphere	0.09 ± 0.07	0.12 ± 0.03	0.31
CVR non-symptomatic hemisphere	0.12 ± 0.08	0.14 ± 0.06	0.71
CVR ACA symptomatic	0.08 ± 0.08	0.09 ± 0.05	0.62
CVR ACA non-symptomatic	0.11 ± 0.08	0.13 ± 0.06	0.46
CVR MCA symptomatic	0.03 ± 0.07	0.07 ± 0.06	0.09
CVR MCA non-symptomatic	0.10 ± 0.11	0.10 ± 0.09	0.86
CVR PCA symptomatic	0.23 ± 0.06	0.26 ± 0.07	0.29
CVR PCA non-symptomatic	0.25 ± 0.06	0.28 ± 0.10	0.37

ACA = anterior cerebral artery; BOLD = blood oxygenation-level dependent; CO_2 = carbon dioxide; CVR = cerebrovascular reactivity; MCA = middle cerebral artery; PCA = posterior cerebral artery; SD = standard deviation.

3.4. *qMRA-NOVA Values after Surgical Revascularization*

Comparing hemispheric pre-bypass and post-bypass volume flow-rate values, a significant improvement after surgical revascularization is noted in the VFRs of the affected hemisphere (affected hemisphere preOP vs. postOP (mL/min): 282.77 ± 89.70 vs. 383.70 ± 40.37; $p < 0.003$). This increase in volume flow rate is attributed to the bypass flow (qMRA-NOVA bypass VFR (mL/min): 86.70 ± 30.32) (Table 5). Figure 3 visually depicts the change in the volume flow rate of the affected hemisphere for each patient before and after the bypass. All but one patient exhibited an increase in the volume flow rate of the affected hemisphere after surgical revascularization. This patient also showed no improvement in the CVR values following revascularization but exhibited the most relevant affected-hemisphere CVR worsening, as shown in the individual data in Figure 2.

Table 5. Comparison of pre- and post-revascularization qMRA-NOVA values.

qMRA-NOVA (mL/min)			
(Mean ± SD)	**Pre-Bypass (n = 10)**	**Post-Bypass (n = 10)**	***p*-Value**
VFR A2 affected	96.69 ± 53.94	117.10 ± 56.90	0.39
VFR A2 unaffected	97.23 ± 70.46	112.40 ± 60.58	0.59
VFR M1 affected	16.15 ± 18.45	11.00 ± 16.07	0.49
VFR M1 unaffected	101.38 ± 86.97	115.10 ± 111.99	0.74
VFR P2 affected	164.69 ± 63.20	175.40 ± 32.49	0.63
VFR P2 unaffected	123.54 ± 61.59	113.30 ± 32.69	0.64
VFR affected hemisphere *	282.77 ± 89.70	383.70 ± 40.37	0.003
VFR unaffected hemisphere	322.15 ± 109.05	349.00 ± 102.96	0.56
VFR bypass	/	86.70 ± 30.32	/

A2 = second segment of the anterior cerebral artery; M1 = first segment of the middle cerebral artery; P2 = second segment of the posterior cerebral artery; VFR = volume flow rate. * indicates a statistically significant difference between pre- and post-bypass values.

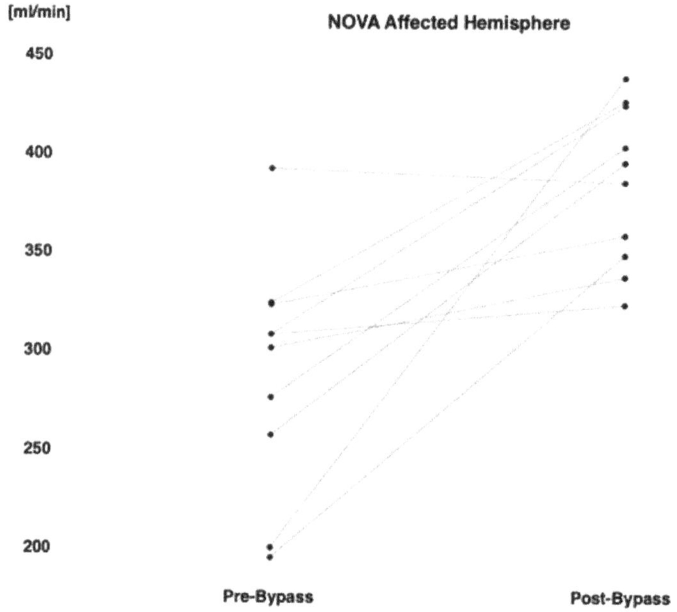

Figure 3. Graphical representation of hemispheric volume flow rates before and after STA-MCA bypass.

4. Discussion

Our cohort study revealed a significant improvement in the volume flow rate within the symptomatic hemisphere and a trend towards significant improvement in the BOLD-CVR values of the affected MCA territory, as well as of the affected hemisphere, following combined (direct and indirect) bypass in Moyamoya vasculopathy patients. The improved flow in the affected hemisphere stemmed from the efficacy of the flow-augmentation bypass. The BOLD-CVR analyses demonstrated an interesting trend, with an improvement in the absolute cerebrovascular reactivity values in all vascular territories of the symptomatic hemisphere.

4.1. Cerebral Hemodynamics in Patients with Moyamoya Vasculopathy

In individuals with Moyamoya vasculopathy, the gradual narrowing of the supraclinoidal ICA and its proximal branches, coupled with the development of numerous delicate collateral vessels, leads to compromised and often negative cerebrovascular reactivity, elevating the risk of recurrent ischemic stroke events [1,8,27]. The vasodilatation of arterioles and the establishment of collateral flow pathways serve as compensatory mechanisms to maintain regional cerebral blood flow [28–30]. Previous studies have utilized impaired BOLD-CVR, along with (recurrent) clinical symptoms, to identify patients who could benefit from surgical revascularization. These studies showed that bypass surgery improved cerebrovascular reactivity in the revascularized hemisphere [31–33].

In our cohort, the observed improvement in cerebrovascular reactivity did not reach statistical significance. This can be attributed to three key factors: the timepoint of the advanced neuroimaging, the size of the patient sample, as well as the inclusion of both patients with ischemic and hemorrhagic presentations. In our investigation, which focused on post-operative BOLD-CVR analysis, we considered the initial BOLD-CVR images following surgical revascularization that were obtained approximately three months after the surgery. Given that Moyamoya vasculopathy involves chronic vascular impairment [2], it may take several months for the effects of the surgical revascularization on brain hemodynamics to become more evident. This could explain the lack of significant improvement if the initial post-revascularization BOLD-CVR imaging was conducted "too early" after surgery. However, nine out of twelve patients (75%) showed an improvement in the absolute CVR values of the affected hemisphere and the affected (symptomatic) MCA territory.

Moreover, one important aspect is that the patients underwent a combined (direct + indirect) revascularization. It is known that the impact of revascularization with an indirect bypass promotes neoangiogenesis over time, resulting in more delayed benefits. It could be that the three patients with CVR worsening relied more on the indirect bypass rather than the direct bypass, and therefore, there was no CVR improvement in the first postoperative BOLD-CVR study, since an indirect bypass requires time before its positive effects become apparent. Conversely, in cases where BOLD-CVR images were acquired later after surgical revascularization, an eventual natural progression of Moyamoya disease might lead to a worsening in the hemodynamic status of the contralateral hemisphere, potentially influencing the cerebrovascular reactivity of the revascularized hemisphere. The second factor involves the patient sample. Our study comprised 12 patients, and it is conceivable that a study with a larger cohort could yield statistically significant results.

Our findings align with previous studies, supporting the efficacy of cerebrovascular revascularization surgery in enhancing cerebrovascular reactivity in the affected hemisphere. A study conducted by Han et al. [31] emphasized that extracranial-to-intracranial bypass resulted in a normalized or improved cerebrovascular reactivity in 52 out of 55 impaired hemispheres [31]. Another study by Sam and colleagues demonstrated a post-revascularization improvement in cerebrovascular reactivity in both the affected and unaffected middle cerebral artery territory [34]. In our study, we similarly observed a post-revascularization improvement in the CVR of the affected middle cerebral artery territory. However, we did not observe improvement in the CVR of the unaffected middle cerebral artery territory. Notably, the anterior cerebral artery territory exhibited the lowest improvement in the cerebrovascular reactivity after bypass surgery. This can be attributed to the fact that the STA-MCA bypass directly revascularizes only the MCA territory and does not directly enhance perfusion in the ACA territory. Our results, coupled with the existing literature, affirm that STA-MCA bypass surgery in Moyamoya patients effectively increases the cerebrovascular reactivity and restores cerebrovascular impairment in the middle cerebral artery territory.

4.2. Quantitative Flow Analysis in Patients with Moyamoya Vasculopathy

The preoperative findings from the qMRA-NOVA analysis reveal that the posterior cerebral arteries exhibit the highest VFR values compared to other arteries in the circle of Willis. This observation is attributed to the predominant involvement of stenosis in Moyamoya vasculopathy in the anterior circulation, while the posterior circulation possesses a significant compensatory mechanism due to leptomeningeal collateral engagement. A study conducted by Khan et al. indicates that the flow in the affected posterior circulation decreases six months after STA-MCA bypass surgery [35].

The increase in the post-operative volume flow rate in the affected hemisphere is attributed to the STA-MCA bypass, which demonstrated an average flow of 86.70 ± 30.32 mL/min in our study cohort. Notably, two patients exhibited bypass volume flow rates exceeding 100 mL/min (111 mL/min and 152 mL/min, respectively), highlighting the principle that the bypass flow is contingent on the flow demand of the revascularized vascular territory [8,36]. As noted in Table 5, there is a decrease in the mean value of the volume flow rate of the affected M1, which could be due to some backflow caused by strong bypass flow.

4.3. Uncovering the Link between Impaired Hemodynamics and Blood Flow in Moyamoya Vasculopathy

Preoperative diagnostic angiography of all 12 enrolled patients with Moyamoya vasculopathy revealed leptomeningeal collaterals in the middle cerebral artery territory originating from both the anterior cerebral artery and posterior cerebral artery. These collaterals serve to compensate for the flow deficit in the middle cerebral artery region. The risk of hemorrhage or ischemic manifestation is contingent upon the efficacy of these collaterals, emphasizing the need to quantify collateral flow [37]. While angiography allows us to demonstrate the cerebrovascular anatomy and to detect the occluded vessels and illustrates the presence of collaterals, it does not assess the impact of collateral vessels on the perfusion of a specific vascular territory, i.e., there is no information about the functionality of these vessels and the flow they provide [27,35,38]. In our study, some patients, despite the bilateral involvement of the supraclinoid ICA and its branches, presented with fewer symptoms compared to other patients with stenosis in a single artery. This once again highlights that angiography alone is insufficient for predicting clinical symptoms (i.e., future stroke events) and functional outcomes in individuals affected by Moyamoya vasculopathy.

BOLD-CVR and qMRA-NOVA serve as complementary techniques for quantifying the cerebral hemodynamics and flow rate. BOLD-CVR enables the measurement of the cerebrovascular reserve capacity, while qMRA-NOVA provides information about the collateral vessel status and quantitative flow through the intracranial arteries and the bypass [39]. Our BOLD-CVR and qMRA-NOVA values indicated a correlation between impaired BOLD-CVR values and the low-flow areas defined by qMRA-NOVA values. Brain territories exhibiting a lower BOLD-CVR are those perfused by stenotic vessels with a reduced volume flow rate. Abnormal BOLD-CVR values were predominantly observed in the anterior and middle cerebral artery territories, whereas the BOLD-CVR in posterior territories was relatively spared. In all the included patients, the BOLD-CVR of the PCA territory remained preserved. As previously mentioned, this preservation is attributed to the fact that intracranial stenosis in Moyamoya patients primarily involves the anterior circulation, and the posterior circulation possesses a compensatory mechanism, especially through leptomeningeal collaterals [37]. Given that impaired CVR is an important risk factor for future cerebral infarction and can serve as an indication for surgical revascularization [31,40,41], regular monitoring of the cerebrovascular reserve capacity and quantitative blood flow has an important role for patients with Moyamoya vasculopathy.

4.4. Limitations

Moyamoya vasculopathy is relatively rare in Switzerland. Our study specifically focused on the adult population, even though a significant proportion comprises children. The limitations of our study stem from the small size of the patient sample along with the considerable diversity among the included patients (unilateral and bilateral vasculopathy). The indirect revascularization techniques varied among the patients: nine underwent EDS, two underwent EDMS, and one underwent EDPS. These variations in indirect revascularization should not significantly impact hemodynamic and flow outcomes, as indirect bypass takes time to develop. Our BOLD-CVR imaging was conducted around 3 months post-surgery and qMRA-NOVA a few days post-surgery. Additionally, the timing of the advanced quantitative MRI performed after surgical revascularization varied, with NOVA conducted immediately after the surgery and BOLD-CVR conducted approximately 3 months after surgery.

4.5. Future Directions

Our results emphasize the significance of advanced quantitative hemodynamic and flow studies in patients with Moyamoya vasculopathy. Our future objectives involve expanding the patient cohort for analysis, validating our findings in an external cohort, and introducing the BOLD-CVR as a hemodynamic marker and qMRA-NOVA as a flow marker in the decision-making process for determining whether a conservative or surgical treatment is more suitable for individual patients with Moyamoya vasculopathy. Furthermore, our goal is to conduct larger multi-center studies and randomized clinical trials using BOLD-CVR for the hemodynamic assessment of patients with Moyamoya vasculopathy. It is important to note that the BOLD-CVR technique can be easily implemented across different MRI vendors, and the sequence itself takes only a few minutes.

5. Conclusions

Our findings affirm the existence of hemodynamic and flow impairments in patients with Moyamoya vasculopathy. Bypass surgery emerges as an effective treatment strategy, demonstrating (non-significant) improvements in impaired BOLD-CVR and an increase in cumulative cerebral blood flow.

Supplementary Materials: The following supporting information can be downloaded at: https://www.mdpi.com/article/10.3390/brainsci14080762/s1, Table S1: Overview of clinical and quantitative imaging data for all included patients.

Author Contributions: Conceptualization: L.G.N., J.F., M.S. and G.E.; methodology: L.G.N., J.B., L.M.H., M.S. and G.E.; software: L.G.N. and M.S.; validation: L.M.H., T.S. and M.S., formal analysis: L.G.N., J.B., L.M.H. and M.S.; investigation; J.B., L.M.H., V.S., T.S., M.S. and G.E. resources, J.F., M.S. and G.E.; data curation, J.F., M.S. and G.E.; writing—original draft preparation, L.G.N. and M.S.; writing—review and editing, J.B., E.C., C.H.B.v.N., S.W., M.S., G.E., Z.K., A.L. and L.R.; visualization, L.G.N. and M.S.; supervision, M.S. and G.E.; project administration, M.S. and G.E.; funding acquisition, J.F., M.S. and G.E. All authors have read and agreed to the published version of the manuscript.

Funding: This research was funded by the Clinical Research Priority Program of the University of Zurich (UZH CRPP Stroke).

Institutional Review Board Statement: The study was conducted in accordance with the Declaration of Helsinki and approved by the Ethics Committee of the Canton of Zurich under the reference number KEK 2020-02314 (Date of approval: 17 November 2020).

Informed Consent Statement: Informed consent was obtained from all subjects involved in the study.

Data Availability Statement: The original contributions presented in the study are included in the article; further inquiries can be directed to the corresponding author.

Conflicts of Interest: The authors declare no conflicts of interest.

Abbreviations

ACA = anterior cerebral artery; BOLD = blood oxygenation-level dependent; CVR = cerebrovascular reactivity; ICA = internal cerebral artery; M1 = first segment of the middle cerebral artery; MCA = middle cerebral artery; NOVA = non-invasive optimal vessel analysis; qMRA = quantitative magnetic resonance angiography; PCA = posterior cerebral artery; STA = superficial temporal artery.

References

1. Scott, R.M.; Smith, E.R. Moyamoya disease and moyamoya syndrome. *N. Engl. J. Med.* **2009**, *360*, 1226–1237. [CrossRef] [PubMed]
2. Shang, S.; Zhou, D.; Ya, J.; Li, S.; Yang, Q.; Ding, Y.; Ji, X.; Meng, R. Progress in moyamoya disease. *Neurosurg. Rev.* **2020**, *43*, 371–382. [CrossRef] [PubMed]
3. Burke, G.M.; Burke, A.M.; Sherma, A.K.; Hurley, M.C.; Batjer, H.H.; Bendok, B.R. Moyamoya disease: A summary. *Neurosurg. Focus* **2009**, *26*, E11. [CrossRef]
4. Liu, J.J.; Steinberg, G.K. Direct Versus Indirect Bypass for Moyamoya Disease. *Neurosurg. Clin. N. Am.* **2017**, *28*, 361–374. [CrossRef] [PubMed]
5. Finkenstaedt, S.; Guida, L.; Regli, L.; Esposito, G. Surgical revascularization of frontal areas in pediatric Moyamoya vasculopathy: A systematic review. *J. Neurosurg. Sci.* **2021**, *65*, 287–304. [CrossRef] [PubMed]
6. Esposito, G.; Kronenburg, A.; Fierstra, J.; Braun, K.P.; Klijn, C.J.; van der Zwan, A.; Regli, L. "STA-MCA bypass with encephalo-duro-myo-synangiosis combined with bifrontal encephalo-duro-periosteal-synangiosis" as a one-staged revascularization strategy for pediatric moyamoya vasculopathy. *Childs Nerv. Syst.* **2015**, *31*, 765–772. [CrossRef]

7. Esposito, G.; Amin-Hanjani, S.; Regli, L. Role of and Indications for Bypass Surgery After Carotid Occlusion Surgery Study (COSS)? *Stroke* **2016**, *47*, 282–290. [CrossRef]
8. Esposito, G.; Sebök, M.; Amin-Hanjani, S.; Regli, L. Cerebral Bypass Surgery: Level of Evidence and Grade of Recommendation. *Acta Neurochir. Suppl.* **2018**, *129*, 73–77.
9. Grüter, B.E.; Tosic, L.; Voglis, S.; Vasella, F.; Mutschler, V.; Bichsel, O.; Scherrer, N.; Regli, L.; Esposito, G. Trends in Literature on Cerebral Bypass Surgery: A Systematic Review. *Cerebrovasc. Dis.* **2022**, *51*, 102–113. [CrossRef]
10. Bersano, A.; Khan, N.; Fuentes, B.; Acerbi, F.; Canavero, I.; Tournier-Lasserve, E.; Vajcoczy, P.; Zedde, M.L.; Hussain, S.; Lémeret, S.; et al. European Stroke Organisation (ESO) Guidelines on Moyamoya angiopathy Endorsed by Vascular European Reference Network (VASCERN). *Eur. Stroke J.* **2023**, *8*, 55–84. [CrossRef]
11. Lehman, V.T.; Cogswell, P.M.; Rinaldo, L.; Brinjikji, W.; Huston, J.; Klaas, J.P.; Lanzino, G. Contemporary and emerging magnetic resonance imaging methods for evaluation of moyamoya disease. *Neurosurg. Focus* **2019**, *47*, E6. [CrossRef]
12. Du, L.; Jiang, H.; Li, J.; Duan, T.; Zhou, C.; Yan, F. Imaging methods for surgical revascularization in patients with moyamoya disease: An updated review. *Neurosurg. Rev.* **2022**, *45*, 343–356. [CrossRef]
13. Fierstra, J.; van Niftrik, C.; Warnock, G.; Wegener, S.; Piccirelli, M.; Pangalu, A.; Esposito, G.; Valavanis, A.; Buck, A.; Luft, A.; et al. Staging Hemodynamic Failure With Blood Oxygen-Level-Dependent Functional Magnetic Resonance Imaging Cerebrovascular Reactivity: A Comparison Versus Gold Standard (^{15}O-)H_2O-Positron Emission Tomography. *Stroke* **2018**, *49*, 621–629. [CrossRef]
14. Yuxue, S.; Yan, W.; Bingqian, X.; Hao, L.; Chaoyue, L. Arterial spin labeling for moyamoya angiopathy: A preoperative and postoperative evaluation method. *Transl. Neurosci.* **2023**, *14*, 20220288. [CrossRef]
15. Sebök, M.; Esposito, G.; Niftrik, C.; Fierstra, J.; Schubert, T.; Wegener, S.; Held, J.; Kulcsár, Z.; Luft, A.R.; Regli, L. Flow augmentation STA-MCA bypass evaluation for patients with acute stroke and unilateral large vessel occlusion: A proposal for an urgent bypass flowchart. *J. Neurosurg.* **2022**, *137*, 1047–1055. [CrossRef]
16. Sebök, M.; van Niftrik, C.H.B.; Winklhofer, S.; Wegener, S.; Esposito, G.; Stippich, C.; Luft, A.; Regli, L.; Fierstra, J. Mapping Cerebrovascular Reactivity Impairment in Patients with Symptomatic Unilateral Carotid Artery Disease. *J. Am. Heart Assoc.* **2021**, *10*, e020792. [CrossRef]
17. Sebök, M.; van der Wouden, F.; Mader, C.; Pangalu, A.; Treyer, V.; Fisher, J.A.; Mikulis, D.J.; Hüllner, M.; Regli, L.; Fierestra, J.; et al. Hemodynamic Failure Staging With Blood Oxygenation Level-Dependent Cerebrovascular Reactivity and Acetazolamide-Challenged (^{15}O-)H_2O-Positron Emission Tomography Across Individual Cerebrovascular Territories. *J. Am. Heart Assoc.* **2023**, *12*, e029491. [CrossRef]
18. White, T.; Gandhi, S.; Langer, D.J.; Katz, J.M.; Dehdashti, A.R. Does Advanced Imaging Aid in the Preoperative Evaluation of Patients with Moyamoya Disease? *Cureus* **2022**, *14*, e29816. [CrossRef]
19. Amin-Hanjani, S.; Singh, A.; Rifai, H.; Thulborn, K.R.; Alaraj, A.; Aletich, V.; Charbel, F.T. Combined direct and indirect bypass for moyamoya: Quantitative assessment of direct bypass flow over time. *Neurosurgery* **2013**, *73*, 962–967; discussion 967–968. [CrossRef]
20. Sebök, M.; van Niftrik, C.H.B.; Piccirelli, M.; Bozinov, O.; Wegener, S.; Esposito, G.; Pangalu, A.; Valavanis, A.; Buck, A.; Luft, A.R.; et al. BOLD cerebrovascular reactivity as a novel marker for crossed cerebellar diaschisis. *Neurology* **2018**, *91*, e1328–e1337. [CrossRef]
21. Sebök, M.; van Niftrik, C.H.B.; Piccirelli, M.; Muscas, G.; Pangalu, A.; Wegener, S.; Stippich, C.; Regli, L.; Fierstra, J. Crossed Cerebellar Diaschisis in Patients with Symptomatic Unilateral Anterior Circulation Stroke Is Associated with Hemodynamic Impairment in the Ipsilateral MCA Territory. *J. Magn. Reson. Imaging* **2021**, *53*, 1190–1197. [CrossRef]
22. Sebök, M.; van Niftrik, C.H.B.; Wegener, S.; Luft, A.; Regli, L.; Fierstra, J. Agreement of novel hemodynamic imaging parameters for the acute and chronic stages of ischemic stroke: A matched-pair cohort study. *Neurosurg. Focus* **2021**, *51*, E12. [CrossRef] [PubMed]
23. Slessarev, M.; Han, J.; Mardimae, A.; Prisman, E.; Preiss, D.; Volgyesi, G.; Ansel, C.; Duffin, J.; Fisher, J.A. Prospective targeting and control of end-tidal CO_2 and O_2 concentrations. *J. Physiol.* **2007**, *581 Pt 3*, 1207–1219. [CrossRef] [PubMed]
24. Sebök, M.; Höbner, L.M.; Fierstra, J.; Schubert, T.; Wegener, S.; Kulcsár, Z.; Luft, A.R.; Regli, L.; Esposito, G. Flow-augmentation STA-MCA bypass for acute and subacute ischemic stroke due to internal carotid artery occlusion and the role of advanced neuroimaging with hemodynamic and flow-measurement in the decision-making: Preliminary data. *Quant. Imaging Med. Surg.* **2024**, *14*, 777–788. [CrossRef] [PubMed]
25. Kronenburg, A.; Esposito, G.; Fierstra, J.; Braun, K.P.; Regli, L. Combined Bypass Technique for Contemporary Revascularization of Unilateral MCA and Bilateral Frontal Territories in Moyamoya Vasculopathy. *Acta Neurochir. Suppl.* **2014**, *119*, 65–70. [PubMed]
26. Esposito, G.; Burkhardt, J.K.; Bozinov, O.; Regli, L. Indocyanine green videoangiography for the identification of superficial temporal artery branches in EC-IC bypass surgery. *Acta Neurochir.* **2016**, *158*, 565–570. [CrossRef] [PubMed]
27. van Niftrik, C.H.B.; Sebök, M.; Nicholson, P.; Olijnyk, L.; Thurner, P.; Venkatraghavan, L.; Schaafsma, J.; Radovanovic, I.; Fisher, J.A.; Krings, T.; et al. A dual-center validation of the PIRAMD scoring system for assessing the severity of ischemic Moyamoya disease. *Quant. Imaging Med. Surg.* **2023**, *13*, 4618–4632. [CrossRef]
28. Nemoto, E.M.; Yonas, H.; Kuwabara, H.; Pindzola, R.R.; Sashin, D.; Meltzer, C.C.; Price, J.C.; Chang, Y.; Johnson, D.W. Identification of hemodynamic compromise by cerebrovascular reserve and oxygen extraction fraction in occlusive vascular disease. *J. Cereb. Blood Flow Metab.* **2004**, *24*, 1081–1089. [CrossRef] [PubMed]

29. Derdeyn, C.P. Hemodynamics and oxygen extraction in chronic large artery steno-occlusive disease: Clinical applications for predicting stroke risk. *J. Cereb. Blood Flow Metab.* **2018**, *38*, 1584–1597. [CrossRef]
30. Zhu, F.; Qian, Y.; Xu, B.; Gu, Y.; Karunanithi, K.; Zhu, W.; Chen, L.; Mao, Y.; Morgan, M.K. Quantitative assessment of changes in hemodynamics of the internal carotid artery after bypass surgery for moyamoya disease. *J. Neurosurg.* **2018**, *129*, 677–683. [CrossRef]
31. Han, J.S.; Abou-Hamden, A.; Mandell, D.M.; Poublanc, J.; Crawley, A.P.; Fisher, J.A.; Mikulis, D.J.; Tymianski, M. Impact of extracranial-intracranial bypass on cerebrovascular reactivity and clinical outcome in patients with symptomatic moyamoya vasculopathy. *Stroke* **2011**, *42*, 3047–3054. [CrossRef] [PubMed]
32. Conklin, J.; Fierstra, J.; Crawley, A.P.; Han, J.S.; Poublanc, J.; Mandell, D.M.; Silver, F.L.; Tymianski, M.; Fisher, J.A.; Mikulis, D.J. Impaired cerebrovascular reactivity with steal phenomenon is associated with increased diffusion in white matter of patients with Moyamoya disease. *Stroke* **2010**, *41*, 1610–1616. [CrossRef] [PubMed]
33. Mesiwala, A.H.; Sviri, G.; Fatemi, N.; Britz, G.W.; Newell, D.W. Long-term outcome of superficial temporal artery-middle cerebral artery bypass for patients with moyamoya disease in the US. *Neurosurg. Focus* **2008**, *24*, E15. [CrossRef] [PubMed]
34. Sam, K.; Poublanc, J.; Sobczyk, O.; Han, J.S.; Battisti-Charbonney, A.; Mandell, D.M.; Tymianski, M.; Crawley, A.P.; A Fisher, J.; Mikulis, D.J. Assessing the effect of unilateral cerebral revascularisation on the vascular reactivity of the non-intervened hemisphere: A retrospective observational study. *BMJ Open* **2015**, *5*, e006014. [CrossRef] [PubMed]
35. Khan, N.; Lober, R.M.; Ostergren, L.; Petralia, J.; Bell-Stephens, T.; Navarro, R.; Feroze, A.; Steinberg, G.K. Measuring Cerebral Blood Flow in Moyamoya Angiopathy by Quantitative Magnetic Resonance Angiography Noninvasive Optimal Vessel Analysis. *Neurosurgery* **2017**, *81*, 921–927. [CrossRef]
36. Kim, T.; Oh, C.W.; Bang, J.S.; Kim, J.E.; Cho, W.S. Moyamoya Disease: Treatment and Outcomes. *J. Stroke* **2016**, *18*, 21–30. [CrossRef]
37. Sebök, M.; Niftrik, C.; Lohaus, N.; Esposito, G.; Amki, M.E.; Winklhofer, S.; Wegener, S.; Regli, L.; Fierstra, J. Leptomeningeal collateral activation indicates severely impaired cerebrovascular reserve capacity in patients with symptomatic unilateral carotid artery occlusion. *J. Cereb. Blood Flow Metab.* **2021**, *41*, 3039–3051. [CrossRef]
38. Strother, M.K.; Anderson, M.D.; Singer, R.J.; Du, L.; Moore, R.D.; Shyr, Y.; Ladner, T.; Arteaga, D.; Day, M.; Clemmons, P.; et al. Cerebrovascular collaterals correlate with disease severity in adult North American patients with Moyamoya disease. *Am. J. Neuroradiol.* **2014**, *35*, 1318–1324. [CrossRef]
39. Heyn, C.; Poublanc, J.; Crawley, A.; Mandell, D.; Han, J.S.; Tymianski, M.; Terbrugge, K.; Fisher, J.; Mikulis, D. Quantification of cerebrovascular reactivity by blood oxygen level-dependent MR imaging and correlation with conventional angiography in patients with Moyamoya disease. *Am. J. Neuroradiol.* **2010**, *31*, 862–867. [CrossRef]
40. Hauser, T.K.; Seeger, A.; Bender, B.; Klose, U.; Thurow, J.; Ernemann, U.; Tatagiba, M.; Meyer, P.T.; Khan, N.; Roder, C. Hypercapnic BOLD MRI compared to $H_2{}^{15}O$ PET/CT for the hemodynamic evaluation of patients with Moyamoya Disease. *Neuroimage Clin.* **2019**, *22*, 101713. [CrossRef]
41. Mikulis, D.J.; Krolczyk, G.; Desal, H.; Logan, W.; Deveber, G.; Dirks, P.; Tymianski, M.; Crawley, A.; Vesely, A.; Kassner, A.; et al. Preoperative and postoperative mapping of cerebrovascular reactivity in moyamoya disease by using blood oxygen level-dependent magnetic resonance imaging. *J. Neurosurg.* **2005**, *103*, 347–355. [CrossRef] [PubMed]

brain sciences

MDPI

Article

Microsurgical Clipping of Unruptured Middle Cerebral Artery Bifurcation Aneurysms: A Single-Center Experience

Nico Stroh-Holly [1], Philip Rauch [1,*], Harald Stefanits [1], Philipp Hermann [2,3], Helga Wagner [2,3], Michael Sonnberger [4], Maria Gollwitzer [1], Stefan Aspalter [1], Andreas Gruber [1,5] and Matthias Gmeiner [1,5]

1 Department of Neurosurgery, Kepler University Hospital, Johannes Kepler University Linz, Wagner-Jauregg-Weg 15, A-4020 Linz, Austria
2 Center for Clinical Studies (CCS Linz), Johannes Kepler University Linz, A-4040 Linz, Austria
3 Institute of Applied Statistics, Johannes Kepler University Linz, A-4040 Linz, Austria
4 Institute of Neuroradiology, Kepler University Hospital, Johannes Kepler University Linz, A-4040 Linz, Austria
5 Clinical Research Institute for Neuroscience, Johannes Kepler University Linz, A-4040 Linz, Austria
* Correspondence: philip-rudolf.rauch@kepleruniklinikum.at

Abstract: Background/Objectives: Microsurgical clipping has traditionally been considered a standard treatment for middle cerebral artery (MCA) aneurysms. Recently, a caseload reduction related to improved endovascular treatment options has occurred in cerebrovascular neurosurgery. Therefore, studies that report the clinical and radiological outcomes after clipping are highly warranted. Methods: Patients with an unruptured MCA bifurcation aneurysm, who were surgically treated at the Department of Neurosurgery in Linz between 2002 and 2019, were included in this study. Clinical and radiological outcome parameters were evaluated for each patient. Results: Overall, 272 patients were eligible for inclusion. Complete aneurysm occlusion was demonstrated in 266 (99.3%) of the 268 (98.5%) patients who underwent postoperative digital subtraction angiography. In six (2.2%) patients, a permanent new neurological deficit (pNND) persisted after treatment. Intraoperative aneurysm rupture was a significant factor ($p = 0.0049$) in the logistic regression. At the last follow-up, only two patients (0.7%) had an unfavorable outcome (mRS > 2). More recent surgeries were associated with fewer cases of pNND ($p = 0.009$). A transient new neurological deficit occurred in 13 patients (4.8%), with aneurysm size being a significant risk factor ($p = 0.009$). Surgical site infections were reported in four patients (1.5%), with patient age ($p = 0.039$) and time ($p = 0.001$) being significant factors. Two patients died (0.7%) perioperatively and two patients (0.7%) needed a retreatment in the long-term follow-up. Conclusions: The findings indicate that microsurgical clipping is a safe procedure with minimal need for retreatment. It achieves a high occlusion rate while maintaining a very low rate of adverse outcomes. Continuous intraoperative enhancements over time have contributed to a progressive improvement in clinical outcomes in recent years. This trend is exemplified by the absence of detectable pNND in the era of ICG angiography. Consequently, these data support the conclusion that microsurgical clipping should still be considered an appropriate treatment option for unruptured MCA bifurcation aneurysms.

Keywords: intracranial aneurysm; unruptured intracranial aneurysm; middle cerebral artery aneurysm; clipping; microsurgical treatment; outcome

1. Introduction

The prevalence of unruptured intracranial aneurysms (UIAs) is estimated at 3%, and their detection has significantly improved, attributable to advancements in and increased accessibility of intracranial imaging techniques [1–3]. The natural course of UIAs remains inherently uncertain, and approximations of the rupture risk assessment are available in previous studies [4–6]. The risk of aneurysm rupture and consequently of a subarachnoid hemorrhage (SAH) needs to be balanced with the risk of prophylactic aneurysm treatment, regardless of the treatment modality. For predicting clinical and functional outcomes after microsurgical treatment of UIAs, Machine Learning (ML)-based models have been published recently [7]. A multidisciplinary consensus on which aneurysms have a higher rupture risk and therefore which ones need to be treated has already been discussed in several consensus papers [8,9]. The question of the most appropriate treatment method becomes more debatable due to the increasing number of endovascular options [10,11].

Approximately one third of UIAs are middle cerebral artery (MCA) aneurysms [5]. Microsurgical clipping has long been the exclusive treatment strategy for unruptured intracranial aneurysms (UIAs), particularly for those located in the MCA bifurcation [12]. Rapidly emerging modern endovascular therapy approaches, such as coiling, stent- or balloon-assisted coiling, Flow Diverter (FD) or WovenEndoBridge (WEB) Implantation, now aim to compete with the results of the gold standard of microsurgical clipping [13–18].

The discourse surrounding the optimal future treatment method for unruptured intracranial aneurysms is dynamic and ongoing. Recent cohort studies highlight the potential of endovascular techniques, pointing to their enhanced long-term occlusion rates and minimally invasive nature as reasons for their increasing adoption [18–20].

In terms of occlusion rate, permanent repair, or thromboembolic events, a number of cohort studies still show superior results with microsurgical clipping for unruptured MCA aneurysms [10,21–25]. The anatomical characteristics of unruptured MCA aneurysms, including their wide-necked bases, trifurcated anatomy, and involvement of M2 branches, have traditionally been viewed as challenges for endovascular treatment, making microsurgical clipping a preferred approach for these specific situations [22].

In the context of evolving therapeutic techniques, the need for a detailed evaluation of outcomes and complications across a comprehensive cohort becomes paramount. This retrospective explorative study, by focusing on the microsurgical treatment of 272 unruptured MCA bifurcation aneurysms at a high-volume center over an extended duration of 18 years, aims to contribute valuable insights to the scientific discourse on the most effective treatment modalities for these aneurysms, enhancing our understanding of patient outcomes in the long term.

2. Material and Methods

2.1. Overview

The retrospective explorative study obtained ethical approval from the local Ethics Committee of the Federal State Upper Austria (EK-No.: 1255/2019). This investigation centered on patients with an unruptured MCA bifurcation aneurysm who received microsurgical clipping treatment at the Department of Neurosurgery, Kepler University Hospital Linz, from January 2002 to October 2019. The patient cohort was derived from our hospital's surgical database, which is maintained for clinical purposes and quality assurance. Patient data were systematically collected and collated in a retrospective database for subsequent analysis.

2.2. Patient-Specific Parameters

Fundamental patient demographics, encompassing age and gender, were extracted from the medical records of the Department of Neurosurgery at the Kepler University Hospital Linz. Additionally, a comprehensive assessment of individual medical histories was carried out, which included an investigation into any previous occurrences of SAH and the confirmed diagnosis of autosomal dominant polycystic kidney disease (ADPKD).

2.3. Aneurysm-Specific Parameters

Angiographic imaging was systematically conducted for all patients as a preoperative measure, utilizing either digital subtraction angiography (DSA) or computed tomography angiography (CTA). A meticulous evaluation of various aneurysm-related parameters was undertaken based on the radiographic reports. In the case of missing reports, experienced neuroradiologists conducted a thorough reassessment of the radiographic images.

The size of each aneurysm was stratified into three categories: small (<10 mm), large (10–25 mm), and giant aneurysms (>25 mm) [26]. Additionally, the study evaluated various factors, including the aneurysm's specific location, the presence of blebs, evidence of calcification or thrombosis, any previous attempts at coiling, and the detection of concurrent aneurysms. The presence of coincident aneurysms was not considered as an exclusion criterion. Only MCA bifurcation aneurysms were included in this study. Thus, aneurysms of the M1 segment, as well as peripheral MCA aneurysms of the M3 and M4 segments, were excluded.

2.4. Intraoperative Parameters

The microsurgical procedures were executed by experienced senior neurosurgeons. Intraoperative metrics, including the quantity of clips used, the utilization of intraoperative neuromonitoring through somatosensory evoked potentials (SSEP) and motor evoked potentials (MEP), the application of intraoperative indocyanine green (ICG) angiography, instances of intraoperative aneurysm rupture, and the need for clip repositioning or temporary clipping for proximal vascular control, were systematically extracted from the surgical reports. The surgical technique employed was uniform across all cases, ensuring a standardized and comparable basis for analysis.

2.5. Radiological Outcome Parameters

Aneurysm occlusion was rigorously assessed through either intraoperative or postoperative DSA (Figure 1). Occlusion levels were determined using the Raymond Roy Occlusion Classification (RROC), which organizes occlusion results into three specific categories: Class I, which represents complete occlusion without any remaining aneurysm; Class II, which denotes the presence of a residual neck; and Class III, which indicates the continued existence of a residual aneurysm [27].

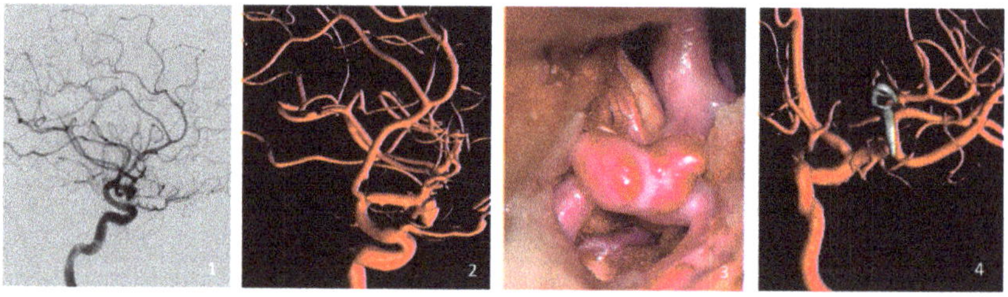

Figure 1. Illustration of a representative case of the cohort (clipping of a left-sided MCA bifurcation aneurysm). Preoperative Digital Subtraction Angiography (**1**) and the reconstructed 3D Rotational Angiography (**2**). Intraoperative view of the MCA aneurysm with its blebs just before the clipping (**3**), and the intraoperative reconstructed 3D Rotational Angiography (**4**).

This categorization framework provided a nuanced evaluation of the effectiveness of the surgical intervention and was pivotal for discerning the extent of aneurysm closure in a standardized manner.

2.6. Clinical Outcome Parameters

To assess morbidity and mortality, an array of postoperative parameters was extracted from the medical records in accordance with the current literature [21,27,28]. These parameters included postoperative intracerebral hemorrhage (ICH), incidents of postoperative epileptic seizures, and occurrences of postoperative surgical site infection (SSI).

New postoperative neurological deficits (NND) were categorized into transient (tNND) and permanent (pNND) categories—with pNND persisting beyond hospital discharge. Additional outcome parameters included chronic subdural hematoma (cSDH), pulmonary embolism (PE), and perioperative mortality.

Reoperations necessitated by the primary surgical procedure were systematically documented as critical outcome variables. Moreover, longitudinal monitoring was employed to assess aneurysm recurrence and the incidence of subarachnoid hemorrhage (SAH) during the follow-up. These measures facilitated a nuanced understanding of postoperative and long-term patient outcomes, crucial for evaluating the procedure's efficacy and safety.

2.7. Statistical Analysis

The statistical analysis was conducted at the Center for Clinical Studies (CCS) of the Johannes Kepler University in Linz. Statistical analysis included descriptive statistics for all valid observations. For nominal variables, absolute and relative frequencies, and for metric variables, mean and standard deviation (SD) as well as median and range were computed. To analyze the association between two nominal variables, Fisher's exact test was used. Logistic regression models were fitted to model the effects of patient-specific, aneurysm-specific, and intraoperative parameters on the probability of the following outcomes: NND, pNND, tNND, postoperative epileptic seizures, and SSI. For each of these outcomes, a model with all potential regressors not leading to separation was first fitted. Then, stepwise variable selection using the Akaike Information Criterion (AIC) was performed. In all regression analyses, observations with missing values in any of the relevant variables were excluded. All statistical analyses were performed using the statistical software R (R Foundation for Statistical Computing, Version 4.4.1, Vienna, Austria).

3. Results

In the analysis, 272 aneurysms were evaluated in total. The patient cohort had a mean age of 55 years, with 76 (27.9%) males and 196 (72.1%) females. Additionally, 42 (15.4%) patients presented with a documented history of SAH, although the origin of the bleeding was not linked to the MCA bifurcation aneurysms being studied. All patient-specific preoperative data are succinctly summarized in Table 1.

Table 1. Descriptive statistics of preoperative patient- and aneurysm-specific parameters. For categorial variables, absolute frequencies (percent) are reported. There were no missing values. ADPKD = autosomal dominant polycystic kidney disease, SAH = subarachnoidal haemorrhage, max. = maximal, mm = millimeter, prev. = previously.

Preoperative Parameters		**Value**
Number of aneurysms (n)		272
Patient-specific parameters		
Sex	female	196 (72.06%)
	male	76 (27.94%)
Mean Age in years (standard deviation)		55.08 (10.4)
ADPKD		5 (1.84%)
Unrelated SAH in anamnesis		42 (15.44%)
Aneurysm-specific parameters		
Side	right	151 (55.51%)
	left	121 (44.49%)
Size	Small (<10 mm)	242 (88.97%)
	Large (10–25 mm)	29 (10.66%)
	Giant (>25 mm)	1 (0.37%)
Max. Diameter mean in mm (range)		5.81 (2–25)
Prev. Coiled	No	265 (97.43%)
	Yes	7 (2.57%)

Table 1. *Cont.*

Preoperative Parameters		Value
Thrombosed	No	263 (96.69%)
	Yes	9 (3.31%)
Blebs	No	219 (80.51%)
	Yes	53 (19.49%)
Fusiform	No	268 (98.53%)
	Yes	4 (1.47%)

Analysis of aneurysm-specific parameters revealed that 151 (55.5%) of the aneurysms were located in the right MCA bifurcation, whereas 121 (44.5%) were found in the left MCA bifurcation. The majority of these aneurysms, accounting for 242 (89%) cases, exhibited a maximum diameter size of the aneurysm smaller than 10 mm, whereas 29 (10.7%) aneurysms measured between 10 and 25 mm. Remarkably, only one (0.4%) aneurysm characterized as giant—with a diameter exceeding 25 mm—was documented within the registry. The calculated average diameter across all aneurysms was 5.8 mm (range 2–25 mm).

Notably, in seven (2.6%) instances, aneurysms were initially treated with coiling and then necessitated subsequent microsurgical intervention due to recurrence. Additionally, preoperative angiography revealed the presence of a daughter aneurysm, resembling a bleb, in 53 (19.5%) cases. It is important to highlight that preoperative DSA was accessible for 241 (88.6%) patients, whereas 31 patients (11.4%) underwent preoperative assessment using CTA. Comprehensive details of the aneurysm-specific preoperative parameters are also summarized in Table 1.

3.1. Intraoperative Parameters

The intraoperative parameters are detailed in Table 2. The average number of clips used for aneurysm treatment was 1.5, ranging from 1 to 8. Notably, the repositioning of clips became necessary in 60 (22.4%) cases, and 8 (3.0%) aneurysms experienced rupture during the surgical approach. Temporary clipping of the parenteral vessel was required in 38 (14.1%) instances. Intraoperative monitoring, encompassing MEP and SSEP, was available in 68 (25%) procedures, while intraoperative ICG angiography was used in 102 (37.5%) cases.

Table 2. Intraoperative parameters. For categorical variables, absolute frequencies (percent of non-missing values) are reported. MEP = motor evoked potentials, SSEP = somatosensory evoked potentials, ICG = indocyanine green angiography.

Intraoperative Parameters	Value (%)
Reposition of clips	60 (22.39%)
Average number of clips	1.46
Intraoperative Rupture of aneurysm	8 (2.96%)
Temporary Clipping	38 (14.13%)
Intraoperative Neuromonitoring (MEP, SSEP)	68 (25%)
Intraoperative ICG angiography	102 (37.5%)

3.2. Outcome Parameters

In 268 (98.5%) patients, either intraoperative or postoperative DSA was conducted. In 99.3% of cases, the DSA demonstrated a RROC Class I occlusion—a complete occlusion without any evidence of a residual neck or aneurysmal remnants. Three patients (1.1%) were identified with an ICH necessitating surgical revision. These hemorrhages were associated with the surgical approach, and aneurysm-related secondary bleeding was conclusively ruled out in all instances.

Postoperatively, NND was observed in 19 (7%) patients, with 6 (2.2%) patients exhibiting pNND and 13 (4.8%) patients experiencing tNND. Eleven (4%) patients presented with epileptic seizures for the first time postoperatively. SSI necessitating revision occurred in four (1.7%) cases, and cSDH requiring burr hole trepanation at follow-up was observed in three (1.1%) cases. Two patients died postoperatively, and therefore overall mortality was 0.7% (fulminant sepsis, pulmonary embolism). Additionally, two (0.7%) patients experienced recurrent aneurysms in the subsequent follow-up—both underwent surgical retreatment. Details of all postoperative radiological and clinical parameters are presented in Tables 3 and 4.

Table 3. Radiological and Clinical Outcome Parameters. For categorical variables, absolute frequencies (percent of non-missing values) are reported; DSA = digital subtraction angiography, RROC = Raymond–Roy occlusion classification, ICH = intracerebral hematoma, NND = new neurological deficit, MRI = magnetic resonance imaging, SSI = surgical site infection, cSDH = chronic subdural hematoma, SAH = subarachnoidal haemorrhage; a = data missing for four patients.

Radiological Outcome Parameters	Absolut Frequency (%)
Intra-/Postoperative DSA	268 (98.53%)
Postoperative occlusion rate (a)	
RROC Class I	266 (99.25%)
RROC Class II	0
RROC Class III	2 (0.75%)
Clinical outcome parameters	**Absolut frequency (%)**
Postoperative ICH	3 (1.1%)
New neurological deficit (NND)	19 (6.99%)
permanent NND	6 (2.21%)
mRS 0–2 („favorable outcome")	4 (1.47%)
mRS 3–5 („unfavorable outcome")	2 (0.74%)
transient NND	13 (4.78%)
Epileptic seizure postoperative	11 (4.04%)
Surgical site infection (SSI)	4 (1.47%)
Chronic subdural hematoma (cSDH)	3 (1.1%)
Pulmonary embolism	2 (0.74%)
Recurrent Aneurysm (follow-up)	2 (0.74%)
Retreatment (follow-up)	2 (0.74%)
SAH in follow-up	1 (0.37%)
Perioperative Death	2 (0.74%)

Table 4. This table reports the results of the logistic regression model for the outcome parameter NND. Stepwise variable selection was performed using the Akaike Information Criterion (AIC). Fusiform is not used as regressor due to separation. NND = new neurological deficit; ADPKD = autosomal dominant polycystic kidney disease, ICG = indocyanine green angiography, No. = number.

	Estimate	Std. Error	z-Value	*p*-Value
New neurological Deficit (NND)				
Intercept	−2.546	0.860	−2.961	0.003
Sex (male)	−0.243	0.628	−0.387	0.699
Age (in years)	0.046	0.029	1.596	0.111
ADPKD (yes)	0.753	1.935	0.389	0.697
Side (left)	0.837	0.559	1.499	0.134
Previously Coiled (yes)	0.947	1.195	0.792	0.428
Size—max. Diameter mean in mm	0.064	0.085	0.756	0.450
Thrombosed (yes)	1.399	1.164	1.202	0.230
Blebs (yes)	−0.575	0.756	−0.761	0.447
Intraoperative Neuromonitoring (yes)	0.499	0.912	0.548	0.584
Intraoperative ICG angiography (yes)	0.325	1.030	0.315	0.753
No. of Clips	0.176	0.289	0.610	0.542
Reposition of clips (yes)	0.545	0.642	0.849	0.396
Intraoperative Rupture of aneurysm (yes)	0.122	1.398	0.087	0.930
Temporary Clipping (yes)	0.121	0.747	0.161	0.872
Year of Surgery	−0.149	0.098	−1.527	0.127
	Logistic regression model after stepwise variable selection:			
Intercept	−3.388	0.432	−7.836	<0.001
Side (left)	0.897	0.531	1.689	0.091
Size—max. Diameter mean in mm	0.168	0.052	3.246	0.001

3.3. Logistic Regression for Outcome Parameters

Logistic regression analyses were conducted for the outcome parameters (NND, pNND, tNND, epileptic seizures postoperative and SSI). For all these models, at least 265 (97.43%) valid observations without any missing values were used for model fitting. Tables 4–8 present the results from the full logistic regression models (with all covariates except those leading to separation) and after stepwise variable selection using the AIC. The key findings of the logistic regression models after stepwise variable selection are described here.

The size of the aneurysm exhibited an association with postoperative NND ($p = 0.001$), particularly with tNND ($p = 0.009$). Intraoperative temporary clipping was associated with the occurrence of postoperative epileptic seizures ($p = 0.037$). The occurrence of intraoperative aneurysm rupture is associated with the development of pNND ($p = 0.049$). Risk of pNND is lower in more recent surgeries ($p = 0.009$), but higher with interoperative neuromonitoring ($p = 0.023$). For the association between ICG angiography and pNND, Fisher's exact test yields a p-value of $p = 0.087$.

Table 5. This table reports the results of the logistic regression model for the outcome parameter pNND. Previously coiled, fusiform and intraoperative ICG angiography were not used as regressors due to separation. Stepwise variable selection was performed using the Akaike Information Criterion (AIC). NND = new neurological deficit; pNND = permanent new neurological deficit, ADPKD = autosomal dominant polycystic kidney disease, No. = number.

	Estimate	Std. Error	z-Value	*p*-Value
Permanent NND (pNND)				
Intercept	−1.618	1.701	−0.951	0.342
Sex (male)	−2.033	1.722	−1.181	0.238
Age (in years)	0.047	0.066	0.719	0.472
ADPKD (yes)	3.212	4.541	0.707	0.479
Side (left)	0.500	1.033	0.484	0.628
Size—max. Diameter mean in mm	−0.098	0.200	−0.490	0.624
Thrombosed (yes)	2.157	1.944	1.110	0.267
Blebs (yes)	0.424	1.277	0.332	0.740
Intraoperative Neuromonitoring (yes)	3.068	1.834	1.673	0.094
No. of Clips	−0.119	0.740	−0.160	0.873
Reposition of clips (yes)	1.547	1.238	1.250	0.211
Intraoperative Rupture of aneurysm (yes)	2.517	2.341	1.075	0.282
Temporary Clipping (yes)	−2.920	2.393	−1.220	0.222
Year of Surgery	−0.461	0.205	−2.249	0.025
	Logistic regression model after stepwise variable selection:			
Intercept	−1.255	1.012	−1.240	0.215
Sex (male)	−1.999	1.399	−1.429	0.153
Intraoperative Neuromonitoring (yes)	3.093	1.356	2.281	0.023
Intraoperative Rupture of aneurysm (yes)	3.196	1.622	1.971	0.049
Temporary Clipping (yes)	−2.448	1.892	−1.294	0.196
Year of Surgery	−0.403	0.154	−2.615	0.009

Table 6. This table reports the results of the logistic regression model for the outcome parameter tNND. ADPKD, fusiform, and intraoperative rupture of the aneurysm were not used as regressors due to separation. Stepwise variable selection was performed using the Akaike Information Criterion (AIC). NND = new neurological deficit; tNND = transient new neurological deficit, ADPKD = autosomal dominant polycystic kidney disease, ICG = indocyanine green angiography, No. = Number.

	Estimate	Std. Error	z-Value	*p*-Value
Transient NND (tNND)				
Intercept	−3.507	1.048	−3.346	0.001
Sex (male)	0.227	0.709	0.320	0.749
Age (in years)	0.064	0.036	1.790	0.073
Side (left)	0.828	0.667	1.241	0.215
Previously Coiled (yes)	1.428	1.214	1.177	0.239
Size—max. Diameter mean in mm	0.079	0.104	0.763	0.446

Table 6. *Cont.*

	Estimate	Std. Error	z-Value	p-Value
Thrombosed (yes)	1.432	1.458	0.982	0.326
Blebs (yes)	−1.207	1.160	−1.040	0.298
Intraoperative Neuromonitoring (yes)	−0.964	1.072	−0.899	0.368
Intraoperative ICG angiography (yes)	1.675	1.155	1.449	0.147
No. of Clips	0.315	0.364	0.865	0.387
Reposition of clips (yes)	0.022	0.857	0.025	0.980
Temporary Clipping (yes)	0.527	0.871	0.605	0.545
Year of Surgery	−0.147	0.123	−1.194	0.232
	Logistic regression model after stepwise variable selection:			
Intercept	−3.305	0.343	−9.637	<0.001
Size—max. Diameter mean in mm	0.149	0.057	2.600	0.009

Table 7. This table reports the results of the logistic regression model for the outcome parameter epileptic seizures postoperative. Previously coiled and thrombosed were not used as regressors due to separation. Stepwise variable selection was performed using the Akaike Information Criterion (AIC). ADPKD = autosomal dominant polycystic kidney disease, ICG = indocyanine green angiography, No. = number.

	Estimate	Std. Error	z-Value	p-Value
Epileptic seizures postoperative				
Intercept	−2.457	1.098	−2.237	0.025
Sex (male)	1.994	0.763	2.614	0.009
Age (in years)	0.019	0.038	0.498	0.619
ADPKD (yes)	4.381	2.026	2.162	0.031
Side (left)	−0.667	0.795	−0.839	0.402
Size—max. Diameter mean in mm	0.098	0.128	0.770	0.441
Fusiform (yes)	2.610	1.683	1.551	0.121
Blebs (yes)	−0.532	0.943	−0.564	0.573
Intraoperative Neuromonitoring (yes)	0.749	1.149	0.652	0.515
Intraoperative ICG angiography (yes)	3.130	1.618	1.934	0.053
No. of Clips	−0.658	0.604	−1.090	0.276
Reposition of clips (yes)	0.552	0.866	0.638	0.523
Intraoperative Rupture of aneurysm (yes)	−2.704	2.507	−1.079	0.281
Temporary Clipping (yes)	1.674	0.877	1.909	0.056
Year of Surgery	−0.312	0.149	−2.092	0.036
	Logistic regression model after stepwise variable selection:			
Intercept	−3.447	0.872	−3.953	<0.001
Sex (male)	1.736	0.729	2.381	0.017
ADPKD (yes)	3.227	1.555	2.076	0.038
Fusiform (yes)	3.358	1.484	2.263	0.024
Intraoperative ICG angiography (yes)	2.779	1.439	1.932	0.053
Temporary Clipping (yes)	1.560	0.747	2.089	0.037
Year of Surgery	−0.258	0.121	−2.125	0.034

Table 8. This table reports the results of the logistic regression model for the outcome parameter SSI. Stepwise variable selection was performed using the Akaike Information Criterion (AIC). ADPKD, previously coiled, thrombosed, fusiform, temporary clipping, and intraoperative rupture of the aneurysm were not used as regressors due to separation. SSI = surgical site infection, ADPKD = autosomal dominant polycystic kidney disease, ICG = indocyanine green angiography, No. = number.

	Estimate	Std. Error	z-Value	*p*-Value
Surgical Site Infection (SSI)				
Intercept	−1.153	1.204	−0.957	0.338
Sex (male)	0.804	0.885	0.908	0.364
Age (in years)	0.119	0.052	2.267	0.023
Side (left)	−0.871	0.896	−0.972	0.331
Size—max. Diameter mean in mm	−0.165	0.144	−1.144	0.253
Blebs (yes)	0.360	0.930	0.387	0.699
Intraoperative Neuromonitoring (yes)	3.127	1.267	2.468	0.014
Intraoperative ICG angiography (yes)	5.600	2.269	2.467	0.014
No. of Clips	0.174	0.680	0.256	0.798
Reposition of clips (yes)	0.753	1.078	0.698	0.485
Year of Surgery	−0.776	0.245	−3.173	0.002
	Logistic regression model after stepwise variable selection:			
Intercept	−1.046	0.682	−1.534	0.125
Age (in years)	0.091	0.044	2.069	0.039
Intraoperative Neuromonitoring (yes)	2.309	1.013	2.280	0.023
Intraoperative ICG angiography (yes)	4.914	1.969	2.496	0.013
Year of Surgery	−0.662	0.200	−3.305	0.001

4. Discussion

In this study, we report on a cohort of 272 unruptured MCA bifurcation aneurysms treated with microsurgical techniques, marking it as one of the largest datasets from a single institution examined to date. This study reports a high (99,3%) aneurysm occlusion rate and a low unfavorable outcome rate concerning pNND. Furthermore, the results show a low retreatment rate of 0.7% after microsurgical clipping of unruptured MCA bifurcation aneurysms.

Compared to other series of unruptured MCA bifurcation aneurysms, Nussbaum et al. published a large monocentric, single-surgeon experience, including 716 patients [21]. Further large monocentric case series of microsurgically treated patients with unruptured MCA aneurysms have been presented by Rodriguez et al. (n = 261), Metayer et al. (n = 158), and Morgan et al. (n = 263) [22,28,29].

Our angiographic assessment revealed an aneurysm occlusion rate of 99.3%, aligning closely with the range of 92% to 98.9% reported in the existing literature [11,21–24,30–32]. It is well known from prior benchmark studies that microsurgically treated MCA aneurysms generally exhibit extremely low recurrence rates and very high occlusion rates in angiographic long-term follow-ups. Spetzler et al. demonstrated a long-term occlusion rate of 93% in angiographic controls after 10 years, while Mooney et al. reported an occlusion rate of 95% after 6 years with a mean angiographic follow-up of 3.7 years [33,34]. Rodriguez et al. even reported a long-term recurrence rate of 0% with a mean angiographic follow-up of 3.9 years [22].

Recently published data reveals that complete occlusion rates for MCA aneurysms treated with coiling, with or without adjunctive stent- or balloon-assistance, stands at 29.4% [35]. Further, Bracard et al.'s subanalysis on coiling of unruptured MCA aneurysms indicates a complete occlusion rate of 31.6% [13]. With regard to emerging endovascular approaches, the literature cites initial occlusion rates for WEB devices from 17.7% to 53.8%, with an increase of up to 59.4% observed after a 3-year follow-up [15,19,20]. Meanwhile, for flow diverters (FD), initial occlusion rates are documented at 5–10%, with a subsequent rise to 55.6–82.1% after a period exceeding 12 months [17,18,36,37]. A recent meta-analysis by Tocacelli et al. reported an average occlusion rate of 31.5% in the initial phase and 60% in the long term (beyond 12 months) for all endovascular treatment modalities [10].

The findings of this study validate the conclusions of prior research, indicating that microsurgical intervention for unruptured aneurysms tends to provide superior rates of closure, both in the initial phase and throughout the follow-up period, when contrasted with endovascular treatment modalities [11,24,25,38,39].

The outcomes reveal an exceptionally low retreatment rate, observed in only two (0.7%) patients. Both cases demonstrated complete occlusion in their initial postoperative angiographic evaluations. Recurrence was observed in one aneurysm through routine follow-up imaging, necessitating surgical intervention for correction. The second recurrence led to a more severe outcome, presenting as a ruptured aneurysm resulting in SAH, which also required surgical retreatment. The low retreatment rate observed in this study aligns with the existing literature [21,22,29,30,40]. In contrast, endovascular alternatives show device-dependent retreatment rates ranging from 8.7% to 21.1% for WEB [15,19,20,41] and 2.3% to 9.3% for FD [17,18].

Within this cohort, six (2.2%) patients experienced a permanent deficit postoperatively. The modified Rankin Score is a frequently used evaluation tool for the clinical outcome after neurosurgical interventions; we therefore performed a subanalysis, which indicated that only two (0.7%) patients should be classified as having an unfavorable outcome (mRS > 2), while the remaining four (1.5%) with a permanent deficit should be classified as having a favorable outcome (mRS 0–2) [22]. Procedure-related complications are also observed in endovascularly treated MCA aneurysms: Iosif et al. [36] reported a 6.9% incidence of procedure-related ischemic events in FD, while De Leacy et al. [20] documented a 6.8% occurrence of permanent deficits in cases involving WEB. In the context of FD for treating MCA aneurysms, thromboembolic events have been reported to occur with a frequency ranging from 8% to ~17% according to findings by Diestro et al. and Salem et al. [17,18]

The mortality rate of 0.7% is attributed to two postoperative deaths unrelated to the clipping procedure. Patient A experienced a fulminant pulmonary embolism, while Patient B developed fatal sepsis, both ultimately resulting in death.

Although Fisher's exact test did not identify an association between ICG angiography and pNND, it is noteworthy—as highlighted in Table 9—that no cases of pNND were reported when ICG angiography was used in conjunction with conventional angiography. The additional intraoperative benefit of ICG angiography has already been demonstrated several times [42,43].

Table 9. Subanalysis of the effect of ICG on permanent neurological deficits (pNND). Crosstable of absolute frequencies and p-value of Fisher's exact test (right column). ICG = indocyanine green angiography, pNND = permanent new neurological deficit.

		pNND		p-Value
		Yes	No	
ICG Angiography	yes	0	102	0.087
	no	6	163	

The logistic regression analysis indicates that patients operated on more recently (year of operation) tend to experience fewer instances of pNND (p = 0.009). This temporal trend can likely be attributed to the increasing experience and continuous improvement in both surgical techniques and the ongoing enhancement of technical capabilities in the intraoperative setup. The consistent integration of intraoperative neuromonitoring—high-resolution intraoperative angiography in the hybrid operating room—combined with ICG angiography, is a possible contributor to this advancement. In addition to the continuous progress in endovascular treatment methods, the results demonstrate that microsurgical treatment is also progressively improving in its outcomes in recent years. The incidence of postoperative SSI exhibited a similar trend after stepwise variable selection, with a reduction in cases ($p = 0.001$) over time. Furthermore, the results indicate that older patients are more likely to experience postoperative SSI ($p = 0.04$). This finding suggests that the probability of developing postoperative SSI increases with each additional year of age within this cohort. This is a critical consideration for clinical practice, particularly when evaluating risk factors in the treatment and monitoring of elderly patients. Compared to the multicenter analysis of Drexler et al., the incidence of postoperative SSI with 1.5% (benchmark cutoff: $\leq$2.7%) is lower than in the benchmark study [44].

With regard to the occurrence of postoperative epileptic seizures, our result of 4.0% is comparable with the available literature (between 2.6% and 15.7%) [45]. Postoperative epileptic seizures are associated with prolonged hospitalization, and the rate of epileptic seizures after endovascular treatment of UIAs is likely to be lower than after microsurgical clipping according to Hoh et al. (6.2% vs. 9.2%), although no distinction was made between the respective endovascular treatment methods [46].

The results of this cohort show that postoperative ICH occurred in 1.1% of the cases as a consequence of the surgical approach employed, necessitating postoperative surgical revision. Importantly, in each of these cases, aneurysm-related secondary bleeding could be ruled out. When comparing our findings to a similar large series published by Metayer et al., the incidences are comparable (1.1% vs. 1.0%), reinforcing the consistency of our results with the existing literature [28].

In summary, our results demonstrate a remarkably high rate of aneurysm occlusion and a notably low rate of retreatment, exceeding the efficacy of endovascular therapy approaches described in the existing literature. This is corroborated by a recent meta-analysis by Tocacelli et al., which compared microsurgical clipping with endovascular techniques for MCA aneurysms, reinforcing our findings [10]. Consequently, these data support the position that microsurgical clipping should be considered the treatment of choice for unruptured MCA bifurcation aneurysms.

5. Limitations

The retrospective nature of data collection represents a notable limitation of this study, inherently allowing for potential confounding variables or biases. Although all patients underwent surgery performed by various experienced neurosurgeons, it remains a single-center experience and therefore carries the risk of selection or performance bias. Additionally, the surgeons' experience over time might have influenced outcomes, although this factor was not systematically assessed. The study exclusively focused on microsurgical interventions, thus omitting any cases from the registry that were treated with endovascular approaches. This decision was made to maintain the study's focus on providing insights into the current microsurgical management of unruptured MCA bifurcation aneurysms, rather than aiming to demonstrate therapeutic superiority. The representation of large or giant aneurysms in the registry appears to be lower compared to other databases, making it difficult to generalize the findings to more complex MCA bifurcation cases. Further, the evaluation of postoperative neurocognitive outcomes would be of interest, but this information could not be obtained from the retrospective data. Another limitation of this study is the lack of an independent audit or external data collection, which carries a substantial risk of reporting bias.

6. Conclusions

The favorable outcomes observed in our study align well with existing benchmarks. This includes a low retreatment rate (0.7%), coupled with a high occlusion rate (99.3%) and a notably low incidence of unfavorable outcomes (0.7%). Continuous enhancements over time, aided by the integration of intraoperative adjuncts (such as intraoperative ICG angiography or intraoperative neuromonitoring), have contributed to a consistent improvement in clinical outcomes. This trend is exemplified by the absence of detectable pNND in the era of ICG angiography. Further prospective investigations, particularly randomized studies comparing the outcomes of microsurgical and endovascular interventions, are warranted.

Author Contributions: N.S.-H.: Conceptualization, Methodology, Formal Analysis, Project Administration, Writing—Original Draft, Writing—Review and Editing, and Visualization; P.R.: Methodology, Writing—Review and Editing, and Validation; H.S.: Validation; P.H.: Formal Analysis and Visualization; H.W.: Formal Analysis and Writing—Original Draft; M.S.: Investigation; M.G. (Maria Gollwitzer): Investigation; S.A.: Data Curation; A.G.: Methodology, Review and Editing; M.G. (Matthias Gmeiner): Conceptualization, Validation, Supervision, and Writing—Review and Editing. All authors have made substantial contributions to all of the following: revising the manuscript critically for important intellectual content; final approval of the version to be submitted. All authors have read and agreed to the published version of the manuscript.

Funding: This research received no external funding.

Institutional Review Board Statement: The retrospective study obtained ethical approval from the local Ethics Committee of the Federal State Upper Austria (EK-No.: 1255/2019, 15 January 2020).

Informed Consent Statement: Not applicable.

Data Availability Statement: The data that support the findings of this study are available on reasonable request from the corresponding author Philip Rauch. The data are not publicly available due to privacy and ethical restrictions.

Acknowledgments: Supported by Johannes Kepler University Open Access Publishing Fund.

Conflicts of Interest: The authors declare that there are no conflicts of interest or financial disclosures related to this work.

Abbreviations

cSDH	chronic subdural hematoma
DSA	Digital Subtraction Angiography
FD	Flow-Diverter
ICG	Indocyanine green angiography
ICH	intracerebral hematoma
MCA	middle cerebral artery
MEP	motor evoked potential
MRI	Magnetic Resonance Imaging
NND	new neurological deficit
pNND	permanent new neurological deficit
RROC	Raymond–Roy occlusion classification
SAH	subarachnoid hemorrhage
SD	standard deviation (SD)
SSEP	somatosensory evoked potential
SSI	surgical site infection
tNND	transient new neurological deficit
UIA	unruptured intracranial aneurysm
WEB	Woven Endo Bridge

References

1. Laukka, D.; Kivelev, J.; Rahi, M.; Vahlberg, T.; Paturi, J.; Rinne, J.; Hirvonen, J. Detection Rates and Trends of Asymptomatic Unruptured Intracranial Aneurysms From 2005 to 2019. *Neurosurgery* **2024**, *94*, 297–306. [CrossRef]
2. Imaizumi, Y.; Mizutani, T.; Shimizu, K.; Sato, Y.; Taguchi, J. Detection rates and sites of unruptured intracranial aneurysms according to sex and age: An analysis of MR angiography–based brain examinations of 4070 healthy Japanese adults. *J. Neurosurg.* **2018**, *130*, 1–6. [CrossRef]
3. Vlak, M.H.; Algra, A.; Brandenburg, R.; Rinkel, G.J. Prevalence of unruptured intracranial aneurysms, with emphasis on sex, age, comorbidity, country, and time period: A systematic review and meta-analysis. *Lancet Neurol.* **2011**, *10*, 626–636. [CrossRef]
4. Juvela, S.; Poussa, K.; Lehto, H.; Porras, M. Natural history of unruptured intracranial aneurysms: A long-term follow-up study. *Stroke* **2013**, *44*, 2414–2421. [CrossRef]
5. Greving, J.P.; Wermer, M.J.H.; Brown, R.D.; Morita, A.; Juvela, S.; Yonekura, M.; Ishibashi, T.; Torner, J.C.; Nakayama, T.; E Rinkel, G.J.; et al. Development of the PHASES score for prediction of risk of rupture of intracranial aneurysms: A pooled analysis of six prospective cohort studies. *Lancet Neurol.* **2013**, *13*, 59–66. [CrossRef]
6. The UCAS Japan Investigators. The natural course of unruptured cerebral aneurysms in a Japanese cohort. *N. Engl. J. Med.* **2012**, *366*, 2474–2482. [CrossRef]
7. Stroh, N.; Stefanits, H.; Maletzky, A.; Kaltenleithner, S.; Thumfart, S.; Giretzlehner, M.; Drexler, R.; Ricklefs, F.L.; Dührsen, L.; Aspalter, S.; et al. Machine learning based outcome prediction of microsurgically treated unruptured intracranial aneurysms. *Sci. Rep.* **2023**, *13*, 22641. [CrossRef]
8. Etminan, N.; Brown, R.D.; Beseoglu, K.; Juvela, S.; Raymond, J.; Morita, A.; Torner, J.C.; Derdeyn, C.P.; Raabe, A.; Mocco, J.; et al. The unruptured intracranial aneurysm treatment score. *Neurology* **2015**, *85*, 881–889. [CrossRef]
9. Etminan, N.; Beseoglu, K.; Barrow, D.L.; Bederson, J.; Brown, R.D.; Connolly, E.S.; Derdeyn, C.P.; Hänggi, D.; Hasan, D.; Juvela, S.; et al. Multidisciplinary consensus on assessment of unruptured intracranial aneurysms. *Stroke* **2014**, *45*, 1523–1530. [CrossRef]
10. Toccaceli, G.; Diana, F.; Cagnazzo, F.; Cannizzaro, D.; Lanzino, G.; Barbagallo, G.M.; Certo, F.; Bortolotti, C.; Signorelli, F.; Peschillo, S. Microsurgical Clipping Compared with New and Most Advanced Endovascular Techniques in the Treatment of Unruptured Middle Cerebral Artery Aneurysms: A Meta-Analysis in the Modern Era. *World Neurosurg.* **2020**, *137*, 451–464.e1. [CrossRef]
11. Alreshidi, M.; Cote, D.J.; Dasenbrock, H.H.; Acosta, M.; Can, A.; Doucette, J.; Simjian, T.; Hulou, M.M.; A Wheeler, L.; Huang, K.; et al. Coiling Versus Microsurgical Clipping in the Treatment of Unruptured Middle Cerebral Artery Aneurysms: A Meta-Analysis. *Neurosurgery* **2018**, *83*, 879–889. [CrossRef]
12. Sturiale, C.L.; Scerrati, A.; Ricciardi, L.; Rustemi, O.; Auricchio, A.M.; Norri, N.; Piazza, A.; Ranieri, F.; Tomatis, A.; Albanese, A.; et al. Clipping versus coiling for treatment of middle cerebral artery aneurysms: A retrospective Italian multicenter experience. *Neurosurg. Rev.* **2022**, *45*, 3179–3191. [CrossRef]
13. Bracard, S.; Abdel-Kerim, A.; Thuillier, L.; Klein, O.; Anxionnat, R.; Finitsis, S.; Lebedinsky, A.; de Freitas, C.M.; Pinheiro, N.; de Andrade, G.C.; et al. Endovascular coil occlusion of 152 middle cerebral artery aneurysms: Initial and midterm angiographic and clinical results. *J. Neurosurg.* **2010**, *112*, 703–708. [CrossRef]
14. Duan, G.; Zhang, Y.; Yin, H.; Wu, Y.; Zhang, X.; Zhao, R.; Yang, P.; Zuo, Q.; Feng, Z.; Zhang, L.; et al. Predictors of recurrence and complications for the endovascular treatment of unruptured middle cerebral artery aneurysm: A high-volume center experience over 12 years. *Eur. J. Radiol.* **2023**, *163*, 110833. [CrossRef]
15. Pierot, L.; Szikora, I.; Barreau, X.; Holtmannspoetter, M.; Spelle, L.; Herbreteau, D.; Fiehler, J.; Costalat, V.; Klisch, J.; Januel, A.-C.; et al. Aneurysm treatment with WEB in the cumulative population of two prospective, multicenter series: 3-year follow-up. *J. Neurointerv. Surg.* **2021**, *13*, 363–368. [CrossRef]
16. Zhang, S.-M.; Liu, L.-X.; Ren, P.-W.; Xie, X.-D.; Miao, J. Effectiveness, Safety and Risk Factors of Woven EndoBridge Device in the Treatment of Wide-Neck Intracranial Aneurysms: Systematic Review and Meta-Analysis. *World Neurosurg.* **2020**, *136*, e1–e23. [CrossRef]
17. Salem, M.M.; Khorasanizadeh, M.; Lay, S.V.; Renieri, L.; Kuhn, A.L.; Sweid, A.; Massari, F.; Moore, J.M.; Tjoumakaris, S.I.; Jabbour, P.; et al. Endoluminal flow diverting stents for middle cerebral artery bifurcation aneurysms: Multicenter cohort. *J. Neurointerv. Surg.* **2022**, *14*, 1084–1089. [CrossRef]
18. Diestro, J.D.B.; Adeeb, N.; Dibas, M.; Boisseau, W.; Harker, P.; Brinjikji, W.; Xiang, S.; Joyce, E.; Shapiro, M.; Raz, E.; et al. Flow Diversion for Middle Cerebral Artery Aneurysms: An International Cohort Study. *Neurosurgery* **2021**, *89*, 1112–1121. [CrossRef]
19. Arthur, A.S.; Molyneux, A.; Coon, A.L.; Saatci, I.; Szikora, I.; Baltacioglu, F.; Sultan, A.; Hoit, D.; Almandoz, J.E.D.; Elijovich, L.; et al. The safety and effectiveness of the Woven EndoBridge (WEB) system for the treatment of wide-necked bifurcation aneurysms: Final 12-month results of the pivotal WEB Intrasaccular Therapy (WEB-IT) Study. *J. Neurointerv. Surg.* **2019**, *11*, 924–930. [CrossRef]
20. A De Leacy, R.; Fargen, K.M.; Mascitelli, J.R.; Fifi, J.; Turkheimer, L.; Zhang, X.; Patel, A.B.; Koch, M.J.; Pandey, A.S.; Wilkinson, D.A.; et al. Wide-neck bifurcation aneurysms of the middle cerebral artery and basilar apex treated by endovascular techniques: A multicentre, core lab adjudicated study evaluating safety and durability of occlusion (BRANCH). *J. Neurointerv. Surg.* **2019**, *11*, 31–36. [CrossRef]
21. Nussbaum, E.S.; Madison, M.T.; Goddard, J.K.; Lassig, J.P.; Kallmes, K.M.; Nussbaum, L.A. Microsurgical treatment of unruptured middle cerebral artery aneurysms: A large, contemporary experience. *J. Neurosurg.* **2018**, *130*, 1498–1504. [CrossRef]

22. Rodríguez-Hernández, A.; Sughrue, M.E.; Akhavan, S.; Habdank-Kolaczkowski, J.; Lawton, M.T. Current management of middle cerebral artery aneurysms: Surgical results with a "clip first" policy. *Neurosurgery* **2013**, *72*, 415–427. [CrossRef]
23. Güresir, E.; Schuss, P.; Berkefeld, J.; Vatter, H.; Seifert, V. Treatment results for complex middle cerebral artery aneurysms. A prospective single-center series. *Acta Neurochir.* **2011**, *153*, 1247–1252. [CrossRef]
24. Smith, T.R.; Cote, D.J.; Dasenbrock, H.H.; Hamade, Y.J.; Zammar, S.G.; El Tecle, N.E.; Batjer, H.H.; Bendok, B.R. Comparison of the Efficacy and Safety of Endovascular Coiling Versus Microsurgical Clipping for Unruptured Middle Cerebral Artery Aneurysms: A Systematic Review and Meta-Analysis. *World Neurosurg.* **2015**, *84*, 942–953. [CrossRef]
25. Dammann, P.; Schoemberg, T.; Müller, O.; Özkan, N.; Schlamann, M.; Wanke, I.; Sandalcioglu, I.E.; Forsting, M.; Sure, U. Outcome for unruptured middle cerebral artery aneurysm treatment: Surgical and endovascular approach in a single center. *Neurosurg. Rev.* **2014**, *37*, 643–651. [CrossRef]
26. International Study of Unruptured Intracranial Aneurysms Investigators. Unruptured intracranial aneurysms—Risk of rupture and risks of surgical intervention. *N. Engl. J. Med.* **1998**, *339*, 1725–1733. [CrossRef]
27. Mascitelli, J.R.; Moyle, H.; Oermann, E.K.; Polykarpou, M.F.; A Patel, A.; Doshi, A.H.; Gologorsky, Y.; Bederson, J.B.; Patel, A.B. An update to the Raymond–Roy Occlusion Classification of intracranial aneurysms treated with coil embolization. *J. Neurointerv. Surg.* **2015**, *7*, 496–502. [CrossRef]
28. Metayer, T.; Leclerc, A.; Borha, A.; Derrey, S.; Langlois, O.; Barbier, C.; Aldea, S.; le Guerinel, C.; Piotin, M.; Vivien, D.; et al. Microsurgical Clipping of Middle Cerebral Artery Aneurysms: Complications and Risk Factors for Complications. *World Neurosurg.* **2022**, *168*, e87–e96. [CrossRef]
29. Morgan, M.K.; Mahattanakul, W.; Davidson, A.; Reid, J. Outcome for middle cerebral artery aneurysm surgery. *Neurosurgery* **2010**, *67*, 755–761; discussion 761. [CrossRef]
30. Choi, S.W.; Ahn, J.S.; Park, J.C.; Kwon, D.H.; Kwun, B.D.; Kim, C.J. Surgical treatment of unruptured intracranial middle cerebral artery aneurysms: Angiographic and clinical outcomes in 143 aneurysms. *J. Cerebrovasc. Endovasc. Neurosurg.* **2012**, *14*, 289–294. [CrossRef]
31. Choi, J.H.; Park, J.E.; Kim, M.J.; Kim, B.S.; Shin, Y.S. Aneurysmal Neck Clipping as the Primary Treatment Option for Both Ruptured and Unruptured Middle Cerebral Artery Aneurysms. *J. Korean Neurosurg. Soc.* **2016**, *59*, 269–275. [CrossRef]
32. Yang, K.; Begley, S.L.; Lynch, D.; Turpin, J.; Aminnejad, M.; Farrokhyar, F.; Dehdashti, A.R. Long-term outcomes of surgical clipping of saccular middle cerebral artery aneurysms: A consecutive series of 92 patients. *Neurosurg. Rev.* **2023**, *46*, 271. [CrossRef]
33. Spetzler, R.F.; McDougall, C.G.; Zabramski, J.M.; Albuquerque, F.C.; Hills, N.K.; Nakaji, P.; Karis, J.P.; Wallace, R.C. Ten-year analysis of saccular aneurysms in the Barrow Ruptured Aneurysm Trial. *J. Neurosurg.* **2019**, *132*, 771–776. [CrossRef]
34. Mooney, M.A.; Simon, E.D.; Brigeman, S.; Nakaji, P.; Zabramski, J.M.; Lawton, M.T.; Spetzler, R.F. Long-term results of middle cerebral artery aneurysm clipping in the Barrow Ruptured Aneurysm Trial. *J. Neurosurg.* **2018**, *130*, 895–901. [CrossRef]
35. Abla, A.A.; Jahshan, S.; Kan, P.; Mokin, M.; Dumont, T.M.; Eller, J.L.; Snyder, K.V.; Hopkins, L.N.; Siddiqui, A.H.; Levy, E.I. Results of endovascular treatment of middle cerebral artery aneurysms after first giving consideration to clipping. *Acta Neurochir.* **2013**, *155*, 559–568. [CrossRef]
36. Iosif, C.; Mounayer, C.; Yavuz, K.; Saleme, S.; Geyik, S.; Cekirge, H.; Saatci, I. Middle Cerebral Artery Bifurcation Aneurysms Treated by Extrasaccular Flow Diverters: Midterm Angiographic Evolution and Clinical Outcome. *Am. J. Neuroradiol.* **2017**, *38*, 310–316. [CrossRef]
37. Michelozzi, C.; Darcourt, J.; Guenego, A.; Januel, A.-C.; Tall, P.; Gawlitza, M.; Bonneville, F.; Cognard, C. Flow diversion treatment of complex bifurcation aneurysms beyond the circle of Willis: Complications, aneurysm sac occlusion, reabsorption, recurrence, and jailed branch modification at follow-up. *J. Neurosurg.* **2018**, *131*, 1751–1762. [CrossRef]
38. Schwartz, C.; Aster, H.-C.; Al-Schameri, R.; Müller-Thies-Broussalis, E.; Griessenauer, C.J.; Killer-Oberpfalzer, M. Microsurgical clipping and endovascular treatment of middle cerebral artery aneurysms in an interdisciplinary treatment concept: Comparison of long-term results. *Interv. Neuroradiol.* **2018**, *24*, 608–614. [CrossRef]
39. Steklacova, A.; Bradac, O.; Charvat, F.; De Lacy, P.; Benes, V. "Clip first" policy in management of intracranial MCA aneurysms: Single-centre experience with a systematic review of literature. *Acta Neurochir.* **2016**, *158*, 533–546. [CrossRef]
40. Munich, S.A.; Vakharia, K.; McPheeters, M.J.; Tso, M.K.; Waqas, M.; Snyder, K.V.; Siddiqui, A.H.; Davies, J.M.; Levy, E.I. Make Clipping Great Again: Microsurgery for Cerebral Aneurysms by Dual-Trained Neurosurgeons. *World Neurosurg.* **2020**, *137*, e454–e461. [CrossRef] [PubMed]
41. Hagen, F.; Maurer, C.; Berlis, A. Endovascular Treatment of Unruptured MCA Bifurcation Aneurysms Regardless of Aneurysm Morphology: Short- and Long-Term Follow-Up. *Am. J. Neuroradiol.* **2019**, *40*, 503–509. [CrossRef] [PubMed]
42. Dashti, R.; Laakso, A.; Niemelä, M.; Porras, M.; Hernesniemi, J. Microscope-integrated near-infrared indocyanine green videoangiography during surgery of intracranial aneurysms: The Helsinki experience. *Surg. Neurol.* **2009**, *71*, 543–550; discussion 550. [CrossRef] [PubMed]
43. Raabe, A.; Nakaji, P.; Beck, J.; Kim, L.J.; Hsu, F.P.K.; Kamerman, J.D.; Seifert, V.; Spetzler, R.F. Prospective evaluation of surgical microscope—Integrated intraoperative near-infrared indocyanine green videoangiography during aneurysm surgery. *J. Neurosurg.* **2005**, *103*, 982–989. [CrossRef] [PubMed]

44. Drexler, R.; Sauvigny, T.; Pantel, T.F.; Ricklefs, F.L.; Catapano, J.S.; Wanebo, J.E.; Lawton, M.T.; Sanchin, A.; Hecht, N.; Vajkoczy, P.; et al. Global Outcomes for Microsurgical Clipping of Unruptured Intracranial Aneurysms: A Benchmark Analysis of 2245 Cases. *Neurosurgery* **2023**, *94*, 369–378. [CrossRef]
45. Fushihara, G.; Kamide, T.; Kimura, T.; Takeda, R.; Ikeda, T.; Kikkawa, Y.; Araki, R.; Kurita, H. Factors associated with early seizures after surgery of unruptured intracranial aneurysms. *Clin. Neurol. Neurosurg.* **2019**, *178*, 93–96. [CrossRef]
46. Hoh, B.L.; Nathoo, S.; Chi, Y.-Y.; Mocco, J.; Barker, F.G. Incidence of seizures or epilepsy after clipping or coiling of ruptured and unruptured cerebral aneurysms in the nationwide inpatient sample database: 2002–2007. *Neurosurgery* **2011**, *69*, 644–650. [CrossRef]

brain sciences

MDPI

Article

Radiological Outcome of Middle Meningeal Artery Embolization in Relation to Chronic Subdural Hematoma Cause and Architecture

Ahmed Abdelghafar [1,*], Andrew Falzon [2], Eef J. Hendriks [1,3], Ivan Radovanovic [4,5], Hugo Andrade [4,5], Joanna D. Schaafsma [6] and Pascal J. Mosimann [1,3,4,5,*]

1 Division of Neuroradiology, Joint Department of Medical Imaging, Toronto Western Hospital, University Health Network, Toronto, ON M5T 2S8, Canada
2 Atkinson Morley Regional Neuroscience Centre, St George's University Hospital, Tooting, London SW17 0QT, UK
3 Department of Medical Imaging, University of Toronto, Toronto, ON M5T 1W7, Canada
4 Division of Neurosurgery, Toronto Western Hospital, Toronto, ON M5T 2S8, Canada
5 Sprott Department of Surgery, University of Toronto, Toronto, ON M5G 2C4, Canada
6 Department of Neurology, University of Toronto, Toronto, ON M5S 3H2, Canada
* Correspondence: aabdelghafar.workacc@gmail.com (A.A.); pascal.mosimann@uhn.ca (P.J.M.)

Abstract: Background/Objectives: MMAE (middle meningeal artery embolization) has emerged as a potential effective treatment for cSDH (chronic subdural hematoma). In this study, MMAE efficiency with regards to cSDH cause and architecture was explored. The comparability of cSDH thickness and volume as parameters for cSDH pre- and post-MMAE assessment was also analyzed. **Methods**: In this retrospective cohort study, 52 consecutive cSDH patients treated with MMAE in a single tertiary center were included. The cohort was divided into two group pairs pertaining to cSDH cause (spontaneous or traumatic) and cSDH architecture (non-mature or mature). The radiological outcome was compared in each group before and after MMAE and between each group pair using CT imaging. A correlation analysis between cSDH thickness and volume before and after MMAE was also performed. **Results**: A statistically significant positive linear association between cSDH thickness and volume at admission and at each follow-up interval (1–3, 3–6, 6–12 months) was noticed. cSDH thickness and volume reduction in each group was statistically significant, except for a traumatic cSDH volume reduction at 6–12 months. There was no statistically significant difference between each group pair in the cSDH thickness and volume reduction difference at all the follow-up intervals. **Conclusions**: A comparable efficiency of MMAE may be achieved in non-mature and mature as well as in spontaneous and traumatic cSDH, with an advantage for spontaneous cSDH at 6–12 months follow-up compared to traumatic cSDH. Traumatic cSDH may require a relatively long-term follow-up post-MMAE. cSDH thickness and volume, as parameters for pre- and post-MMAE cSDH evaluation, appear similar.

Keywords: middle meningeal artery embolization; chronic subdural hematoma; chronic subdural hematoma architecture; chronic subdural hematoma cause

1. Introduction

cSDH (chronic subdural hematoma) is a relatively common condition associated with increased morbidity and mortality [1,2]. It has an increased propensity to persist or grow, if left untreated, due to a potentially ongoing neurovascular inflammatory cascade [3–5]. cSDH growth may be associated with poor functional outcome and high mortality rates [2,6]. The appropriate diagnosis and management of cSDH are therefore important to hinder its progression.

cSDH may be managed conservatively, if grossly asymptomatic. It may be managed with surgical drainage via a twist drill, craniotomy, burr hole craniotomy, or mini craniotomy in those who are symptomatic [7–9].

MMAE (middle meningeal artery embolization) is increasingly considered for cSDH treatment [10–13]. It was postulated that MMAE interrupts the blood supply of the neovascular membrane of cSDH, thought to be responsible for cSDH formation and growth [14,15]. Multiple studies have demonstrated a favorable cSDH outcome after MMAE [16,17].

The study goals are to analyze and compare MMAE efficiency in specific cohort groups with regards to cSDH cause and architecture and to assess the similarity between cSDH thickness and volume as radiological parameters for cSDH evaluation before and after MMAE.

2. Materials and Methods

This retrospective cohort study included 52 consecutive cases, diagnosed with cSDH and treated with MMAE between January 2020 and December 2023 in a single tertiary center.

The STROBE checklist was used throughout.

The inclusion criteria were as follows:

1. Patients diagnosed with cSDH, treated with MMAE and followed up for at least 1 month;
2. Available clinical data, procedural details, pre-procedural and follow-up CT scans.

Exclusion criteria included the following:

1. Insufficient DICOM (Digital Imaging and Communications in Medicine);
2. Post-MMAE surgical evacuation.

Post-MMAE surgical evacuation was thought to possibly overestimate or underestimate cSDH measurements at follow-up.

Clinical and imaging data were extracted from the center's research database and electronic medical records.

2.1. MMAE Procedural Details

MMAE was performed in a sterile condition in a biplane neuroangiography suite. The procedure was performed either under general anesthesia or conscious sedation and the arterial access was either through the right femoral or the right radial artery.

Selective catheterization was carried out using a coaxial or tri-axial technique. The anatomical origin of the ipsilateral ophthalmic artery was confirmed through CCA or ICA angiography. Further anatomy was confirmed through selective microcatheter angiography of the middle meningeal artery trunk, frontal, and parietal branches.

The embolization technique entailed either PVA (polyvinyl alcohol) particles, PVA particles–microcoils, liquid embolic agents (Onyx), microcoils, or Onyx–microcoils. The technique used was determined based on collateralization and anatomy.

2.2. Imaging Assessment

CT imaging was performed before MMAE and at follow-up, in compliance with the center's guidelines for cSDH patient management.

cSDH volume was measured using the ABC/2 method [18]. The cSDH thickness was the same as that used in calculating cSDH volume.

In cases with pre-MMAE surgical evacuation, the last CT scan before MMAE and after surgical evacuation was considered for hematoma thickness and volume assessment at admission.

2.3. Statistics

Statistical analysis was carried out using IBM SPSS statistics 29.0.2.0. Continuous variables were described with mean, median, standard deviation, and/or confidence interval.

Categorical variables were described with frequency and/or percentage.

The correlation between the cSDH thickness and the volumes at admission and at each follow-up interval was evaluated. Shapiro–Wilk test was performed for all variables. Correlation test results were described with Pearson's correlation coefficient (r) for direction and strength and *p*-value for significance of the association.

The cohort was divided into 2 group pairs in relation to cSDH cause and architecture.

cSDH is defined as hematoma collection in the subdural space with outer and inner membranes [19].

cSDH cause is either spontaneous or traumatic [20].

cSDH architecture at admission is either type 1 homogenous/laminar (non-mature cSDH) or type 2 separated/trabecular (mature cSDH) [21].

In each group, pre- and post-MMAE cSDH thickness and volume were compared. Paired *t*-test and Wilcoxon signed-rank test were used.

Post-MMAE radiological outcome was defined as cSDH thickness/volume difference, which is the difference between cSDH thickness/volume at follow-up and at admission. Furthermore, 1–3, 3–6, 6–12 months' follow-up intervals were included.

cSDH thickness/volume difference was compared between each group pair at each follow-up interval. Univariate analysis was conducted with an independent *t*-test, Mann–Whitney U test, ANCOVA, and/or generalized linear model (GLM).

The Shapiro–Wilk test was performed for the compared variables in each group to assess normal distribution. Levene's test was performed to evaluate the equality of variance for the variables compared between each group pair.

The following possible covariates were compared between groups: age, sex, antiplatelet therapy, anticoagulant therapy, hepatic comorbidity, alcohol intake, dementia, previous surgical evacuation, MMAE technique, and PVA particle size. Hematoma architecture type was additionally considered for cSDH cause group comparison.

Current antiplatelets and/or anticoagulant therapy have been defined as concomitant treatment by antiplatelet or anticoagulant at admission. Hepatic comorbidity has been defined as the diagnosis of any hepatic digestive, synthetic, metabolic or excretory dysfunction at admission [22]. Current alcohol intake was defined as lifetime drinking of $\geq$12 drinks and an average of >7 drinks per week for women and >14 drinks per week for men in the previous year to admission [23]. Dementia was defined as a decline in memory, executive functions, and behavioral changes with functional impairment [24].

The comparison between each group pair was performed with a Chi-Squared test for the categorical covariates, and the independent *t*-test and/or Mann–Whitney U test for the continuous covariate.

The Shapiro–Wilk test and Levene's test were carried out for the continuous covariate.

Statistical significance was defined as p-value < 0.05.

2.4. Ethics, Informed Consent and Confidentiality

Research ethics board approval was obtained (ID 24-5029). Written consent was waived due to the retrospective type of study. Data were anonymized.

3. Results

3.1. cSDH Volume and Thickness Correlation

The association between cSDH thickness and volume at admission was evaluated. This was also evaluated at each follow-up interval.

Pearson's correlation yielded a statistically significant strong positive linear association ($p < 0.001$, r = 1) between the thickness and volume at admission and at each follow-up interval.

All compared variables were normally distributed.

3.2. cSDH Cause Groups

The cohort was divided into 21 spontaneous cSDH cases (group 1) and 31 traumatic cSDH cases (group 2).

The mean age in the first group was 71, with a range of 62 and standard deviation of 15. Up to 7/21 (33.3%) were females and 14/21 (66.7%) were males. The embolization technique used was PVA in 12 cases, PVA–microcoils in 7 cases, Onyx in 1 case, and microcoils in 1 case.

In the second group, the mean age was 73, while the age range was 37 with a standard deviation of 10. Up to 6/31 (19.4%) cases were females, and 25/31 (80.6%) cases were males. The embolization technique used was PVA in 12 cases, PVA–microcoils in 17 cases, Onyx in 1 case, and Onyx–microcoils in 1 case.

Hepatic disease ($p = 0.022$), antiplatelets ($p = 0.01$), and particle type ($p = 0.005$) showed statistically significant difference between the groups.

The results showed statistically significant lower values of cSDH thickness and volume at each follow-up interval for each group compared to the admission values, except for the traumatic cSDH volume at 6–12 months. The traumatic cSDH volume reduction at 6–12 months was not statistically significant (Table 1a,b).

Table 1. (**a**) Comparison of cSDH (chronic subdural hematoma) thickness/volume before and after MMAE (middle meningeal artery embolization) in relation to cSDH cause and architecture type, using paired *t*-test. $p < 0.05$ was considered statistically significant. (**b**) Comparison of cSDH thickness/volume before and after MMAE with regards to cSDH cause and architecture type, using Wilcoxon signed-rank test. $p < 0.05$ was considered statistically significant.

(a)

Thickness (T) and Volume (V) at Admission (0) and at Interval Follow-Up	***T*-Test Significance ($p < 0.05$)**			
	cSDH Cause		**cSDH Architecture**	
	Spontaneous	**Traumatic**	**Non-Mature**	**Mature**
T 0—at 1–3 months (mm)	<0.001	<0.001	<0.001	<0.001
V 0—at 1–3 months (cm^3)	<0.001	<0.001	<0.001	<0.001
T 0—at 3–6 months (mm)	<0.001	<0.001	<0.001	<0.001
V 0—at 3–6 months (cm^3)	0.001	<0.001	<0.001	<0.001
T 0—at 6–12 months (mm)	<0.001	<0.001	<0.001	0.025
V 0—at 6–12 months (cm^3)	<0.001	<0.001	<0.001	0.003

(b)

Thickness (T) and Volume (V) at Admission (0) and at Interval Follow-Up	**Wilcoxon Signed-Rank Test Significance ($p < 0.05$)**			
	cSDH Cause		**cSDH Architecture**	
	Spontaneous	**Traumatic**	**Non-Mature**	**Mature**
T 0—at 1–3 months (mm)	<0.001	<0.001	<0.001	<0.001
V 0—at 1–3 months (cm^3)	<0.001	<0.001	<0.001	<0.001
T 0—at 3–6 months (mm)	0.012	<0.001	0.008	0.001
V 0—at 3–6 months (cm^3)	0.012	<0.001	0.008	0.001
T 0—at 6–12 months (mm)	0.002	0.068	0.008	0.018
V 0—at 6–12 months (cm^3)	0.002	0.068	0.008	0.018

The mean thickness and volume reduction difference at 1–3 and 3–6 months in the traumatic cSDH was higher than the spontaneous cSDH. However, this was higher at 6–12 months in the spontaneous cSDH compared to the traumatic cSDH.

The thickness/volume reduction differences between the group pairs were statistically significant at 3–6 months.

The thickness/volume reduction difference between the groups was not statistically significant at all the follow-up intervals after the correction for covariates (Table 2).

Table 2. Comparison of thickness and volume reduction differences at follow-up between spontaneous and traumatic cSDH groups. $p < 0.05$ was considered statistically significant.

Spontaneous–Traumatic cSDH Groups Differences	Mean Difference	95% CI		Significance ($p < 0.05$)			
		Lower	Upper	*T*-Test	MWU *	ANCOVA	GLM *
T Difference at 1–3 Months (mm) *	−0.37	−5.13	4.40	0.438	0.910	0.145	0.119
V Difference at 1–3 Months (cm^3) *	−1.68	−32.37	29.01	0.456	0.860	0.187	0.172
T Difference at 3–6 months (mm)	−7.32	−13	−1.63	0.007	0.044	0.329	0.536
V Difference at 3–6 Months (cm^3)	−34.21	−74.07	5.63	0.044	0.048	0.559	0.670
T Difference at 6–12 Months (mm)	0.67	−8.84	10.18	0.44	0.626	0.253	0.138
V Difference at 6–12 Months (cm^3)	18.46	−37.88	74.8	0.247	0.716	0.467	0.354

* GLM, generalized linear model MWU; Mann-Whitney U test; T, cSDH thickness; V, cSDH volume.

3.3. cSDH Architecture Groups

A total of 23 cases had type 1 cSDH, and 29 had type 2 at admission (Figure 1).

In the type 1 group, the mean age was 74 with a range of 34 and standard deviation of 9.

Up to 8/23 cases (34.8%) were females and 15/23 (65.2%) were males. A total of 8 cases had PVA particles, while 15 had combined PVA–microcoils.

In type 2 group, the mean age was 71 with a standard deviation of 14 and a range of 64. Approximately 5/29 cases (17.2%) were females and 24/29 (82.8%) were males.

The embolization results for type 2 group were as follows: 16 PVA, 9 PVA–microcoils, 2 Onyx, 1 with microcoils, and 1 combined Onyx–microcoils.

None of the covariates showed a statistically significant difference between the groups.

There were statistically significant lower values of cSDH thickness/volume at each follow-up interval for each group compared to the admission values (Table 1a,b).

The mean thickness and volume reduction difference in the type 1 hematoma was higher than the type 2 at all follow-up intervals.

The thickness/volume reduction difference between groups was not statistically significant at all the follow-up intervals (Table 3).

Table 3. Hematoma type 1 and 2 groups thickness and volume reduction differences comparison at follow-up. $p < 0.05$ was considered statistically significant.

Hematoma Type 1–Type 2 Groups Differences	Mean Difference	95% CI		Significance ($p < 0.05$)	
		Lower	Upper	*T*-Test	MWU *
T Difference at 1–3 Months (mm) *	0.1	−4.52	4.76	0.479	0.816
V Difference at 1–3 Months (cm^3) *	2.8	−27.06	32.68	0.425	0.864
T Difference at 3–6 Months (mm)	4	−2.97	11.01	0.122	0.198
V Difference at 3–6 Months (cm^3)	23	−17.06	63.06	0.122	0.356
T Difference at 6–12 Months (mm)	5.7	−1.92	13.35	0.065	0.089
V Difference at 6–12 Months (cm^3)	7.7	−42.13	57.56	0.372	0.368

* MWU, Mann–Whitney U test; T, cSDH thickness; V, cSDH volume.

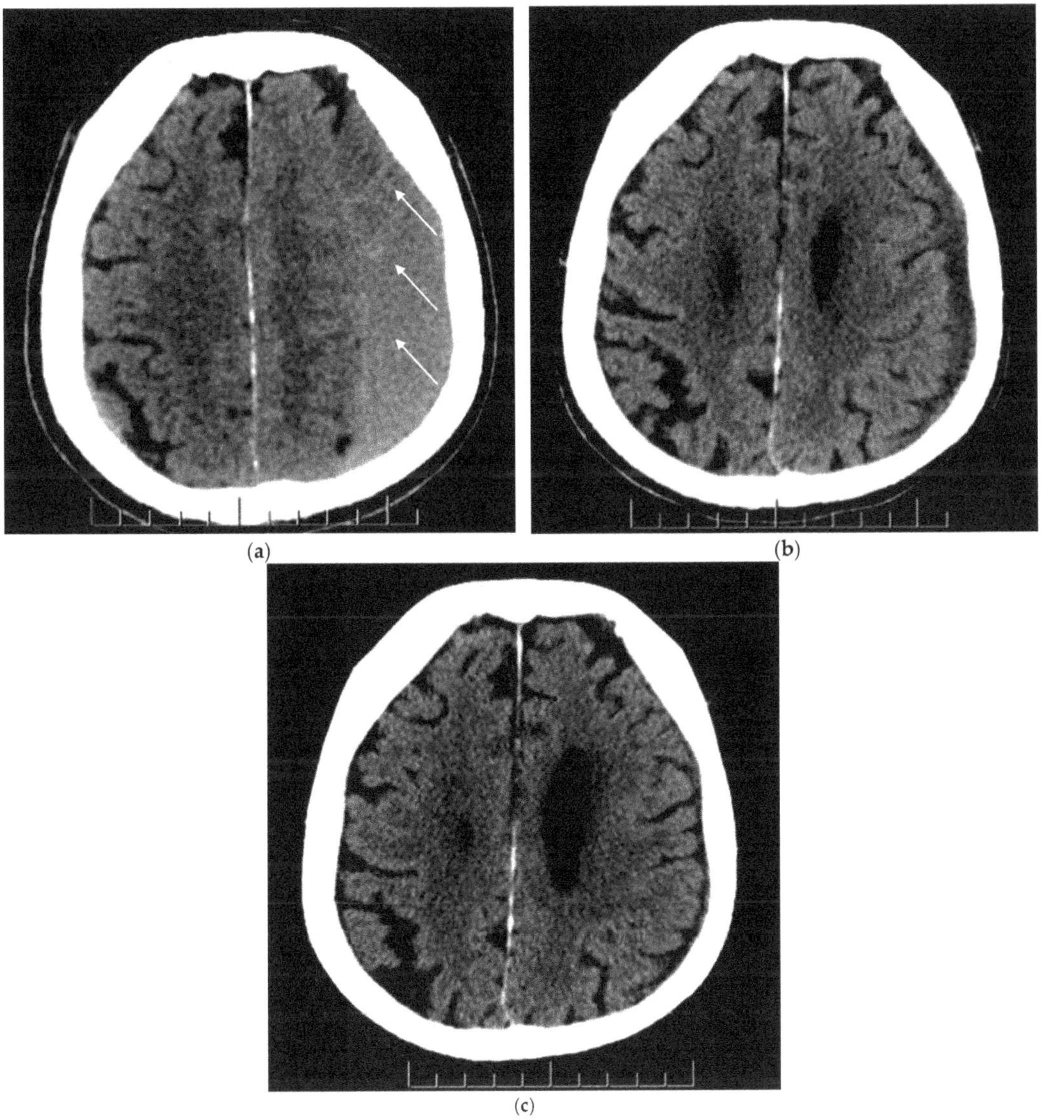

Figure 1. (**a**–**c**) Axial view of non-contrast CT head scans before and after MMAE (middle meningeal artery embolization) for the same patient. Figure parts a, b and c represent chronic subdural hematoma (cSDH) pre-MMAE (baseline), at 1–3 months and 3–6 months post-MMAE, respectively. (**a**) A non-mature mixed cSDH was noticed at baseline on the left cerebral hemisphere with sulcal effacement, obliteration of the left lateral ventricle and slight midline shift to the right. The white arrows demonstrate the mixed cSDH nature; (**b**) Improvement of the cSDH and mass effect was noticed in 6-week CT scan post-MMAE; (**c**) A near-complete resolution of cSDH and mass effect was noticed in 5-month CT scan.

4. Discussion

4.1. Imaging Parameters for Post-MMAE cSDH Change Assessment

The cSDH volume and thickness are frequently used parameters in assessing cSDH size [25,26]. Multiple techniques for thickness and volume measurements have been proposed [27,28].

The initial evaluation of cSDH thickness and volume appeared effective in cSDH prognosis prediction after surgery [29,30]. The question was whether both parameters were comparable in evaluating cSDH change after MMAE.

The results showed a very strong positive correlation between the cSDH thickness and volume before and after the MMAE. cSDH thickness and volume appear to be comparable parameters in evaluating the cSDH radiological outcomes after the MMAE.

4.2. cSDH Cause

cSDH develops as a result of chronic inflammatory neovascularization bleeding within the hematoma membrane in the subdural space [31]. Trauma and spontaneous bleeding have been described as potential causes that may provoke this inflammatory and neoangiogenic process [32,33]. cSDH is not necessarily preceded by an acute subdural hematoma or traumatic event [34,35].

The results suggest that the cSDH volume/thickness reduction in each group was statistically significant, except for the cSDH volume reduction at 6–12 months in the traumatic cSDH group (Table 1a,b). Additionally, the cSDH volume/thickness reduction difference between groups was not statistically significant (Table 2).

MMAE appears to have similar efficiency in hematoma reduction when comparing both groups. Traumatic cSDH may need a relatively long-term follow-up to monitor the radiological outcomes (Tables 1a,b and 2).

4.3. cSDH Architecture

Different hematoma architecture types were suggested, including homogenous, laminar, separated, and trabecular [21,36,37]. cSDH trajectory was thought to initially start with homogenous/laminar types and then develop into mature separated/trabecular types [21].

The initial cSDH types were associated with a relatively faster rate of hematoma volume reduction compared to the mature cSDH types after MMAE [38].

For each group, the results showed a significant cSDH thickness and volume reduction post-MMAE (Table 1a,b). When comparing both groups, cSDH thickness and volume reduction difference was higher in the type 1 hematoma compared to type 2 at all follow-up intervals. This difference was not statistically significant (Table 3).

Both the non-mature and mature cSDH types appeared to have a comparable efficient radiological outcome after the MMAE (Tables 1a,b and 3).

4.4. Limitations

The retrospective nature of the study may be associated with recall bias. We therefore assessed the clinical information in detail and in variable encounters.

To ensure accuracy and tackle potential bias, double blinded measurements were performed by two experienced researchers for imaging data evaluation. A review from an experienced independent reviewer was added in case of any discrepancy.

5. Conclusions

MMAE appears similarly efficient in cSDH thickness and volume reduction pertaining to both non-mature and mature hematoma architectures. It appears to have a comparable, efficient radiological outcome for both spontaneous and traumatic cSDH, with an edge for the spontaneous type on a long-term follow-up. Traumatic cSDH may require a relatively long follow-up time to assess the radiological outcomes. cSDH thickness and volume appear to be comparable radiological parameters in the evaluation of cSDH before and after MMAE.

Author Contributions: Conceptualization, P.J.M. and A.A.; Methodology, A.A.; Validation, P.J.M.; E.J.H., I.R., H.A. and J.D.S.; Formal Analysis, A.A.; Investigation, A.A.; Resources, P.J.M.; Writing—Original Draft Preparation, A.A. and A.F.; Writing—Review and Editing, P.J.M., E.J.H., I.R., H.A. and J.D.S.; Supervision, P.J.M.; Project Administration, A.A. and A.F. All authors have read and agreed to the published version of the manuscript.

Funding: This research received no external funding.

Institutional Review Board Statement: The study was conducted according to the guidelines of the Declaration of Helsinki and approved by the Institutional Review Board of University Health Network (protocol code 24-5029, approved in January 2024).

Informed Consent Statement: Patient consent was waived due to the retrospective nature of the study.

Data Availability Statement: The data presented in this study are available on request from the corresponding authors due to ethical restrictions.

Conflicts of Interest: The authors declare no conflicts of interest.

References

1. Miranda, L.B.; Braxton, E.; Hobbs, J.; Quigley, M.R. Chronic Subdural Hematoma in the Elderly: Not a Benign Disease: Clinical Article. *J. Neurosurg.* **2011**, *114*, 72–76. [CrossRef] [PubMed]
2. Feghali, J.; Yang, W.; Huang, J. Updates in Chronic Subdural Hematoma: Epidemiology, Etiology, Pathogenesis, Treatment, and Outcome. *World Neurosurg.* **2020**, *141*, 339–345. [CrossRef] [PubMed]
3. Weigel, R.; Schilling, L.; Schmiedek, P. Specific Pattern of Growth Factor Distribution in Chronic Subdural Hematoma (CSH): Evidence for an Angiogenic Disease. *Acta Neurochir.* **2001**, *143*, 811–819. [CrossRef] [PubMed]
4. Ducruet, A.F.; Grobelny, B.T.; Zacharia, B.E.; Hickman, Z.L.; DeRosa, P.L.; Anderson, K.; Sussman, E.; Carpenter, A.; Connolly, E.S. The Surgical Management of Chronic Subdural Hematoma. *Neurosurg. Rev.* **2012**, *35*, 155–169. [CrossRef] [PubMed]
5. Tamura, R.; Sato, M.; Yoshida, K.; Toda, M. History and Current Progress of Chronic Subdural Hematoma. *J. Neurol. Sci.* **2021**, *429*, 118066. [CrossRef]
6. Yang, W.; Huang, J. Chronic Subdural Hematoma. *Neurosurg. Clin. N. Am.* **2017**, *28*, 205–210. [CrossRef]
7. Kolias, A.G.; Chari, A.; Santarius, T.; Hutchinson, P.J. Chronic Subdural Haematoma: Modern Management and Emerging Therapies. *Nat. Rev. Neurol.* **2014**, *10*, 570–578. [CrossRef]
8. Blaauw, J.; Jacobs, B.; Den Hertog, H.M.; Van Der Gaag, N.A.; Jellema, K.; Dammers, R.; Lingsma, H.F.; Naalt, J.V.D.; Kho, K.H.; Groen, R.J.M. Neurosurgical and Perioperative Management of Chronic Subdural Hematoma. *Front. Neurol.* **2020**, *11*, 550. [CrossRef]
9. Foppen, M.; Bandral, H.V.; Slot, K.-A.M.; Vandertop, W.P.; Verbaan, D. Success of Conservative Therapy for Chronic Subdural Hematoma Patients: A Systematic Review. *Front. Neurol.* **2023**, *14*, 1249332. [CrossRef]
10. Link, T.W.; Rapoport, B.I.; Paine, S.M.; Kamel, H.; Knopman, J. Middle Meningeal Artery Embolization for Chronic Subdural Hematoma: Endovascular Technique and Radiographic Findings. *Interv. Neuroradiol.* **2018**, *24*, 455–462. [CrossRef]
11. Srivatsan, A.; Mohanty, A.; Nascimento, F.A.; Hafeez, M.U.; Srinivasan, V.M.; Thomas, A.; Chen, S.R.; Johnson, J.N.; Kan, P. Middle Meningeal Artery Embolization for Chronic Subdural Hematoma: Meta-Analysis and Systematic Review. *World Neurosurg.* **2019**, *122*, 613–619. [CrossRef] [PubMed]
12. Fiorella, D.; Arthur, A.S. Middle Meningeal Artery Embolization for the Management of Chronic Subdural Hematoma. *J. Neurointerv. Surg.* **2019**, *11*, 912–915. [CrossRef] [PubMed]
13. Haldrup, M.; Ketharanathan, B.; Debrabant, B.; Schwartz, O.S.; Mikkelsen, R.; Fugleholm, K.; Poulsen, F.R.; Jensen, T.S.R.; Thaarup, L.V.; Bergholt, B. Embolization of the Middle Meningeal Artery in Patients with Chronic Subdural Hematoma—A Systematic Review and Meta-Analysis. *Acta Neurochir.* **2020**, *162*, 777–784. [CrossRef] [PubMed]
14. Ishihara, H.; Ishihara, S.; Kohyama, S.; Yamane, F.; Ogawa, M.; Sato, A.; Matsutani, M. Experience in Endovascular Treatment of Recurrent Chronic Subdural Hematoma. *Interv. Neuroradiol.* **2007**, *13*, 141–144. [CrossRef]
15. Ban, S.P.; Hwang, G.; Byoun, H.S.; Kim, T.; Lee, S.U.; Bang, J.S.; Han, J.H.; Kim, C.-Y.; Kwon, O.-K.; Oh, C.W. Middle Meningeal Artery Embolization for Chronic Subdural Hematoma. *Radiology* **2018**, *286*, 992–999. [CrossRef]
16. Catapano, J.S.; Ducruet, A.F.; Nguyen, C.L.; Baranoski, J.F.; Cole, T.S.; Majmundar, N.; Wilkinson, D.A.; Fredrickson, V.L.; Cavalcanti, D.D.; Albuquerque, F.C. Middle Meningeal Artery Embolization for Chronic Subdural Hematoma: An Institutional Technical Analysis. *J. Neurointerv. Surg.* **2021**, *13*, 657–660. [CrossRef]
17. Ironside, N.; Nguyen, C.; Do, Q.; Ugiliweneza, B.; Chen, C.-J.; Sieg, E.P.; James, R.F.; Ding, D. Middle Meningeal Artery Embolization for Chronic Subdural Hematoma: A Systematic Review and Meta-Analysis. *J. Neurointerv. Surg.* **2021**, *13*, 951–957. [CrossRef]

18. Gebel, J.M.; Sila, C.A.; Sloan, M.A.; Granger, C.B.; Weisenberger, J.P.; Green, C.L.; Topol, E.J.; Mahaffey, K.W. Comparison of the ABC/2 Estimation Technique to Computer-Assisted Volumetric Analysis of Intraparenchymal and Subdural Hematomas Complicating the GUSTO-1 Trial. *Stroke* **1998**, *29*, 1799–1801. [CrossRef]
19. Robinson, R.G. Chronic Subdural Hematoma: Surgical Management in 133 Patients. *J. Neurosurg.* **1984**, *61*, 263–268. [CrossRef]
20. Lee, K.-S. ReviewNatural History of Chronic Subdural Haematoma. *Brain Inj.* **2004**, *18*, 351–358. [CrossRef]
21. Nakaguchi, H.; Tanishima, T.; Yoshimasu, N. Factors in the Natural History of Chronic Subdural Hematomas That Influence Their Postoperative Recurrence. *J. Neurosurg.* **2001**, *95*, 256–262. [CrossRef] [PubMed]
22. Tennant, B.C. Hepatic Function. In *Clinical Biochemistry of Domestic Animals*; Elsevier: Amsterdam, The Netherlands, 1997; pp. 327–352, ISBN 978-0-12-396305-5.
23. Schoenborn, C.A.; Adams, P.E. Health Behaviors of Adults: United States, 2005–2007. In *Vital Health Statistics*; Series 10; Number 245; U.S. Department of Health and Human Services: Washington, DC, USA, 2010; pp. 1–132.
24. World Health Organization (Ed.) *The ICD-10 Classification of Mental and Behavioural Disorders: Clinical Descriptions and Diagnostic Guidelines*; World Health Organization: Geneva, Switzerland, 1992; ISBN 978-92-4-154422-1.
25. Omura, Y.; Ishiguro, T. Middle Meningeal Artery Embolization for Chronic Subdural Hematoma: A Systematic Review. *Front. Neurol.* **2023**, *14*, 1259647. [CrossRef] [PubMed]
26. Levitt, M.R.; Hirsch, J.A.; Chen, M. Middle Meningeal Artery Embolization for Chronic Subdural Hematoma: An Effective Treatment with a Bright Future. *J. Neurointerv. Surg.* **2024**, *16*, 329–330. [CrossRef] [PubMed]
27. Won, S.-Y.; Zagorcic, A.; Dubinski, D.; Quick-Weller, J.; Herrmann, E.; Seifert, V.; Konczalla, J. Excellent Accuracy of ABC/2 Volume Formula Compared to Computer-Assisted Volumetric Analysis of Subdural Hematomas. *PLoS ONE* **2018**, *13*, e0199809. [CrossRef] [PubMed]
28. Bechstein, M.; McDonough, R.; Fiehler, J.; Zanolini, U.; Rai, H.; Siddiqui, A.; Shotar, E.; Rouchaud, A.; Goyal, M.; Gellissen, S. Radiological Evaluation Criteria for Chronic Subdural Hematomas: Review of the Literature. *Clin. Neuroradiol.* **2022**, *32*, 923–929. [CrossRef] [PubMed]
29. Yamamoto, H.; Hirashima, Y.; Hamada, H.; Hayashi, N.; Origasa, H.; Endo, S. Independent Predictors of Recurrence of Chronic Subdural Hematoma: Results of Multivariate Analysis Performed Using a Logistic Regression Model. *J. Neurosurg.* **2003**, *98*, 1217–1221. [CrossRef]
30. Stanišić, M.; Hald, J.; Rasmussen, I.A.; Pripp, A.H.; Ivanović, J.; Kolstad, F.; Sundseth, J.; Züchner, M.; Lindegaard, K.-F. Volume and Densities of Chronic Subdural Haematoma Obtained from CT Imaging as Predictors of Postoperative Recurrence: A Prospective Study of 107 Operated Patients. *Acta Neurochir.* **2013**, *155*, 323–333; discussion 333. [CrossRef]
31. Edlmann, E.; Giorgi-Coll, S.; Whitfield, P.C.; Carpenter, K.L.H.; Hutchinson, P.J. Pathophysiology of Chronic Subdural Haematoma: Inflammation, Angiogenesis and Implications for Pharmacotherapy. *J. Neuroinflamm.* **2017**, *14*, 108. [CrossRef]
32. Lucke-Wold, B.P.; Turner, R.C.; Josiah, D.; Knotts, C.; Bhatia, S. Do Age and Anticoagulants Affect the Natural History of Acute Subdural Hematomas? *Arch. Emerg. Med. Crit. Care* **2016**, *1*, 1010.
33. Weigel, R.; Schilling, L.; Krauss, J.K. The Pathophysiology of Chronic Subdural Hematoma Revisited: Emphasis on Aging Processes as Key Factor. *Geroscience* **2022**, *44*, 1353–1371. [CrossRef]
34. Holl, D.C.; Volovici, V.; Dirven, C.M.F.; Peul, W.C.; van Kooten, F.; Jellema, K.; van der Gaag, N.A.; Miah, I.P.; Kho, K.H.; den Hertog, H.M.; et al. Pathophysiology and Nonsurgical Treatment of Chronic Subdural Hematoma: From Past to Present to Future. *World Neurosurg.* **2018**, *116*, 402–411.e2. [CrossRef] [PubMed]
35. Edlmann, E.; Whitfield, P.C.; Kolias, A.; Hutchinson, P.J. Pathogenesis of Chronic Subdural Hematoma: A Cohort Evidencing De Novo and Transformational Origins. *J. Neurotrauma* **2021**, *38*, 2580–2589. [CrossRef] [PubMed]
36. Chon, K.-H.; Lee, J.-M.; Koh, E.-J.; Choi, H.-Y. Independent Predictors for Recurrence of Chronic Subdural Hematoma. *Acta Neurochir.* **2012**, *154*, 1541–1548. [CrossRef] [PubMed]
37. Miah, I.P.; Tank, Y.; Rosendaal, F.R.; Peul, W.C.; Dammers, R.; Lingsma, H.F.; den Hertog, H.M.; Jellema, K.; van der Gaag, N.A.; Dutch Chronic Subdural Hematoma Research Group. Radiological Prognostic Factors of Chronic Subdural Hematoma Recurrence: A Systematic Review and Meta-Analysis. *Neuroradiology* **2021**, *63*, 27–40. [CrossRef]
38. Uttam, B.K.; Yuanyuan, L.; Bizhan, A.; Thorsten, F.R.; Mazhar, K.; Marco, C.; Dheeraj, G. Short-Term Follow-up Pilot Study of Sole Middle Meningeal Artery Embolization for Chronic Subdural Hematoma: Influence of Internal Architecture on the Radiological Outcomes. *Neuroradiology* **2023**, *65*, 1143–1153. [CrossRef]

brain sciences

MDPI

Article

Clinical and Anatomical Characteristics of Perforator Aneurysms of the Posterior Cerebral Artery: A Single-Center Experience

Anahita Malvea [1], Shigeta Miyake [1,2], Ronit Agid [1], Hugo Andrade Barazarte [1,3], Richard Farb [1], Timo Krings [1,3], Pascal John Roger Mosimann [1,3], Patrick Joseph Nicholson [4], Ivan Radovanovic [3], Karel Terbrugge [1], Robert Willinsky [1], Joanna Danielle Schaafsma [5] and Eef J. Hendriks [1,*]

1 Division of Neuroradiology, Joint Department of Medical Imaging, Toronto Western Hospital, University Health Network, 399 Bathurst St, Toronto, ON M5T 2S8, Canada
2 Department of Neurosurgery, Yokohama City University School of Medicine, Yokohama 236-0027, Japan
3 Department of Neurosurgery, Toronto Western Hospital, University Health Network, Toronto, ON M5G 2C4, Canada
4 Department of Neuroradiology, Beaumont Hospital, BL6 4LA Dublin, Ireland
5 Department of Neurology, University Health Network, Toronto, ON M5G 2C4, Canada
* Correspondence: eef.hendriks@uhn.ca

Abstract: Introduction: Posterior cerebral artery (PCA) aneurysms represent up to 1% of all cerebral aneurysms. P1-P2 perforator aneurysms are thought to be even less prevalent and often require complex treatment strategies due to their anatomical and morphological characteristics, with risk of a perforator infarct. We studied the treatment of P1-P2 perforator aneurysms in a single-center cohort from a high-volume tertiary center, reporting clinical and anatomical characteristics, treatment strategies, and outcomes. Methods: A retrospective analysis of adult patients with a P1-P2 perforator aneurysm who presented at our institution between January 2000 and January 2023 was performed. The patients were analyzed for demographics, clinical presentation, imaging findings, treatment techniques, outcomes, and complications. Subgroup analyses between ruptured versus non-ruptured cases were included. Results: Out of 2733 patients with a cerebral aneurysm, 14 patients (0.5%) presented with a P1-P2 perforator aneurysm. All six patients with a ruptured aneurysm were treated by endovascular coiling, of whom one patient (16.7%) required surgical clipping of a recurrence. One out of eight (12.5%) patients with unruptured aneurysms was treated by surgical clipping. P1-P2 perforator aneurysms predominantly affected middle-aged individuals (median 59.5 years), with 10/14 (71.4%) being female. Endovascular coiling was the primary treatment modality overall, yielding favorable technical outcomes, however, it was complicated by a perforator infarct in two patients (33.3%) without new permanent morbidity or mortality secondary to treatment. Conclusions: P1-P2 perforator aneurysms are a rare subtype of intracranial aneurysm. Endovascular coiling could present an effective treatment modality; however, care should be taken for ischemic complications in the dependent perforator territory. Larger studies are required to provide more insights.

Keywords: cerebral aneurysm; posterior cerebral artery; perforator artery; endovascular coiling

1. Introduction

In general terms, posterior cerebral artery (PCA) aneurysms account for 1% of all intracranial aneurysms [1] and for 7% of aneurysms in the posterior circulation [2]. Up to 54% of patients present with a rupture [3]. Saccular aneurysms are found in 46% and 52% (ruptured versus unruptured), fusiform aneurysms in 15% and 12%, dissecting aneurysms in 21% and 14%, and serpentine aneurysms in 2% and 4%, respectively [1]. Given the high percentage of dissecting or fusiform aneurysms, endovascular treatment often involves stent-assisted coiling, flow diverter treatment [4], or parent vessel occlusion (PVO) [5], rather than unassisted coiling [6]. Essibayi et al., 2002 reported the treatment modalities of ruptured PCA aneurysms, with microsurgery being used in 35.8%, PVO in 34.9%, and reconstructive endovascular treatment in 24.3% [3]. There is an overall treatment-related complication rate of 15%, with hemorrhagic complications accounting for 3% [5] and ischemic complications occurring in approximately 12% of cases. Treatment-related complications were most commonly seen in the PVO group (38.1%) [3], most frequently leading to hemianopia.

From an embryological perspective, the PCA originates from the anterior circulation [7]; however, it is considered a functional artery of the posterior circulation in adults [8]. The PCA is divided into segments: the P1 segment extends from the basilar artery bifurcation to the posterior communicating artery confluence, the P2A segment runs ventrally to the midbrain, the P2B segment is located lateral to the midbrain, the P3 segment is located in the quadrigeminal cistern, and the P4 segment represents the cortical branches (Figure 1) [9]. Various perforating arteries arise from these segments, including the tuberothalamic arteries from the Pcom segment, the paramedian arteries from the P1 segment, and the inferolateral arteries from the P2 segment (Figure 1) [10,11], each with their characteristic supply to the thalamus and/or the midbrain.

The P1 and P2 segments can give rise to unique and clinically significant perforator arterial variation, namely the artery of Percheron and a dominant collicular artery [12]. The artery of Percheron is the anatomical variant artery replacing the normally present bilateral paramedian P1 perforators with a single dominant unilateral trunk originating of the P1 segment that subsequently divides, providing bilateral supply to the thalamus and/or midbrain. The collicular artery is the anatomical variant replacing the inferolateral P2 perforators, coursing medially and parallel to the main P2 segment around the cerebral peduncle, towards the collicular plate, and originating from the P1 or P2A segment (Figure 1).

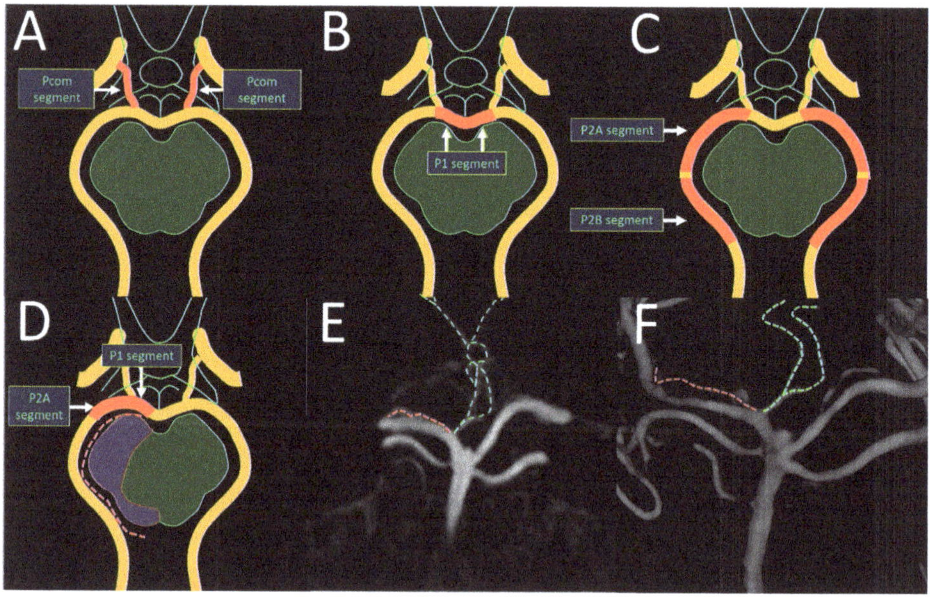

Figure 1. Axial schematic illustrations of the segments of PCA perforators at the level of the midbrain and optic chiasm (**A–C**) representing the 3 major thalamoperforating groups, i.e., Pcom, P1, and P2, supplying different thalamic territories. The tuberothalamic arteries originate from the middle third of the PcomA (**A**), supplying the ventral thalamus. The paramedian P1 perforators originate from the P1 or precommunicating segment (**B**) and supply the medial thalamus and/or rostral midbrain. The

inferolateral perforators, also known as geniculate perforators or direct perforators, originate from the P2 or postcommunicating segment (**C**) and can be divided into the P2A and P2B segments, or crural cistern and ambient cistern segments. The P2A segment supplies the lateral thalamus, whereas the P2B classically supplies the inferolateral pulvinar. An anatomical variant and replacement of the paramedian P1 perforators is the artery of Percheron, representing a single dominant trunk with bilateral supply to the thalamus and/or midbrain ((**E**,**F**); green dotted lines) and originating of the P1 segment. An anatomical variant replacing the inferolateral P2 perforators is the collicular artery (also known as the quadrigeminal or circumcollicular artery), coursing medially to the main P2 segment around the cerebral peduncle towards the collicular plate ((**D**–**F**); red dotted lines) and originating from the P1 or P2A segment. Its name is derived from the area of supply. An identical origin of the collicular artery and the artery of Percheron is possible (**E**,**F**), in which the nomenclature is defined by the territory of supply. The example case demonstrates the presence of a right P1 perforator aneurysm at the origin of the collicular artery and the artery of Percheron.

The incidence of aneurysms of the artery of Percheron and collicular artery is unknown and treatment outcomes are limited to case reports [13–16]. Retrospective cohort studies on PCA aneurysms lack both demographics and outcomes of perforator aneurysms [2] or mainly focus on perforator aneurysms of the basilar artery [16–18]. In this study, we review the incidence, clinical presentation, and treatment outcomes of P1-P2 perforator aneurysms and further discuss their anatomical characteristics. Further insight into the clinical outcomes and detailed anatomy could improve pattern recognition in daily practice and the treatment of this rare and underreported entity.

2. Methods

Following institutional ethics review board approval, we conducted a retrospective analysis of a prospectively collected cerebral aneurysm database at our institution, a tertiary referral center.

The database containing a list of patients with intracranial aneurysms who presented between January 2000 and January 2023 was manually searched (A.M.) for patients meeting the following criteria. Patients were included in this study if they were: (1) over 17 years of age, (2) diagnosed with a perforator aneurysm of the P1 or P2 segment of the posterior cerebral artery (3) presented or were treated between 2000 and 2023, and (4) had at least cross-sectional CTA and/or MRA imaging available. The identification of P1 or P2 segment aneurysms was made by first excluding the patients whose reports did not include a posterior circulation aneurysm. Following that, the list was narrowed to include only posterior circulation aneurysms, and all patients described to have basilar tip aneurysms were excluded. All images in the shortlist were reviewed by A.M. and E.J.H. to identify patients specifically with a P1 P2 perforator aneurysm.

Data on age, sex, clinical presentation, past medical history (including hypertension, smoking, family history, multiplicity of aneurysms), Modified Rankin Scale (mRS), treatment techniques, complications, and clinical outcomes were collected through a chart review.

Statistical analyses were performed to compare the characteristics of ruptured versus non-ruptured subgroups (Table 1). The results are presented as means for continuous variables and frequency (percentage) for categorical data. Data were analyzed using the *t*-test for continuous variables and Fisher's exact test to compare categorical data between groups. All *p*-values were two-sided, and a *p*-value of <0.05 was considered statistically significant. JMP Pro 15 (SASA Institute, Cary, NC, USA) was used for descriptive statistics.

Table 1. Subgroup analyses of P1-P2 perforator aneurysms.

P1-P2 Perforator Aneurysm	Total No	Treatment Group	Conservative Group	*p*-Value
No of cases	14	7 (50%)	7 (50%)	-
Age	59.5 (35–83)	61 (50–76)	54 (35–83)	0.3
Sex (female)	10 (71.4%)	5 (71.4%)	5 (71.4%)	>0.999
Smoking (current and past)	9 (69.2%)	4 (66.7%)	5 (71.4%)	0.66
Hypertension	8 (66.7%)	5 (83.3%)	3 (50%)	0.55
>1 cerebral aneurysm	8 (57.1%)	2 (28.6%)	6 (85.7%)	0.1
Ruptured	6 (42.9%)	6 (85.7%)	0 (0%)	<0.01
Maximum diameter (mm)	3 (1.5–8.5)	3.6 (1.5–8.5)	2.8 (2–3)	0.04
Outcomes				
Remnant after treatment	-	3 (42.9%)	NA	-
Permanent morbidity after treatment	-	0 (0%)	NA	-
Complications after treatment	-	2 (33.3%)	NA	

3. Results

3.1. Patients

Between 2000 and 2023, 2733 patients with a cerebral aneurysm presented to our institution. Of those, 14 patients (0.5%) had a perforator aneurysm of the P1 or P2 segment of the posterior cerebral artery (Table 2). The median age of these 14 patients was 59.5 years (range 35–83) and 10 (71%) were female. Nine patients (69.2%) had a history of smoking and 8 (66.7%) had a history of hypertension (in five patients it was controlled with medication). None of the patients had a known family history of cerebral aneurysms. Six patients (43%) with a P1 or P2 segment perforator aneurysm had a single cerebral aneurysm, including one with an arteriovenous malformation (AVM), and eight patients presented with more than one cerebral aneurysm.

Table 2. Characteristics of patients with a P1-P2 perforator aneurysm and treatment outcomes.

Patient	Ruptured/Unruptured	Year of Procedure or Presentation	Initial Presentation	Baseline mRS	Post Treatment-mRS	Total AA	Hypertension	Past History Smoking	Treatment Complications	Permanent Morbidity	Treatment of P1-P2 Aneurysm	Remnant	Treatment of Other Aneurysms
1	Unruptured	2003	Asymptomatic	0	NA	1	No	No	NA	None	None	NA	NA
2	Ruptured	2005	Symptomatic	0	0	1	Yes	Yes	No	None	Coiling	Yes *	NA
3	Unruptured (PCom Ruptured)	2005	Asymptomatic (Pcom symptomatic)	0	NA	3	Unknown	Yes	NA	None	None	NA	Coiling Pcom AA
4	Ruptured	2004	Symptomatic	Unknown	Unknown	1 AVM	Unknown	Unknown	Unknown	Unknown	Coiling	Yes *	NA
5	Ruptured	2007	Symptomatic			1	Yes–Tx	Yes	Acute perforator infarct in caudothalamic groove post coiling	Due to history of resected astrocytoma, radiation, hydrocephalus	Coiling followed by clipping	Yes	NA
6	Unruptured	2008	Asymptomatic	0	NA	3	Yes–Tx	Yes	NA	None	Clipping	No	Coiling basilar AA
7	Unruptured	2003	Asymptomatic	0	NA	3	No	Yes	NA	None	None	NA	Clipping MCA and anterior choroidal AA
8	Unruptured	2008	Asymptomatic	0	NA	3	Yes	Yes	NA	None	None	NA	Coiling ICA terminus AA
9	Ruptured	2014	Symptomatic	0	0	4	Yes–Tx	No	Acute infarct right thalamus	Due to cardiac arrest	Coiling	No	Coiling Pcom AA
10	Unruptured	2014	Asymptomatic	5	NA	2	No	No	NA	Due to MoyaMoya related ICH	None	NA	NA
11	Unruptured	2002	Asymptomatic	0	NA	2	Yes–Tx	Yes	NA	No	None	NA	NA
12	Unruptured (Ruptured ACA)	1997	Asymptomatic (Symptomatic ACA)	0	NA	3	Yes–Tx	Yes	NA	None	None	NA	Clipping ACA AA
13	Ruptured	2023	Symptomatic	0	0	1	No	No	No	None	Coiling	No	NA
14	Ruptured	2022	Symptomatic	0	0	1	Yes	Yes	No	None	Coiling	No	NA

* Remnant without indication for retreatment. Abbreviations: AA arterial aneurysm; NA not applicable; Tx treatment.

3.2. *Treatment Modalities and Clinical Outcome*

Six of the P1-P2 perforator aneurysm patients (43%) presented with a rupture, and eight patients (57%) had an unruptured P1-P2 perforator aneurysm. The average diameter of the P1-P2 perforator aneurysms was 3 mm (range 1.5–8.5). In our institution, unruptured posterior circulation aneurysms (including P1-P2 perforator aneurysms) are treated after a multidisciplinary discussion of each individual case, reviewing the size (generally at least 4–5 mm to consider treatment), risk factors (hypertension, smoking, family history, previous SAH, PHACES score), age, and comorbidities. Nowadays, endovascular therapy is the first choice for basilar tip and proximal PCA aneurysms, provided it is technically safe and feasible, with stable arterial access. All six ruptured P1-P2 perforator aneurysms were treated with endovascular coiling, with one requiring surgical clipping of a recurrence during follow-up. Following the multidisciplinary discussion, one unruptured wide-necked P1-P2 aneurysm (patient no 6) was treated with uncomplicated surgical clipping, given its size (4 × 3.5 mm). The remainder of the unruptured aneurysms were treated conservatively. Out of the six acute endovascular coiling cases, two patients suffered from silent perforator infarcts (Table 2: patient no 5 and 9). Patient no 5 had a past medical history of astrocytoma resection, radiation, and hydrocephalus treated with VP-drains and demonstrated an asymptomatic small acute infarct in the left ventral thalamus on day 4 MRI of the brain after endovascular coiling. Patient no 9 presented with a subarachnoid hemorrhage and mild left-sided drift, remaining stable after endovascular coiling, with an acute infarct in the right ventral thalamus on day 10 MRI of the brain. The patient suffered an acute respiratory decompensation due to pulmonary edema on postprocedural day 2 and cardiac arrest on day 4 and was discharged to a long-term care facility on day 90. All patients treated within the last 10 years (patient no. 9, 13, 14) had an immediate post-treatment mRS of 0. Patient no. 9 suffered from a respiratory-related cardiac arrest during hospital admission. Patient no. 10, without aneurysm closure treatment, was wheelchair-bound secondary to a prior moyamoya-related hemorrhage, and the remaining six patients were asymptomatic.

4. Discussion

The main findings of our study are: (1) P1-P2 perforator aneurysms are rare, with an incidence of 0.5% in a large single-center cerebral aneurysm cohort, (2) the technical results of endovascular coiling were good, with one case requiring retreatment, (3) endovascular coiling resulted in perforator infarcts in two patients; however, without new permanent morbidity secondary to treatment.

Compared to perforator aneurysms of the proximal anterior cerebral artery (A1 segment) [19,20], the horizontal segment of the middle cerebral artery (M1 segment) [21] and the basilar artery [17], P1-P2 perforator aneurysms have been less frequently reported on. Aneurysms of the A1 segment account for approximately 1% of all cerebral aneurysms and are associated with treatment-related complications exceeding 15% [19,20]. M1 aneurysms are associated with postprocedural infarcts in up to 22% of cases, a mortality rate of approximately 6% [21], and are often associated with hypertension, moyamoya disease, and AVMs. Chau et al. reported treatment-related complications in 17% of basilar artery perforator aneurysms [22]. As such, one may conclude that perforator aneurysms in any given location are associated with a moderate to high risk of ischemic complications due to treatment.

From a neuroanatomical point of view, recognizing the relationship with a perforator artery is important to reduce the complication risks in P1-P2 perforator aneurysm treatment. Features of this subtype of aneurysm are: (1) its off-midline position in relation to the basilar tip (2) its posterior or posterior medial angulation of the aneurysm dome in relation to the P1 or P2 segment, respectively, (3) the origin of a (dominant) perforator trunk juxtaposed to or at the neck of the aneurysm, as opposed to an infundibulum with a perforator at the tip of the conus, (4) stasis of contrast in the aneurysm dome observed in ruptured cases on angiography (Figure 2). Special consideration should be given to the presence of tuberothalamic arteries, a dominant paramedian artery (the artery of Percheron), and the collicular artery (Figure 1) [12]. The tuburothalamic arteries (TTAs) originate from the middle third of the PcomA and classically supply the ventral thalamus. The paramedian P1 arteries supply the medial thalamus and/or rostral midbrain and may supply the anterior thalamus when the TTA is hypoplastic. The inferolateral perforators or geniculate P2 perforators supply the lateral thalamus and inferolateral pulvinar. Both the artery of Percheron and the collicular artery can have an identical origin, in which the nomenclature is defined by the supplied territory (Figure 2). Thus, the collicular artery may originate from the P1 segment, with perforators branching extensively from the mesencephalon to the midbrain, varying among individuals [23].

Limited case reports on P1-P2 perforator artery aneurysm treatment exist (Table 3). Sparacia et al., 2018 described a ruptured aneurysm of the artery of Percheron treated with flow diversion resulting in closure of the aneurysm and occlusion of the artery of Percheron, with secondary bilateral paramedian thalamic infarcts [14]. Oishi et al., 2016 reported on two large P1 aneurysms in close relationship to the artery of Percheron, treated with parent vessel occlusion, resulting in extensive paramedian artery occlusion in one secondary to occlusion of the artery of Percheron [13]. Given the results of the present study and prior case reports, endovascular treatment with (balloon-assisted) coiling, if technically feasible, could represent a viable and preferred treatment of P1-P2 perforator aneurysms. The treatment of a perforator aneurysm inherently poses a risk of a perforator infarct. Risk reduction measures could be an undercoiling technique if technically feasible (i.e., selectively coiling the dome and rupture point and undercoiling of the neck and origin of the perforator), coiling under full heparinization, and/or starting low dose aspirin following endovascular treatment. Surgical clipping is challenging, given the presence of a perforating artery adherent to the neck of the aneurysm [24,25]. Furthermore, clipping in this region poses challenges due to the deep location near cranial nerves, increasing the risk of complications in a restricted surgical field [26,27]. Consequently, treatment strategies differ from those employed for M1 aneurysms [21]. Moreover, trapping and bypass procedures, commonly used for more distal PCA aneurysms, are not suitable. While FD has been considered beneficial [4], reports of FD for posterior circulation indicate a risk of perforator vessel infarction of approximately 7%, along with a high mortality rate [8], raising safety concerns, particularly in the acute phase of a subarachnoid hemorrhage.

Table 3. Literature on P1-P2 perforator aneurysms.

Author	Year	No. of Patients	Age	Aneurysm Description	Treatment	Technique	Complication	Clinical Outcome
Da Ros et al. [16]	2020	1	Unknown	P1 aneurysm	Endovascular	Flow diversion	None	mRS 0
Sparacia et al. [14]	2018	1	48	Artery of Percheron aneurysm	Endovascular	Flow diversion	Bilateral paramedian thalamic infarcts	Hydrocephalus Discharge to rehab
Giordan et al. [15]	2018	1	47	Pseudoaneurysm P1 perforator	DSA only	NA	None	Bilateral third nerve palsy
Oishi et al. [13].	2016	2	49	P1-P2 aneurysm	Endovascular	Parent vessel occlusion	None	Unchanged
			54	P1 aneurysm	Endovascular	Parent vessel occlusion	Extensive thalamic infarction	Decline post treatment to MRS 3 (pretreatment MRS 0)

Limitations of our study are associated to the retrospective nature of this single-center series with insufficient case numbers for proper statistics. Furthermore, due to the long inclusion period of this study, we were unable to obtain comprehensive clinical data on each patient. Lastly, the primary treatment strategy of basilar tip and P1-P2 aneurysms has shifted since the nineties from primary surgical clipping toward a primary endovascular treatment strategy due to the deep location in the brain with a restricted surgical field, as previously mentioned, as well as the evolution of endovascular therapy, with improved access and materials, such as microcatheters and microcoils. The number of coiling versus clipping patients is unequally distributed in our study, and the cases with perforator infarcts were treated in 2007 and 2014. Therefore, it is difficult to postulate whether a shift in treatment strategy and/or improvements in technology have had an influence.

To the best of our knowledge, this is the first retrospective cohort study on patients with a ruptured or unruptured P1-P2 perforator aneurysm addressing clinical outcomes, technical aspects of treatment modalities, and further pointing out anatomical details that could improve pattern recognition and the treatment of this rare entity.

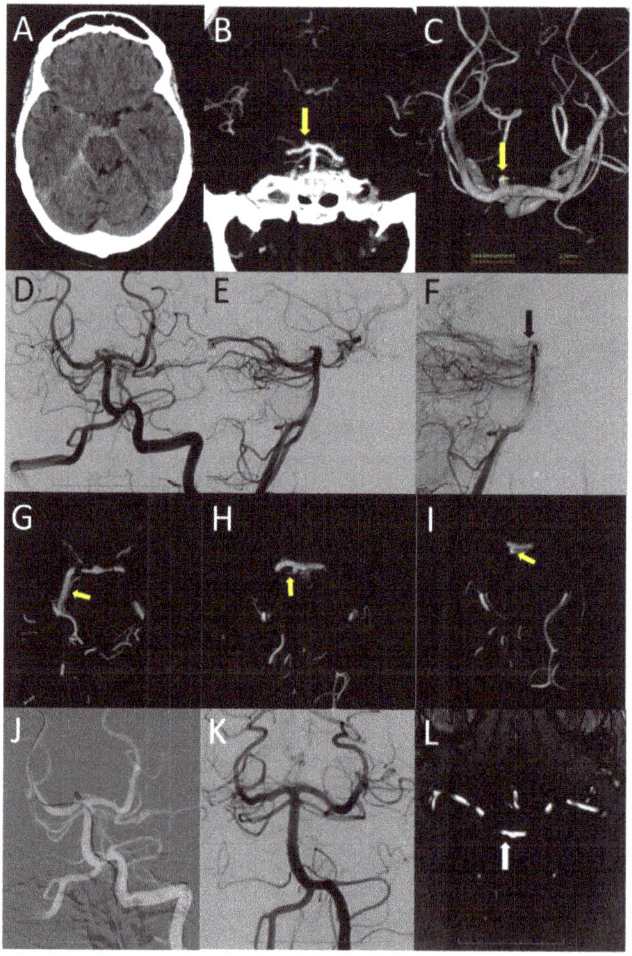

Figure 2. Case no 13 involves a 64-year-old female patient with a subarachnoid hemorrhage (GCS 15, WFNS 1) with the epicenter in the right interpeduncular cistern (**A**), with suspicion of a small superiorly and posteriorly pointing right P1 aneurysm ((**B**,**C**); yellow arrow). AP (**D**) and lateral left

vertebral artery injections (**E**,**F**) confirm a right P1 aneurysm, with stases of contrast in the dome in the late arterial phase ((**F**); black arrow). Axial Xpert CT angiography reconstructions demonstrate the course of the right collicular artery in the crural and ambient cisterns along the posterior cerebral artery ((**G**–**I**); yellow arrows) originating medially from the dome of the aneurysm ((**I**); yellow arrow). An unassisted coiling with balloon presence was performed with two coils (**J**) resulting in direct (**K**) and one-year follow-up closure of the aneurysm on MRA time-of-flight (**L**). There is subtle indentation of the coil mass in the parent artery ((**L**); white arrow).

5. Conclusions

P1-P2 perforator aneurysms are rare and require careful management due to their propensity for ischemic complications. Endovascular coiling could present an effective treatment modality; however, care should be taken for ischemic complications in the dependent perforator territory. Larger studies are required to provide deeper insight.

Author Contributions: Design: E.J.H. Data collection: A.M. and S.M. Writing and figure preparation: A.M., S.M. and E.J.H. prepared the initial draft of the manuscript and figures; all authors re-viewed and edited the manuscript and approved the submitted version. Study supervision: E.J.H. All authors have read and agreed to the published version of the manuscript.

Funding: EJH: PRM: TK thank UMIT (https://universitymedicalimagingtoronto.ca/ accessed on 13 September 2024) for their kind support.

Institutional Review Board Statement: This study was approved by Toronto University REB, Approval no ID: 23-5084 (approved 9 March 2024).

Informed Consent Statement: Informed consent was waived owing to the retrospective nature of this study.

Data Availability Statement: The authors confirm that the data supporting the findings of this study are available within the article.

Conflicts of Interest: EJH is a consultant for Medtronic.

Abbreviations

Posterior cerebral artery (PCA), parent vessel occlusion (PVO), reconstructive endovascular treatment (rEVT), arteriovenous malformation (AVM), posterior communicating artery (PcomA), flow diversion (FD), tuberothalamic artery (TTA)

References

1. Sturiale, C.L.; De Waure, C.; Della Pepa, G.M.; Calabro, G.E.; Albanese, A.; D'Argento, F.; Fernandez, E.; Olivi, A.; Puca, A.; Pedicelli, A. Endovascular Treatment of the Posterior Cerebral Artery Aneurysms: Single-Center Experience and a Systematic Review. *World Neurosurg.* **2016**, *91*, 154–162. [CrossRef] [PubMed]
2. Goehre, F.; Jahromi, B.R.; Hernesniemi, J.; Elsharkawy, A.; Kivisaari, R.; von Und Zu Fraunberg, M.; Jääskeläinen, J.; Lehto, H.; Lehecka, M. Characteristics of posterior cerebral artery aneurysms: An angiographic analysis of 93 aneurysms in 81 patients. *Neurosurgery* **2014**, *75*, 134–144. [CrossRef] [PubMed]
3. Essibayi, M.A.; Oushy, S.H.; Keser, Z.; Lanzino, G. Natural history and management of posterior cerebral artery aneurysms: A systematic review and meta-analysis of individual patient data. *Neurosurg. Rev.* **2022**, *45*, 3595–3608. [CrossRef] [PubMed]
4. MacLean, M.A.; Huynh, T.J.; Schmidt, M.H.; Pereira, V.M.; Weeks, A. Competitive flow diversion of multiple P1 aneurysms: Proposed classification. *BMJ Case Rep.* **2020**, *13*, e015581. [CrossRef] [PubMed]
5. Qin, X.; Xu, F.; Maimaiti, Y.; Zheng, Y.; Xu, B.; Leng, B.; Chen, G. Endovascular treatment of posterior cerebral artery aneurysms: A single center's experience of 55 cases. *J. Neurosurg.* **2017**, *126*, 1094–1105. [CrossRef]
6. Hong, C.-E.; Oh, H.S.; Bae, J.W.; Kim, K.M.; Yoo, D.H.; Kang, H.-S.; Cho, Y.D. Endovascular Treatment in Precommunicating Segment Aneurysms of Posterior Cerebral Artery. *World Neurosurg.* **2024**, *182*, e602–e610. [CrossRef]
7. Ota, T.; Komiyama, M. Cephalic/cardiac neural crest cell and moyamoya disease. *Neuroradiol. J.* **2021**, *34*, 529–533. [CrossRef] [PubMed]
8. Wang, C.-B.; Shi, W.-W.; Zhang, G.-X.; Lu, H.-C.; Ma, J. Flow diverter treatment of posterior circulation aneurysms. A meta-analysis. *Neuroradiology* **2016**, *58*, 391–400. [CrossRef]

9. Ciceri, E.F.; Klucznik, R.P.; Grossman, R.G.; Rose, J.E.; Mawad, M.E. Aneurysms of the posterior cerebral artery: Classification and endovascular treatment. *Am. J. Neuroradiol.* **2001**, *22*, 27–34.
10. Elster, A.D.; Richardson, D.N. Focal high signal on MR scans of the midbrain caused by enlarged perivascular spaces: MR-pathologic correlation. *AJR Am. J. Roentgenol.* **1991**, *156*, 157–160. [CrossRef]
11. Schmahmann, J.D. Vascular syndromes of the thalamus. *Stroke* **2003**, *34*, 2264–2278. [CrossRef] [PubMed]
12. Krings, T.; Geibprasert, S.; Cruz, J.P.; Terbrugge, K.G. Neurovascular Anatomy in Interventional Neuroradiology. In *Neurovascular Anatomy in Interventional Neuroradiology*; Georg Thieme Verlag KG: New York, NY, USA, 2015. Available online: http://www.thieme-connect.de/products/ebooks/lookinside/10.1055/b-0035-129450 (accessed on 5 June 2015).
13. Oishi, H.; Tanoue, S.; Teranishi, K.; Hasegawa, H.; Nonaka, S.; Magami, S.; Yamamoto, M.; Arai, H. Endovascular parent artery occlusion of proximal posterior cerebral artery aneurysms: A report of two cases. *J. Neurointerv. Surg.* **2016**, *8*, 591–593. [CrossRef] [PubMed]
14. Sparacia, G.; Agnello, F.; Midiri, M.; Iaia, A. A rare case of ruptured aneurysm of the paramedian artery of Percheron. *Interv. Neuroradiol.* **2018**, *24*, 509–512. [CrossRef] [PubMed]
15. Giordan, E.; Rabinstein, A.A.; Cloft, H.J.; Lanzino, G. Teaching NeuroImages: Rupture and spontaneous resolution of a P1 perforator pseudoaneurysm. *Neurology* **2018**, *90*, S138–S139. [CrossRef]
16. Da Ros, V.; Diana, F.; Sabuzi, F.; Malatesta, E.; Sanna, A.; Scaggiante, J.; Di Giuliano, F.; Gandini, R.; Floris, R.; Ruggiero, M. Flow diverters for ruptured posterior circulation perforator aneurysms: Multicenter experience and literature review. *J. Neurointerv. Surg.* **2020**, *12*, 688–694. [CrossRef]
17. Ding, D.; Starke, R.M.; E Jensen, M.; Evans, A.J.; Kassell, N.F.; Liu, K.C. Perforator aneurysms of the posterior circulation: Case series and review of the literature. *J. Neurointerv. Surg.* **2013**, *5*, 546–551. [CrossRef] [PubMed]
18. Buell, T.J.; Ding, D.; Raper, D.M.S.; Chen, C.-J.; Hixson, H.R.; Crowley, R.W.; Evans, A.J.; E Jensen, M.; Liu, K.C. Posterior circulation perforator aneurysms: A proposed management algorithm. *J. Neurointerv. Surg.* **2018**, *10*, 55–59. [CrossRef] [PubMed]
19. Chang, H.W.; Youn, S.W.; Jung, C.; Kang, H.-S.; Sohn, C.H.; Kwon, B.J.; Han, M.H. Technical strategy in endovascular treatment of proximal anterior cerebral artery aneurysms. *Acta Neurochir.* **2011**, *153*, 279–285. [CrossRef]
20. Hou, K.; Li, G.; Guo, Y.; Yu, J. Endovascular treatment for aneurysms at the A1 segment of the anterior cerebral artery: Current difficulties and solutions. *Acta Neurol. Belg.* **2021**, *121*, 55–69. [CrossRef]
21. Vargas, J.; Walsh, K.; Turner, R.; Chaudry, I.; Turk, A.; Spiotta, A. Lenticulostriate aneurysms: A case series and review of the literature. *J. Neurointerv. Surg.* **2015**, *7*, 194–201. [CrossRef]
22. Chau, Y.; Sachet, M.; Sédat, J. Should we treat aneurysms in perforator arteries from the basilar trunk? Review of 49 cases published in the literature and presentation of three personal cases. *Interv. Neuroradiol.* **2018**, *24*, 22–28. [CrossRef] [PubMed]
23. O'Reilly, S.T.; Krings, T. Medial Tentorial Meningeal Supply from the Collicular Artery: Anatomy and Endovascular Implications. *Clin. Neuroradiol.* **2023**, *33*, 555–559. [CrossRef] [PubMed]
24. Spiessberger, A.; Strange, F.; Fandino, J.; Marbacher, S. Microsurgical Clipping of Basilar Apex Aneurysms: A Systematic Historical Review of Approaches and their Results. *World Neurosurg.* **2018**, *114*, 305–316. [CrossRef] [PubMed]
25. Li, J.; Azarhomayoun, A.; Nouri, M.; Sakarunchai, I.; Yamada, Y.; Yamashiro, K.; Kato, Y. Surgical Approaches to Basilar Apex Aneurysms: An Illustrative Review. *Asian J. Neurosurg.* **2020**, *15*, 272–277. [CrossRef] [PubMed]
26. Honda, M.; Tsutsumi, K.; Yokoyama, H.; Yonekura, M.; Nagata, I. Aneurysms of the posterior cerebral artery: Retrospective review of surgical treatment. *Neurol. Med. Chir.* **2004**, *44*, 164–169. [CrossRef]
27. Hamada, J.-I.; Morioka, M.; Yano, S.; Todaka, T.; Kai, Y.; Kuratsu, J.-I. Clinical features of aneurysms of the posterior cerebral artery: A 15-year experience with 21 cases. *Neurosurgery* **2005**, *56*, 662–670. [CrossRef]

brain sciences

MDPI

Article

Single-Stage Endovascular Management of Concurrent Intracranial Aneurysms and Arterial Stenoses: Clinical Outcomes, Procedural Strategies, and Predictive Factors

Marat Sarshayev [1], Shayakhmet Makhanbetkhan [1], Aiman Maidan [2,*], Roger Barranco Pons [3], Dimash Davletov [4], Abzal Zhumabekov [1] and Mynzhylky Berdikhojayev [1]

1 National Hospital of the Medical Center of the Presidental Affairs Administration of the Republic of Kazakhstan, Almaty 050060, Kazakhstan; sarshayev_m@snh.kz (M.S.); makhanbetkhan_sh@snh.kz (S.M.); zhumabekov_ash@snh.kz (A.Z.); mynzhyl@gmail.com (M.B.)
2 National Centre for Neurosurgery, Astana 010000, Kazakhstan
3 Al Qassimi Hospital, Dubai 25314, United Arab Emirates; rogerbarrancopons@gmail.com
4 Atchabarov Scientific-Research Institute of Fundamental and Applied Medicine, Asfendiyarov Kazakh National Medical University, Almaty 050000, Kazakhstan; davletovdimash@gmail.com
* Correspondence: maidanaiman@gmail.com; Tel.: +7-701-1110825

Abstract

Background: The coexistence of extracranial arterial stenoses and intracranial aneurysms presents a unique clinical dilemma. While staged interventions are traditionally preferred to reduce procedural risks, recent advances have enabled single-stage endovascular treatment. This study evaluates the clinical outcomes, procedural strategies, and predictive factors associated with such combined interventions. Methods: This retrospective study included 47 patients treated with single-stage endovascular procedures for concurrent extracranial stenosis and intracranial aneurysm between 2016 and 2024. Clinical, angiographic, and procedural data were collected. Outcomes were assessed using the mmodified Rankin Scale (mRS), and statistical analyses were performed to identify associations between clinical variables and functional outcomes. Results: Of the 47 patients, 85.1% achieved favorable outcomes (mRS 0–2) at ≥6-month follow-up. The most commonly treated arteries were the internal carotid artery (70.2%) and the middle cerebral artery (34%). Stent-assisted coiling or flow diversion was performed in 93.6% of aneurysm cases, while 91.5% underwent carotid or vertebral stenting. Lesion laterality (left-sided aneurysms, $p = 0.019$) and stenosis length ($p = 0.0469$) were significantly associated with outcomes. Smoking was linked to multiple stenoses ($p = 0.0191$). Two patients experienced major complications: one aneurysmal rebleed after stenting, and one intraoperative rupture. Conclusions: Single-stage endovascular treatment for patients with concurrent extracranial stenosis and intracranial aneurysm is technically feasible and clinically effective in selected cases. Lesion configuration, anatomical considerations, and individualized planning are critical in optimizing outcomes.

Keywords: intracranial aneurysm; carotid artery stenosis; vertebral artery stenosis; endovascular treatment; single-stage intervention; subarachnoid hemorrhage; modified Rankin Scale; smoking; neurointervention; stroke prevention

1. Introduction

The coexistence of extracranial arterial stenosis and intracranial aneurysm presents a complex therapeutic challenge. Historically, these lesions have been addressed separately, typically beginning with carotid endarterectomy or stenting, followed by delayed aneurysm treatment. However, this sequential approach can result in delays, increased procedural burden, and the risk of aneurysm rupture due to hemodynamic changes following revascularization [1–5].

In the era of modern endovascular techniques, single-stage interventions have emerged as a feasible and potentially safer option for selected patients. This strategy not only minimizes anesthesia exposure and hospital stay but also offers a streamlined solution for resource-limited settings, where repeated access procedures are economically burdensome [6–9].

Despite the increasing application of this approach, there is limited literature addressing patient selection, procedural sequencing, and outcome predictors in such cases. Concerns remain regarding the optimal order of intervention—whether to treat the stenosis first to improve access and reduce ischemic risk, or to secure the aneurysm first to prevent hemorrhagic complications exacerbated by reperfusion [10–13]. Additionally, few studies systematically evaluate the influence of anatomical configuration (ipsilateral vs. contralateral lesions), lesion length, or hemodynamic factors on functional recovery.

This study aims to assess the safety, feasibility, and clinical outcomes of single-stage endovascular treatment in patients with coexisting extracranial stenosis and intracranial aneurysms. We also propose a treatment algorithm based on real-world decision making and lesion-specific characteristics, contributing practical insights for individualized care planning.

2. Materials and Methods

This retrospective study was conducted at the National Hospital of the Medical Center of the Presidential Affairs Administration of the Republic of Kazakhstan in Almaty, Kazakhstan, and included patients treated between January 2016 and December 2024. Eligible patients had coexisting intracranial aneurysms and extracranial arterial stenoses (internal carotid artery [ICA] or vertebral artery [VA]) and underwent single-stage endovascular treatment.

2.1. Inclusion Criteria Were

- Age $\geq$ 18 years.
- Confirmed $\geq$70% extracranial ICA or VA stenosis based on digital subtraction angiography (DSA), CTA, or MRA, evaluated using NASCET criteria.
- At least one saccular or fusiform intracranial aneurysm identified via CTA or DSA.
- Either symptomatic ischemia (e.g., TIA, infarct on DWI) or aneurysm-related symptoms (e.g., headache, SAH).
- Available pre- and post-procedural imaging and clinical records.

Patients with previous intracranial or extracranial interventions, contraindications to dual antiplatelet therapy, or incomplete follow-up were excluded.

2.2. Imaging and Decision Protocol

Pre-treatment imaging included brain MRI with DWI to assess ischemic burden and CTA or DSA to evaluate aneurysm morphology, perfusion patterns, and vessel patency. The decision to treat both lesions in one session was made by a multidisciplinary neurovascular team. In patients with contralateral lesions or ruptured aneurysms, treatment sequencing was individualized. When perfusion through the stenotic segment was severely compromised, revascularization was prioritized. In other cases, aneurysm embolization preceded stenting to minimize rupture risk.

2.3. Procedure

The protocol has remained consistent since 2016; slight updates were implemented in 2020 after the introduction of newer stents. Endovascular procedures were performed under general or local anesthesia using transfemoral access. Aneurysms were treated via coiling, stent-assisted coiling, or flow diversion. Arterial stenoses were treated with balloon angioplasty and/or stenting. In all ICA cases, distal embolic protection devices were employed. Device selection was based on anatomical characteristics and operator preference.

2.4. Periprocedural Management

All patients without subarachnoid hemorrhage (SAH) received dual antiplatelet therapy (aspirin and clopidogrel) at least 5 days before the procedure. In SAH cases, DAPT initiation was delayed or minimized based on hemorrhage severity and urgency of intervention. Intravenous heparin was administered intraoperatively. Postprocedural antiplatelet regimens were adjusted per stent type and patient risk profile.

2.5. Data Collection and Outcomes

Demographic, clinical, radiological, and procedural data were retrospectively collected from electronic health records and imaging archives. Variables included age, sex, comorbidities (hypertension, diabetes, ischemic heart disease, smoking status), aneurysm characteristics (location, size, rupture status), and stenosis features (side, degree, length, symptomatic status).

Procedural details such as stent type, access route, and sequence of interventions were also documented. Modified Rankin Scale (mRS) scores were assessed at baseline and at follow-up by an independent neurologist. The PHASES score was used for aneurysm risk stratification. The primary outcome was a favorable functional outcome at last follow-up, defined as mRS 0–2. Secondary outcomes included periprocedural complications, 30-day mortality, and 30-day re-admission. Complications were categorized as hemorrhagic, ischemic, or technical.

2.6. Statistical Analysis

Descriptive statistics were used for baseline data. Associations between clinical variables and multiple stenoses or aneurysms were assessed using Fisher's exact test. Logistic regression was employed to evaluate the association between smoking and multiple stenoses. The relationship between anatomical factors (e.g., lesion laterality, stenosis length) and functional outcome (mRS 1–2 vs. mRS 3–6) was also tested. A p-value < 0.05 was considered statistically significant. Analyses were performed using SPSS v26 (IBM Corp., Armonk, NY, USA). Regression analysis was used for exploratory purposes; findings should be interpreted cautiously due to small sample size.

2.7. Ethics Statement

This study was approved by the Institutional Ethics Committee (approval #7, dated 12 December 2024). Patient data were anonymized in compliance with the Declaration of Helsinki.

3. Results

A total of 47 patients (mean age: 67.6 $\pm$ 5.9 years; 21 males [44.7%], 26 females [55.3%]) were included. Most patients (95.7%) underwent elective procedures; only two patients (4.3%) presented with ruptured aneurysms requiring urgent intervention. Common presenting symptoms included headache (38.3%), ischemic stroke-related deficits (44.7%), and sensorineural symptoms such as hearing loss (4.3%). One patient presented with Millard–Gubler syndrome.

3.1. Patient Characteristics and Vascular Lesion Profile

In total, 17 patients (36.2%) were active smokers, 11 (23.4%) had diabetes mellitus, and 38 (80.9%) had stage 3 arterial hypertension. Ischemic heart disease was present in 34 patients (72.3%). Aneurysms were most frequently located in the middle cerebral artery (MCA), anterior cerebral artery (ACA), and intracranial ICA segments. The majority of stenoses involved the cervical ICA (57.4%) and vertebral artery (23.4%). Ipsilateral aneurysm–stenosis pairs were observed in 29 patients (61.7%). Patient characteristics can be seen in Table 1.

3.2. Risk Factors and Lesion Characteristics

Smoking was significantly associated with the presence of multiple stenoses (75.0% in smokers vs. 25.0% in non-smokers; $p = 0.0191$, OR = 0.131; 95% CI: 0.023–0.750). Logistic regression confirmed this association, with an odds ratio (OR) of 0.131 (95% CI: 0.023–0.750), indicating that non-smokers were significantly less likely to have multiple stenotic lesions. Other vascular risk factors, including hypertension, diabetes, ischemic heart disease, and obesity, showed no significant association with either multiple stenoses or multiple aneurysms ($p > 0.05$ for all; Table 2).

3.3. Treatment Strategy

The procedural strategy was tailored based on anatomical configuration and clinical presentation. Most cases involved flow diversion or stent-assisted coiling for aneurysm treatment, followed by angioplasty and carotid or vertebral artery stenting. In cases with high-grade ICA stenosis impeding microcatheter navigation, stenting was performed first. In morphologically unstable aneurysms (e.g., wide-neck or high-flow lesions), embolization was prioritized. Dual antiplatelet therapy was used in all elective cases pre- and post-procedurally. No elective patient experienced a deterioration in clinical status postoperatively.

Common devices included Protege (n = 17), ULTIMASTER (n = 8), and CASPER (n = 2). No ischemic periprocedural events were recorded.

3.4. Functional Outcomes and Predictive Factors

At the final follow-up (≥6 months), favorable outcomes (defined as mRS 0–2) were observed in 40 of 47 patients (85.1%). Modified Rankin Scale scores remained stable across the follow-up period for all patients, with no evidence of neurological deterioration. Among the cohort, seven patients (14.9%) had mRS scores of 3–5, indicating moderate to severe disability. No patient experienced mortality or re-admission within 30 days post-procedure.

Notably, left-sided aneurysms were significantly associated with favorable outcomes; all 14 patients with left-sided lesions achieved mRS scores of 1–2 ($p = 0.019$). However, no significant associations were found between outcome and aneurysm-bearing artery ($p = 0.0761$), side of extracranial stenosis ($p = 0.7017$), type of stenotic artery ($p = 0.9497$), or ipsilateral versus contralateral lesion configuration ($p = 0.3108$) (Table 3).

Table 1. Patient Characteristics and Treatment Details for Concurrent Intracranial Aneurysms and Arterial Stenoses.

Patient #	Age	Gender	Presenting Symptoms	Aneurysm (#) and Localization	Stenosis Localization	Ipsilateral Lesion?	Aneurysm Size	Stenosis Length	Stenosis Degree	Stents Used	mRS Before	mRS FU
1	67	m	Persistent headache	(2) A1 left, right MCA bif	M2 left	Yes	Small	20 mm	70%	Ultimaster 3.5× 9;	2	2
2	70	m	Left cerebellar stroke, persistent headache, sensorineural hearing loss	(1) A1 left	V1 left, Left ICA supraclinoid	Yes	Small	15 mm	80%	Destiny 3.0 × 15	1	1
3	75	m	Persistent headache	(1) Right ICA, supraclinoid	V1 right	Yes	Small	15 mm	70%	Ultimaster 3.5 × 9;	2	2
4	72	m	Persistent headache	(1) Right MCA bif	V1 left, V1 right	Yes	Small	30 mm	70%	Ultimaster Nagomi 2.5 × 12; Orsiro 3.5 × 26	1	1
5	65	f	Right frontal and parietal strokes with left-sided hemiparesis	(1) Right MCA bif	Left MCA bif	No	Small	15 mm	70%	LVIS EVO 3.0 × 18	3	3
6	65	m	Left occipital stroke	(1) Right ICA, ophthalmic	V1 left	No	Small	10 mm	70%	Ultimaster 4.0 × 9;	1	1
7	45	f	Persistent headache	(1) Right ICA, supraclinoid	Right ICA, cervical	Yes	Medium	35 mm	80%	X.ACT 8-6 × 30; Carotid WALLSTENT 7–30 × 135	1	1
8	40	f	Persistent headache	(2) Right ICA, supraclinoid, Left ICA ophthalmic	Left ICA supraclinoid	Yes	Small	20 mm	70%	pEGASUS 4.5 × 20	1	1
9	72	f	Persistent headache	(1) Left ICA, communicant	BA	N/A	Small	20 mm	80%	CREDO 5.0 × 20	1	1
10	60	m	Persistent headache	(2) Left M2, left ICA supraclinoid	Right ICA, supraclinoid, cavernous	No	Small	30 mm	80%	Credo 5.0 × 25; Ultimaster 4.0 × 12	2	2
11	69	m	Right frontal and parietal strokes with left-sided hemiparesis	(1) Right ICA, cavernous	Right ICA, supraclinoid	Yes	Small	20 mm	70%	CREDO 4.0 × 20	2	2
12	57	m	Persistent headache	(2) Left ICA, communicant, Left MCA bif	Left ICA, cervical	Yes	Medium	40 mm	99%	X.ACT 10-10 × 30 CASPER 9 × 20 × 143	2	2
13	38	m	Right cerebellar stroke	(1) Left MCA bif	V1 right	No	Small	20 mm	80%	Ultimaster 3.5 × 12	2	1

Table 1. *Cont.*

Patient #	Age	Gender	Presenting Symptoms	Aneurysm (#) and Localization	Stenosis Localization	Ipsilateral Lesion?	Aneurysm Size	Stenosis Length	Stenosis Degree	Stents Used	mRS Before	mRS FU
14	64	f	Left frontal stroke with right-sided hemiparesis	(1) Left MCA bif	Left M2	Yes	Small	20 mm	99%	CREDO 4.0 × 20	2	2
15	60	f	Persistent headache	(1) Right ICA, communicant	Right ICA supraclinoid	Yes	Small	25 mm	75%	CASPER 7 × 30 × 143	1	1
16	43	m	Ruptured aneurysm, left-sided hemiparesis	(3) Right MCA bif, left MCA bif, left ICA choroidal	V1 left, left ICA cervical, right ICA, cervical	Yes	Medium	50 mm	99%	Ultimaster 2.75–9; BioMatrix 3.5 × 9; Wallaby 3.0 × 40; Wallaby 2.5 × 40	3	3
17	56	f	Persistent headache, sensorineural hearing loss	(1) Left MCA bif	Left ICA cervical, right ICA, cervical	Yes	Medium	40 mm	75%	CGuard 10 × 40; CGuard 9 × 30; LEO 2.5 × 25	1	1
18	59	m	Ruptured aneurysm, right parietal strokes, left-sided hemiparesis	(1) BA fusiform	Right ICA, cervical	N/A	Fusiform	25 mm	80%	Mozec 4.5 × 23; CGuard 9 × 40; LEO + 4.5 × 75	3	3
19	68	f	Persistent headache	(1) Right ICA, supraclinoid	V1 left	No	Small	10 mm	90%	Ultimaster Terumo 4.0 × 9.0	1	1
20	57	f	Left temporal stroke	(1) Left MCA bif	Left M1-M2	Yes	Medium	20 mm	70%	Acclino flex 5.0 × 20	2	2
21	66	m	Left frontal stroke	(1) Right MCA bif	Left ICA, cervical	No	Medium	30 mm	70%	Protege 8 × 6–30	1	1
22	64	f	Persistent headache	(1) Right M1	Right ICA, cervical	Yes	Small	30 mm	70%	Protege 8 × 6–30	1	1
23	69	m	Left frontal stroke with right-sided hemiparesis	(1) BA bif	Left ICA, cervical	N/A	Small	30 mm	85%	Protege 8 × 6–30	3	3
24	59	f	Right occipital, cerebellar, and basal ganglia strokes	(1) Acom	V1 Right	N/A	Small	30 mm	95%	AclinoFlex 3.0 × 15	4	4
25	69	m	Right frontal stroke	(1) Left MCA bif	Right ICA cervical	No	Small	40 mm	80%	Protege 8 × 6–40	2	2
26	66	m	Ruptured aneurysm	(1) Left MCA bif	Right ICA supraclinoid	No	Small	30 mm	85%	Protege 8 × 6–30	2	2
27	58	f	Persistent headache	(1) Right ICA supraclinoid	Left ICA, cervical	No	Small	30 mm	80%	Protege 7 × 10–30	2	2

Table 1. *Cont.*

Patient #	Age	Gender	Presenting Symptoms	Aneurysm (#) and Localization	Stenosis Localization	Ipsilateral Lesion?	Aneurysm Size	Stenosis Length	Stenosis Degree	Stents Used	mRS Before	mRS FU
28	61	m	Left occipital and cerebellar strokes	(1) Right M2	V1 Left	No	Small	30 mm	80%	Ultimaster 4.0 × 9; Ultimaster 2.5 × 9; Ultimaster 3.0 × 9	2	2
29	70	f	Right frontal and parietal strokes	(1) Right ICA supraclinoid	Right ICA, cervical	Yes	Small	40 mm	70%	Protege 8-6 × 30	2	2
30	77	f	Right frontal and parietal strokes	(1) Right MCA bif	Right ICA, cervical	Yes	Small	40 mm	85%	Protege 8-6 × 40	2	2
31	65	m	Ruptured aneurysm, left frontal and parietal strokes	(2) Left ICA, ophtalmic, terminus	Left ICA, cervical	Yes	Small	40 mm	80%	Protege 8-6 × 40; LEO 2.0 × 18	2	2
32	75	f	Ruptured aneurysm, right frontal and parietal strokes	(2) Right ICA, communicant, right MCA bif	Right ICA, cervical, left ICA ophtalmic	Yes	Medium	25 mm	70%	Protege 6 × 8–30	3	3
33	56	f	Left temporal stroke	(1) Acom	Left ICA, cervical	N/A	Medium	30 mm	70%	Protege 8-6 × 30	2	2
34	60	f	Ruptured aneurysm, right frontal and parietal strokes	(1) Right MCA bif	Right ICA, cervical	Yes	Small	15 mm	85%	AclinoFlex 3.0 × 15	3	5
35	59	f	Ruptured aneurysm, multiple strokes	(6) Acom, right MCA bif, right ICA ophtalmic, communicant, supraclinoid, left ICA ophtalmic	Right ICA, cervical	Yes	Small	30 mm	80%	Protege 8 × 6–30	3	3
36	55	m	Ruptured aneurysm	(1) Right ICA, communicant	Right ICA cervical	Yes	Medium	30 mm	70%	Protege 8 × 6–30	2	2
37	56	f	Ruptured aneurysm	(1) BA bif	Left ICA cavernous	N/A	Small	30 mm	75%	Orsiro 3.50 × 1; Solitaire AB 6 × 30	2	2
38	63	m	Left frontal stroke	(1) Left MCA bif	Left ICA, cervical	Yes	Small	40 mm	80%	Protege 6 × 8–40 (2)	2	2
39	40	f	Persistent headache	(1) Left ICA, ophtalmic	Left ICA, cervical	Yes	Medium	40 mm	70%	Protege 8 × 6–40; Protege 8 × 6–30	2	2

Table 1. *Cont.*

Patient #	Age	Gender	Presenting Symptoms	Aneurysm (#) and Localization	Stenosis Localization	Ipsilateral Lesion?	Aneurysm Size	Stenosis Length	Stenosis Degree	Stents Used	mRS Before	mRS FU
40	59	f	Right occipital and cerebellar strokes	(1) Right ICA, communicant	V1 right	No	Medium	40 mm	80%	Protege 6 × 8–40	3	4
41	64	f	Left cerebellar stroke	(1) V1 left	V1 left	Yes	Small	10 mm	70%	Resolute ONYX 2.0 × 8	2	2
42	53	m	Right frontal stroke	(2) Acom, left ICA, cavernous	Left ICA, cervical, V1 right, V1 left	Yes	Medium	30 mm	70%	Protege 6 × 8–40	2	2
43	82	f	Persistent headache	(1) Right ICA, cavernous	Right ICA, cervical	Yes	Fusiform	30 mm	70%	Protege 8 × 6–30, Pipeline with Shield 4.5 × 25	2	2
44	63	f	Repeated pontine ischemia, Millard–Gubler syndrome	(1) BA bif	V1 left	N/A	Medium	15 mm	80%	Ultimaster 3.5 × 15	2	2
45	66	m	Right frontal and parietal strokes	(1) Right MCA bif	Right ICA, cervical	Yes	Small	30 mm	85%	CASPER 7-30 × 143	2	2
46	67	f	Persistent headache	(1) Right ICA, ophthalmic	Right ICA, cervical	Yes	Small	40 mm	90%	Protege 6 × 8–40	1	1
47	30	f	Left occipital and cerebellar strokes	(1) V2 right	V3-V4 left	Yes	Small	15 mm	80%	XIENCE Xpedition 4 × 12	3	3

stands for a number.

Table 2. Association between clinical factors and occurrence of multiple stenoses and multiple aneurysms.

	One Stenosis Localization	Multiple Stenosis Localization	Total	p-Value Fisher's
Smoking				
No	28 (71.79%)	2 (25.00%)	30	0.0191
Yes	11 (28.21%)	6 (75.00%)	17	
AH				
AH1	3 (7.69%)	0 (0.00%)	3	0.1217
AH2	3 (7.69%)	3 (37.50%)	6	
AH3	33 (84.62%)	5 (62.50%)	38	
Diabetes				
No	31 (79.49%)	5 (62.50%)	36	0.3673
Yes	8 (20.51%)	3 (37.50%)	11	
IHD				
No	13 (33.33%)	0 (0.00%)	13	0.0855
Yes	26 (66.67%)	8 (100.00%)	34	
Obesity				
Non-obese	29 (74.36%)	7 (87.50%)	36	0.6593
Obese	10 (25.64%)	1 (12.50%)	11	
	One Aneurysm	**Multiple Aneurysms**	**Total**	**p-Value Fisher's**
Smoking				
No	26 (68.42%)	4 (44.44%)	30	0.2516
Yes	12 (31.58%)	5 (55.56%)	17	
AH				
AH1	1 (2.63%)	2 (22.22%)	3	0.1201
AH2	5 (13.16%)	1 (11.11%)	6	
AH3	32 (84.21%)	6 (66.67%)	38	
Diabetes				
No	28 (73.68%)	8 (88.89%)	36	0.6631
Yes	10 (26.32%)	1 (11.11%)	11	
IHD				
No	11 (28.95%)	2 (22.22%)	13	1
Yes	27 (71.05%)	7 (77.78%)	34	
Obesity				
Non-obese	28 (73.68%)	8 (88.89%)	36	0.6631
Obese	10 (26.32%)	1 (11.11%)	11	

Table 3. Relationship between aneurysm/stenosis localization and mRS outcome.

	mRS 1–2	mRS 3–6	Total	*p*-Value Fisher's
Aneurysm side				
Left	14 (37.84%)	0 (0.00%)	14	0.019
Bilateral	6 (16.22%)	5 (50.00%)	11	
Right	17 (45.95%)	5 (50.00%)	22	
Aneurysm arteries				
ACA	1 (2.70%)	0 (0.00%)	1	0.0761
Acom	1 (2.70%)	1 (10.00%)	2	
BA	2 (5.41%)	2 (20.00%)	4	
ICA	15 (40.54%)	1 (10.00%)	16	
MCA	13 (35.14%)	2 (20.00%)	15	
Bilateral	4 (10.81%)	3 (30.00%)	7	
VA	1 (2.70%)	1 (10.00%)	2	
Stenosis side				
Left	17 (45.95%)	3 (30.00%)	20	0.7017
Bilateral	5 (13.51%)	2 (20.00%)	7	
Right	15 (40.54%)	5 (50.00%)	20	
Stenosis arteries				
BA	1 (2.70%)	0 (0.00%)	1	0.9497
ICA	22 (59.46%)	5 (50.00%)	27	
MCA	3 (8.11%)	1 (10.00%)	4	
Multiple	3 (8.11%)	1 (10.00%)	4	
VA	8 (21.62%)	3 (30.00%)	11	
The stenosis side and aneurysm side coincide				
N/A	4 (10.81%)	3 (30.00%)	7	0.3108
No	9 (24.32%)	2 (20.00%)	11	
Yes	24 (64.86%)	5 (50.00%)	29	

Among the anatomical predictors, stenosis length showed a statistically significant association with functional outcome ($p = 0.0469$), with longer stenotic segments correlating with worse mRS scores. In contrast, neither aneurysm size ($p = 0.4291$) nor stenosis severity as measured by percent narrowing ($p = 0.2588$) demonstrated predictive value for clinical outcome (Table 4).

Table 4. Impact of aneurysm size, stenosis length, and degree on mRS outcome.

	mRS 1–2	mRS 3–6	Total	*p*-Value Fisher's
Aneurysm Size				
Fusiform	1 (2.70%)	1 (10.00%)	2	0.4291
Medium	10 (27.03%)	3 (30.00%)	13	
Small	26 (70.27%)	6 (60.00%)	32	
Stenosis length				
10 mm	3 (8.11%)	0 (0.00%)	3	0.0469
15 mm	3 (8.11%)	3 (30.00%)	6	
20 mm	7 (18.92%)	0 (0.00%)	7	
25 mm	1 (2.70%)	2 (20.00%)	3	
30 mm	13 (35.14%)	3 (30.00%)	16	
35 mm	1 (2.70%)	0 (0.00%)	1	
40 mm	9 (24.32%)	1 (10.00%)	10	
50 mm	0 (0.00%)	1 (10.00%)	1	
Stenosis degree				
70	16 (43.24%)	2 (20.00%)	18	0.2588
75	3 (8.11%)	0 (0.00%)	3	
80	11 (29.73%)	4 (40.00%)	15	
85	3 (8.11%)	2 (20.00%)	5	
90	2 (5.41%)	0 (0.00%)	2	
95	0 (0.00%)	1 (10.00%)	1	
99	2 (5.41%)	1 (10.00%)	3	

These findings underscore the importance of lesion morphology—particularly stenosis length—over traditional size-based metrics in predicting recovery. The observed left-side laterality advantage warrants further investigation, potentially reflecting procedural or anatomical factors that influence outcome.

3.5. Complications

Two notable complications were recorded. One patient with a ruptured MCA aneurysm and an ipsilateral critical ICA stenosis developed a subarachnoid hemorrhage after stenting, requiring external ventricular drainage and a decompressive craniectomy; the mRS at 6 months was 5. Another patient experienced an intraoperative aneurysm rupture during coiling (non-ipsilateral), which was managed with intra-arterial nimodipine due to catheter-induced vasospasm; the patient had an mRS of 4 at 4 months.

3.6. Case Examples

Case 1: Simultaneous Treatment of Left MCA Aneurysm and Vertebral Artery Stenosis.

Patient #13 was a 38-year-old male presenting with recurrent occipital headaches, tinnitus, visual disturbances, and transient ischemic attacks. Imaging revealed a saccular aneurysm at the left middle cerebral artery (MCA) bifurcation and an 80% stenosis of the V1 segment of the right vertebral artery. Comorbidities included grade 3 arterial hypertension, impaired glucose tolerance, and grade 1 obesity. A single-stage endovascular procedure was performed. The aneurysm was occluded using balloon-assisted coiling with a LEO stent (2.5 × 18 mm) via the C-stenting technique. In the same session, vertebral artery stenosis was treated with an Ultimaster stent (3.5 × 12 mm). The postoperative course was uneventful, and the patient achieved an mRS of 1 at six months (Figure 1).

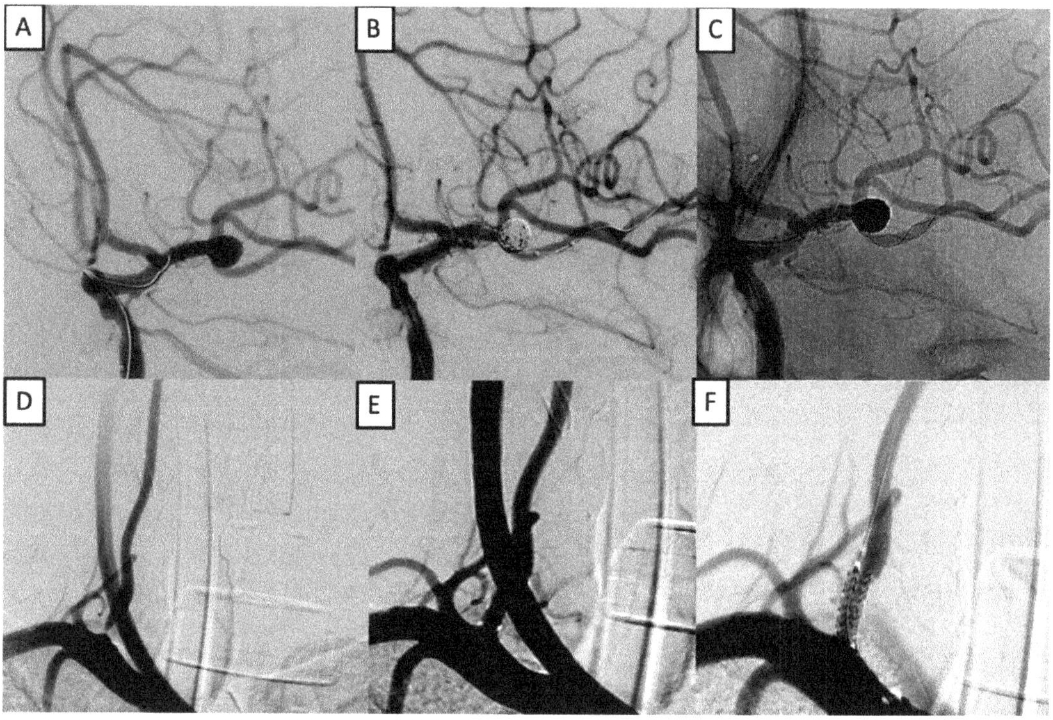

Figure 1. Simultaneous treatment of left MCA aneurysm and right vertebral artery stenosis. (**A–C**): balloon-assisted coiling with LEO stent (2.5 × 18 mm) of a left MCA bifurcation aneurysm. (**D–F**): stenting of right vertebral artery V1 segment using an Ultimaster 3.5 × 12 mm stent.

Case 2: Multivessel Stenosis and Dual Aneurysm Treatment Following SAH.

Patient #12 was a 57-year-old male with a history of smoking and hypertension who initially presented with a subarachnoid hemorrhage (SAH) and a ruptured left ICA aneurysm, treated with coiling. Follow-up imaging showed incomplete occlusion, and additional saccular aneurysms at the left MCA bifurcation and cervical ICA subocclusion were identified.

In a single-stage intervention, balloon angioplasty and stenting of the left cervical ICA were performed using a CASPER 9 × 20 × 143 mm stent, preceded by embolic protection and balloon pre-dilation. Subsequently, the MCA and ICA aneurysms were treated with stent-assisted coiling using a LEO stent (2.5 × 18 mm) and the half-T technique. The final angiography showed successful aneurysm exclusion and vessel patency. At the six-month follow-up, the patient had an mRS of 2 (Figure 2).

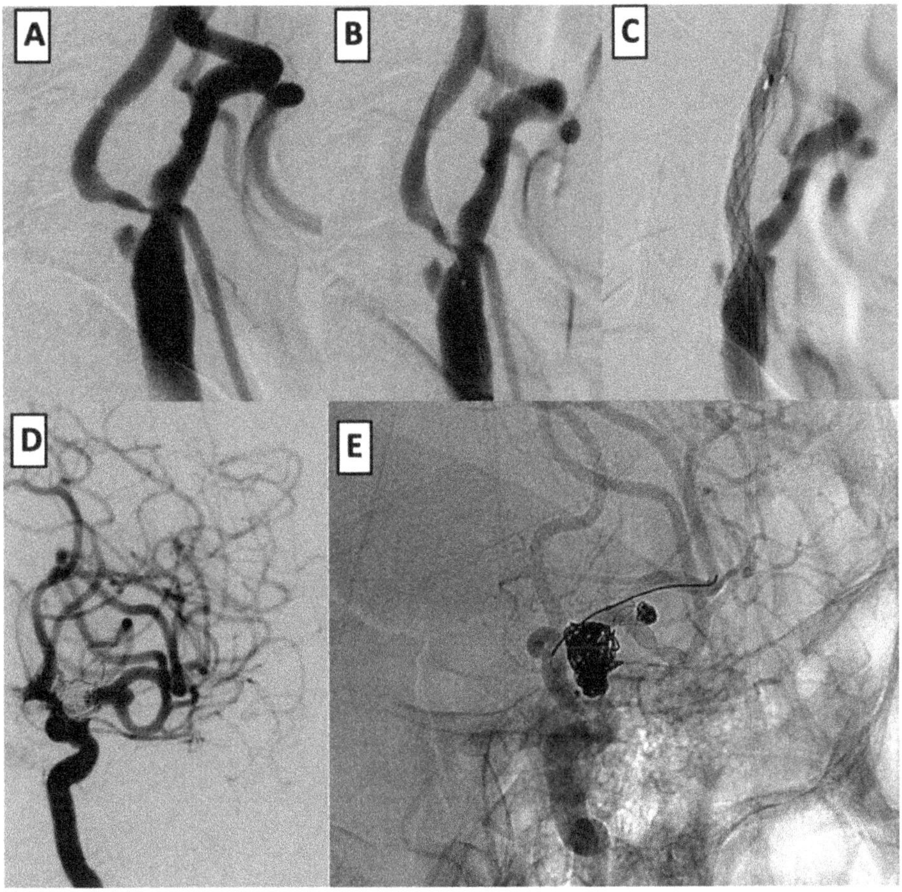

Figure 2. Endovascular management of dual intracranial aneurysms with cervical ICA stenosis. (**A–C**): angioplasty and CASPER stenting of the left cervical ICA after subocclusion and embolic protection. (**D**,**E**): coil embolization of left MCA and ICA aneurysms using half-T stenting technique with LEO stent (2.5 × 18 mm).

4. Discussion

This study adds to the growing body of the literature supporting the feasibility and safety of single-stage endovascular treatment for patients with coexisting intracranial aneurysms and extracranial arterial stenoses [2,4,7]. In the era of precision medicine, such combined interventions align with the shift toward individualized care that balances procedural efficiency with patient-specific anatomical and hemodynamic considerations [5,6].

All patients were followed for a uniform period of 6 months, capturing intermediate-term recovery and early complications such as in-stent thrombosis or aneurysm recurrence. While longer-term surveillance is needed to evaluate durability, this timeframe offers a reliable snapshot of initial outcomes.

In our cohort, smoking was the only factor significantly associated with the presence of multiple stenoses ($p = 0.0191$), reinforcing its role as a systemic atherosclerotic risk factor [8]. This finding aligns with the established literature on smoking's adverse effects on endothelial integrity and vascular remodeling [9]. Other risk factors such as hypertension or ischemic heart disease were not independently predictive, likely reflecting sample size limitations.

Based on our findings and the prior literature, we propose a decision-making algorithm for single-stage intervention, which prioritizes ipsilaterality, symptomatology, lesion size, and anatomical feasibility (Figure 3).

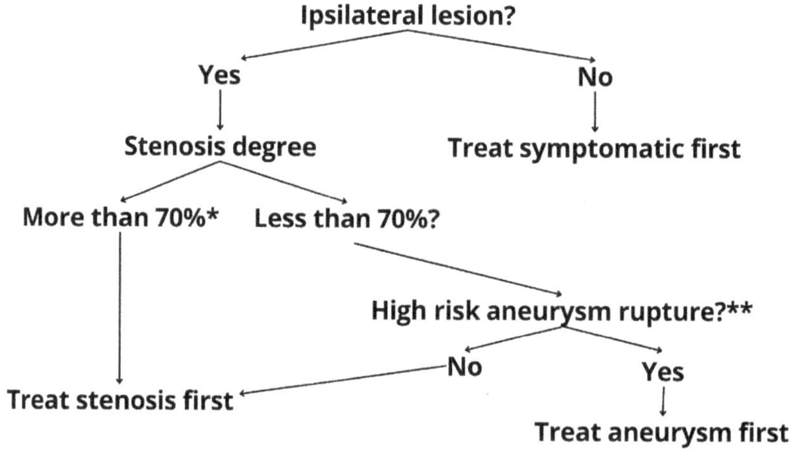

Figure 3. Proposed treatment algorithm for patients with coexisting extracranial stenosis and intracranial aneurysm. The initial step evaluates lesion ipsilaterality. If non-ipsilateral, the symptomatic pathology is prioritized. For ipsilateral lesions, the degree of stenosis is assessed. Stenoses exceeding 70% (as measured by NASCET criteria *) are treated first to ensure safe access and perfusion. If the stenosis is <70%, aneurysm rupture risk is evaluated using the PHASES score **. High-risk aneurysms are prioritized for embolization, while low-risk cases proceed with stenosis treatment. * North American Symptomatic Carotid Endarterectomy Trial (NASCET) criteria. ** Population, hypertension, age, size of aneurysm, earlier SAH, site of aneurysm (PHASES) score.

Our proposed algorithm (Figure 3) also incorporates real-world clinical reasoning suggested by experienced practitioners. Specifically, for symptomatic or >70% asymptomatic stenosis with an unruptured aneurysm—regardless of laterality—ICA stenting is prioritized before aneurysm embolization. The rationale includes the following: (1) reducing hypoperfusion risk during aneurysm navigation, (2) enabling stable catheter positioning distal to the stenosis, and (3) minimizing financial burden in low-resource settings by consolidating procedures and reducing repeated device use. Moreover, treating the aneurysm after stenting may mitigate the risk of pressure-related rupture, also known as normal perfusion breakthrough syndrome. In contrast, in cases of ruptured aneurysm with coexisting symptomatic or severe asymptomatic stenosis, the approach shifts toward initial angioplasty of the ICA to facilitate safe access, followed by aneurysm coiling. If a stent is required for the aneurysm, the ICA stenosis can be addressed concurrently. This sequence minimizes procedural delay in hemorrhagic cases while still preserving cerebral perfusion and catheter stability.

All patients were followed for a uniform period of six months, capturing intermediate-term recovery and procedural complications such as in-stent thrombosis or aneurysm recurrence. Although no patients in our cohort experienced these complications, we have contextualized this in the discussion by referencing the most commonly reported complications—groin hematoma, in-stent thrombosis, and distal embolization—and their incidence rates in the general population. The absence of these events in our group highlights the potential safety of the single-stage strategy, though the relatively small sample limits generalizability.

Balancing ischemic and hemorrhagic risk in these patients remains challenging. Historically, staged approaches like carotid endarterectomy followed by delayed aneurysm embolization were preferred [4,5,7], but they entail logistical and procedural drawbacks. Recent reports suggest that carefully selected patients may benefit from simultaneous interventions [2,8,9].

Case reports highlight the danger of treating carotid stenosis before securing aneurysms. Hartmann et al. [1] described a fatal post-stenting hemorrhage, while Pappada et al. [2] and Adams [5] emphasized the complexity of sequential decisions. Our study supports that, with structured planning, concurrent treatment is not only possible but safe.

Badruddin et al. [8] and Gallego Leon et al. [9] reported strong outcomes in similar cohorts. Our complication rate was low, and factors such as lesion laterality and stenosis length—rather than aneurysm size—were more closely associated with outcome.

We encountered two major complications: aneurysmal rebleeding post-stenting requiring decompressive craniectomy, and intraoperative rupture treated with nimodipine. These underscore the importance of risk stratification, especially in ruptured cases. Hartmann et al. [1] reinforced the theoretical risk of rebleed post-revascularization, validating strategies like coiling first or strict hemodynamic control.

The observed correlation between left-sided aneurysms and favorable outcome was unexpected. Given the complexity of left carotid access and symptomatic burden of left hemispheric strokes [10], this may reflect anatomical variance in our cohort.

These findings suggest that individualized anatomy-driven strategies—potentially aided by AI-based imaging—can enhance procedural outcomes. The lack of correlation between mRS and aneurysm size or stenosis degree suggests that vascular morphology may carry more prognostic value than previously assumed.

Procedurally, our series included patients with ipsilateral, contralateral, symptomatic, and ruptured lesions—all treated in one session. This broad applicability supports single-stage endovascular intervention as a viable alternative to staged approaches in experienced centers [2,4,7,11].

In most cases, CAS was performed first to secure proximal access and reduce embolic load during aneurysm navigation [2,5,12]. When feasible, aneurysm coiling preceded stenting in morphologically unstable lesions. Such flexibility, guided by real-time angiography and preoperative imaging, reflects evolving neurointerventional strategy [6,13].

One high-risk case involved an SAH patient with critical ICA stenosis and impaired perfusion, treated emergently with stenting before embolization. Despite concerns over dual antiplatelet therapy (DAPT) in hemorrhagic states, this decision prioritized cerebral perfusion. Emerging data support cautious DAPT use in such settings [14,15], though we remain conservative and defer stenting when possible in acute SAH.

Limitations

This study has several limitations that must be acknowledged. First, the retrospective and single-center design introduces inherent risks of selection bias and limits the generalizability of the findings. Although our patient population reflects real world clinical complexity, the absence of randomization restricts the ability to draw causal inferences regarding the superiority of single-stage intervention over staged or conservative approaches.

Second, the relatively small sample size (n = 47) constrains the statistical power, particularly in subgroup analyses such as aneurysm location or lesion-specific characteristics. Larger multicenter cohorts would provide more robust evidence to validate the identified associations—such as the impact of stenosis length and aneurysm laterality on functional outcome.

Third, the follow-up duration, with a minimum of three months, may not be sufficient to capture late complications such as in-stent restenosis, delayed aneurysm recurrence, or long-term neurocognitive deficits. A longer follow-up period is essential for assessing the durability and neurological sequelae of the treatment.

Fourth, while the modified Rankin Scale (mRS) is a widely accepted outcome measure, it may not adequately reflect subtle cognitive or functional impairments, particularly in patients with anterior circulation lesions. Future research should incorporate more detailed neuropsychological and quality-of-life assessments.

Finally, the treatment of multiple aneurysms in a single session alongside extracranial stenosis represents a complex and underexplored subgroup. We plan to collect more cases and conduct focused analysis to better understand outcomes in this patient population.

Despite these limitations, our study offers valuable insights into the evolving paradigm of precision-guided single-session endovascular therapy in complex cerebrovascular disease.

5. Conclusions

This study supports the feasibility and safety of single-stage endovascular treatment in patients with concurrent intracranial aneurysms and extracranial arterial stenoses. Our findings suggest that lesion-specific factors—particularly aneurysm laterality and stenosis length—may influence functional outcomes more significantly than aneurysm size or stenosis degree. Smoking emerged as a strong independent predictor of multiple stenoses, underscoring the importance of modifiable risk factor management in cerebrovascular patients.

Future prospective multicenter studies with longer follow-up and expanded functional outcome measures are warranted to refine treatment algorithms and establish evidence-based protocols for this complex patient population.

Author Contributions: Conceptualization, M.S. and M.B.; methodology, D.D.; software, S.M.; validation, R.B.P., A.Z., and M.B.; formal analysis, D.D.; investigation, A.M.; resources, M.B.; data curation, S.M.; writing—original draft preparation, A.M.; writing—review and editing, R.B.P.; visualization, A.Z.; supervision, M.B.; project administration, M.S.; All authors have read and agreed to the published version of the manuscript.

Funding: This research received no external funding.

Institutional Review Board Statement: This study was conducted in accordance with the Declaration of Helsinki, and approved by the Ethics Committee of National Hospital of the Medical Center of the Presidential Affairs Administration of the Republic of Kazakhstan (approval #7, dated 12 December 2024).

Informed Consent Statement: Written informed consent has been obtained from the patients to publish this paper.

Data Availability Statement: The data supporting the findings of this study are available from the corresponding author upon reasonable request. Due to patient privacy regulations and institutional policy, individual-level data cannot be publicly shared but may be provided in anonymized form for academic and research purposes.

Conflicts of Interest: The authors declare no conflicts of interest.

Abbreviations

The following abbreviations are used in this manuscript:

ACA	Anterior Cerebral Artery
Acom	Anterior Communicating Artery
BA	Basilar Artery
CAS	Carotid Artery Stenting
CTA	Computed Tomography Angiography
DAPT	Dual Antiplatelet Therapy
DSA	Digital Subtraction Angiography
DWI	Diffusion-Weighted Imaging
ICA	Internal Carotid Artery
IDH	Isocitrate Dehydrogenase
IHD	Ischemic Heart Disease
MCA	Middle Cerebral Artery
mRS	Modified Rankin Scale
MRI	Magnetic Resonance Imaging
SAH	Subarachnoid Hemorrhage
TIA	Transient Ischemic Attack
VA	Vertebral Artery

References

1. Hartmann, M.; Weber, R.; Zoubaa, S.; Schranz, C.; Knauth, M. Fatal subarachnoid hemorrhage after carotid stenting. *J. Neuroradiol.* **2004**, *31*, 63–66. [CrossRef] [PubMed]
2. Pappada, G.; Fiori, L.; Marina, R.; Vaiani, S.; Gaini, S.M. Management of symptomatic carotid stenoses with coincidental intracranial aneurysms. *Acta Neurochir.* **1996**, *138*, 1386–1390. [CrossRef] [PubMed]
3. Kappelle, L.; Eliasziw, M.; Fox, A.J.; Barnett, H.J. Small, unruptured intracranial aneurysms and management of symptomatic carotid artery stenosis: North American Symptomatic Carotid Endarterectomy Trial Group. *Neurology* **2000**, *55*, 307–309. [PubMed]
4. Ladowski, J.S.; Webster, M.W.; Yonas, H.O.; Steed, D.L. Carotid endarterectomy in patients with asymptomatic intracranial aneurysm. *Ann. Surg.* **1984**, *200*, 70–73. [PubMed]
5. Adams, H.P., Jr. Carotid stenosis and coexisting ipsilateral intracranial aneurysm: A problem in management. *Arch. Neurol.* **1977**, *34*, 515–516. [CrossRef] [PubMed]
6. Kaçar, E.; Nas, Ö.F.; Erdoğan, C.; Hakyemez, B. Single-stage endovascular treatment in patients with severe extracranial large vessel stenosis and concomitant ipsilateral unruptured intracranial aneurysm. *Diagn. Interv. Radiol.* **2015**, *21*, 476–482. [CrossRef] [PubMed] [PubMed Central]
7. Iwata, T.; Mori, T.; Tajiri, H. Successful staged endovascular treatment of a symptomatic cervical bifurcation stenosis coupled with a coincidental unruptured cerebral aneurysm in the carotid distal segment. *AJNR Am. J. Neuroradiol.* **2008**, *29*, 1948–1950. [CrossRef] [PubMed]
8. Badruddin, A.; Teleb, M.S.; Abraham, M.G.; Taqi, M.A.; Zaidat, O.O. Safety and feasibility of simultaneous ipsilateral proximal carotid artery stenting and cerebral aneurysm coiling. *Front. Neurol.* **2010**, *1*, 120. [CrossRef] [PubMed]
9. Gallego León, J.I.; Concepción Aramendía, L.; Ballenilla Marco, F.; Vázquez Suárez, J.C. Concomitant endovascular treatment of concomitant extracranial carotid stenosis and intracranial aneurysm. Our experience. *Interv. Neuroradiol.* **2009**, *15*, 53–59. [CrossRef] [PubMed] [PubMed Central]
10. ACAS Trial Investigators. Endarterectomy for asymptomatic carotid artery stenosis: Executive Committee for the Asymptomatic Carotid Atherosclerosis Study. *JAMA* **1995**, *273*, 1421–1428. [CrossRef]
11. Campos, J.K.; Lin, L.M.; Beaty, N.B.; Bender, M.T.; Jiang, B.; Zarrin, D.A.; Coon, A.L. Tandem cervical carotid stenting for stenosis with flow diversion embolisation for the treatment of intracranial aneurysms. *Stroke Vasc. Neurol.* **2019**, *4*, e000187. [CrossRef]
12. Park, J.C.; Kwon, B.J.; Kang, H.S.; Kim, J.E.; Kim, K.M.; Cho, Y.D.; Han, M.H. Single-stage extracranial carotid artery stenting and intracranial aneurysm coiling: Technical feasibility and clinical outcome. *Interv. Neuroradiol.* **2013**, *19*, 228–234. [CrossRef] [PubMed]
13. Laurent, D.; Lucke-Wold, B.; Leary, O.; Randall, M.H.; Porche, K.; Koch, M.; Chalouhi, N.; Polifka, A.; Hoh, B.L. The evolution of endovascular therapy for intracranial aneurysms: Historical perspective and next frontiers. *Neurosci. Insights* **2022**, *17*, 26331055221117560. [CrossRef] [PubMed]

14. Lee, K.S.; Lee, C.; Dhillon, P.S.; Kirollos, R.; Nga, V.D.W.; Yeo, T.T.; Henkes, H.; Arthur, A.S.; Yeo, L.L.L.; Bhogal, P. Antiplatelet therapy in aneurysmal subarachnoid hemorrhage: An updated meta-analysis. *Neurosurg. Rev.* **2023**, *46*, 221. [CrossRef] [PubMed]
15. Qoorchi Moheb Seraj, F.; Mirbolouk, M.H.; Vaezi, M. Safety of dual antiplatelet therapy in the acute phase of aneurysmal subarachnoid. *Focus* **2023**, *55*, E10. [CrossRef]

brain sciences

MDPI

Article

Ultrasound-Induced Release Profile of Nimodipine from Drug-Loaded Block Copolymers after Singular vs. Repeated Sonication: In Vitro Analysis in Artificial Cerebrospinal Fluid

Katja Döring [1,2], Swetlana Sperling [1], Milena Ninkovic [1], Heinrich Lanfermann [2], Frank Streit [3], Andreas Fischer [3], Veit Rohde [1] and Vesna Malinova [1,4,*]

1 Department of Neurosurgery, University Medical Center Göttingen, 37075 Göttingen, Germany; doering.katja@mh-hannover.de (K.D.); swetlana.sperling@med.uni-goettingen.de (S.S.); milena.ninkovic@med.uni-goettingen.de (M.N.); veit.rohde@med.uni-goettingen.de (V.R.)
2 Department of Interventional and Diagnostic Neuroradiology, Hannover Medical School, 30625 Hannover, Germany; lanfermann.heinrich@mh-hannover.de
3 Department of Clinical Chemistry, University Medical Center Göttingen, 37075 Göttingen, Germany; frank.streit@med.uni-goettingen.de (F.S.); andreas.fischer@med.uni-goettingen.de (A.F.)
4 Department of Neurosurgery, Georg-August-University, Robert-Koch-Straße 40, 37075 Göttingen, Germany
* Correspondence: vesna.malinova@gmail.com; Tel.: +49-551-398798; Fax: +49-551-39-61778

Abstract: Objective: Nimodipine still represents a unique selling point in the prevention of delayed cerebral ischemia (DCI) following aneurysmal subarachnoid hemorrhage (aSAH). Its intrathecal effect is limited by a low oral bioavailability, leading to the development of nanocarrier systems to overcome this limitation. This study investigated the ultrasound-induced release profile of nimodipine from drug-loaded copolymers in artificial cerebrospinal fluid (CSF) within 72 h after a singular versus repeated sonication. Methods: Pluronic® F127 copolymers (Sigma-Aldrich, Taufkirchen, Germany)were loaded with nimodipine by direct dissolution. Spontaneous and on-demand drug release by ultrasound (1 MHz at 1.7 W/cm^2) was determined in artificial cerebrospinal fluid using the dialysis bag method. Nimodipine concentrations were measured at predefined time points within 72 h of sonication. Results: Spontaneous release of nimodipine was enhanced by ultrasound application with significantly increased nimodipine concentrations two hours after a repeated sonication compared to a singular sonication (median 1.62 vs. 17.48 μg/μL, $p = 0.04$). A further trend was observed after four hours (median 1.82 vs. 22.09 μg/μL, $p = 0.06$). There was no difference in the overall nimodipine concentrations between the groups with a singular versus repeated sonication (357.2 vs. 540.3 μg/μL, $p = 0.60$) after 72 h. Conclusions: Repeated sonication resulted in an acceleration of nimodipine release from the drug-loaded copolymer in a CSF medium. These findings confirm the proof of principle of an on-demand guidance of nimodipine release from nimodipine-loaded nanodrugs by means of ultrasound, which suggests that evaluating the concept in an animal model may be appropriate.

Keywords: drug release profile; nimodipine; nanodrug

1. Introduction

Delayed cerebral ischemia (DCI) is a common complication of aneurysmal subarachnoid hemorrhage (aSAH) [1]. The pathophysiology of DCI has been intensively investigated in the past years revealing a multifactorial pathogenesis behind this phenomenon [2]. Despite the continuously growing knowledge regarding the pathophysiology, the treatment options for DCI remain limited [3]. While several drugs have been shown to effectively reverse cerebral vasospasm in patients with aSAH, nimodipine is the only drug that was able to improve the patients' outcome as well [4]. The highest level of evidence exists for the oral administration of nimodipine with six single doses per day [5]. However, first-pass metabolism resulting in an oral bioavailability of only 3–30% limits the intrathecal effect of nimodipine. Additionally, nimodipine-induced side effects after systemic application often led to a reduction or discontinuation of the treatment with nimodipine in clinical practice [6,7]. Addressing these limitations, direct intrathecal nimodipine administration has gained scientific and clinical interest [8]. Nanotechnology is an emerging field of pharmacology that has opened new avenues for direct drug delivery to the site of action [9,10], enabling higher local drug concentrations while circumventing the side effects of the systemic drug administration at the same time. A wide range of synthetic nanostructures (solid lipid nanoparticles, liposomes, nanostructured lipid carriers, nanoshells, quantum dots, and superparamagnetic nanoparticles) has been developed in recent years that can be modulated in size, shape, and surface chemistry and hence provide new solutions for drug delivery [9]. Nanocarriers play an important role in oncology, facilitating the controlled release of anticancer drugs [10].

Polymeric block copolymers consisting of hydrophilic and hydrophobic units, with a hydrophobic core protected by the surrounding hydrophilic chains in aqueous solution, have been already established and proven to be ideal drug carriers for hydrophobic substances such as nimodipine [11,12]. The weak conjugation between the copolymer and the water-insoluble molecule nimodipine is based on hydrophobic interactions, hydrogen bonding and van der Waals forces [13,14]. Several studies on nimodipine-loaded micro- and nanoparticles have been already conducted which have demonstrated a sustained drug release over time immediately after intrathecal administration of drug-loaded nanocarriers [15,16]. In a previous study, we developed a nimodipine-loaded nanodrug and demonstrated a successful on-demand drug release induced by ultrasound [17]. A significantly increased drug release was achieved after a singular sonication. The findings of our previous study gave rise to the question, 'can the release of nimodipine be potentiated by repeated sonications?' In this study, the nimodipine release profile from the nanodrug was explored after repeated sonication and compared to singular sonication in an artificial cerebrospinal fluid (CSF) medium to assess the feasibility of this concept for an upcoming evaluation in animal studies.

2. Materials and Methods

The in vitro experimental setup included three steps: 1—preparation of Pluronic® F-127 (BASF Corporation, Florham Park, Morris, NJ, USA) block copolymers loaded with nimodipine, 2—measurement of the spontaneous continuous release of nimodipine from the Pluronic® F-127 block copolymers, and 3—measurement of the ultrasound-induced release of nimodipine from the Pluronic® F-127 block copolymers after singular and repeated sonication. Pluronic® F-127 block copolymers were used as nanocarriers without further purification. Pluronic® F-127 is a triblock copolymer of polyethylene oxide and polypropylene oxide (PEO-PPO-PEO) with a molecular weight of 12,600 Da and a hydrophilic–lipophilic balance (HLB) of 22 (all data from the manufacturer).

2.1. *Artificial Cerebrospinal Fluid*

Artificial CSF was used to analyze the release profile of nimodipine from drug-loaded Pluronic® F-127 copolymers in a CSF-like medium. Artificial CSF acts as a biological buffer, providing a vital environment by maintaining homeostasis, osmolarity and pH at physiological levels and is commonly used as a laboratory chemical, not only for in vitro but also for in vivo applications. To prepare 1000 mL of artificial CSF solution, 500 mL of Base A was added to a further 500 mL of Base B. Base A is first oxygenated for 10 min; then, 500 mL of Base B is slowly added. The artificial CSF solution prepared in this way is enriched with oxygen throughout its use. With an oxygen enrichment of 95% O_2 and 5% CO_2 (carbogen), the pH is 7.4 (all data from the manufacturer).

2.2. Preparation of Nimodipine-Loaded Pluronic® F-127 Block Copolymers

Pluronic® F-127 copolymers loaded with nimodipine were prepared using the direct dissolution method as previously described by Sotoudegana et al. [18]. The preparation involved the following steps: Briefly, 2 mg of nimodipine powder (Sigma-Aldrich Chemical Company, St. Louis, MO, USA) and a defined amount of Pluronic® F-127 (5%), were added simultaneously to 10 mL of DI at a stirring frequency of 100 U/mL. The suspension was then mixed at 100 rpm for 3 h at room temperature (25 °C). The precipitated nimodipine was separated from the micelle suspension by filtration (pluriStrainer® filter with a mesh size of 1 µm, pluriSelect® Life Science, Leipzig, Germany). The preparation process of nimodipine-loaded Pluronic® F127 block copolymers was reported in detail in an article previously published by our research group [19]. The size of the nimodipine-loaded block copolymers was 122.4 ± 12.3 as measured by transmission electron microscope. The nimodipine-loaded block copolymers had a spherical form with a smooth surface. The size and morphology of the nimodipine-loaded block copolymers remained stable for up to three months [19]. In this previous work, the entrapment efficacy, and the percentage drug load of the nimodipine-loaded block copolymers were evaluated using three different Pluronic® F127 concentrations (5%, 10% and 15%). In this study, the nimodipine-loaded block copolymers with a 5% Pluronic® F127 concentration were used with an entrapment efficacy of 46% and a percentage drug load of 59.58% [19].

2.3. Drug Release from Drug-Loaded-Pluronic® F 127 Block Copolymers

The release of nimodipine from the nimodipine-loaded block copolymers in artificial CSF was evaluated in two steps: 1—spontaneous drug release without external influence and 2—controlled drug release induced by a singular and repeated ultrasound application. The spontaneous and ultrasound-induced release profile setup was repeated five times for every experimental setup (spontaneous, one sonication and two sonications).

2.4. Spontaneous Nimodipine Release without External Influence

The in vitro drug release profile of nimodipine from the Pluronic® F 127 copolymers in artificial CSF was evaluated using the dialysis bag method (Figure 1). For this purpose, the dialysis bags (Spectrum™ Labs Spectra/Por™ 6 3500 D MWCO, Fisher Sientific, Schwarte, Germany) were first soaked in deionized water for 24 h and stored in a cool place at 4 °C until use. For experimental conversion, 10 mL of the nimodipine-loaded micellar solution was added to the dialysis bag. The respective ends of the bags were clamped as intended and placed in 200 mL artificial CSF solution. The whole set-up was stirred at 36.5 °C for 72 h at 100 rpm. At predetermined time points (0, 5, 15 and 30 min and 2, 4, 24, 48 and 72 h) an aliquot of 300 µL was taken from the dissolution medium.

The samples obtained were then immediately frozen at −20 degrees Celsius without further dilution until subsequent analysis using a mass spectrometer. The amount of drug released into the medium was calculated from a calibration curve. A hydroalcoholic solution of nimodipine (Nimodipine Carinopharm, Carinopharm GmbH, Elze, Germany) at a concentration of 0.2 mg/mL was used as a control. For each condition, the analysis was performed five times to determine the mean values and to ensure reproducibility. A Nexera X2 UHPLC, Shimadzu, Duisburg, Germany (Ultra High-Performance Liquid Chromatography) connected to a LCMS-8050 mass spectrometer (Shimadzu, Kyoto, Japan) equipped with an electrospray ion source was used for the determination of nimodipine concentration. A sample volume of 0.1 µL was injected into a Halo 50 × 4.6 × 2.7 µm (Advanced Material Technologies, MZ Analysentechnik, Mainz, Germany). A sharp gradient with mobile phase A (5% ammonium acetate) and mobile phase B (methanol) was used as follows: Initial conditions were 3% B with a flow rate of 0.9 mL/min. Then, 3% B was held for 0.02 min, a linear gradient towards 50% B was used up to 0.8 min and a linear gradient to 95% B was used until 2 min. Column was washed for 0.4 min with 95% B and equilibrated with 3% B from 2.5 to 3 min. For quantification, the MRM (Multiple Reaction Monitoring) transitions 419.2/301.0, CE-22.0, as the quantifier and 343.2, CE-12.0, as a qualifier for nimodipine (rt = 1.27 min) and m/d 3z 295.0/100.0 for internal standard D3-trimipramine (rt 0.65 min) were monitored. Linearity was established in the range of 0.2–200.0 µg/L (0.0108x + 0, r = 0.9999693) (Figures 2 and 3). Within a run, at QC1 (Quality Control 1), 10.0 µg/L CV (cyclic voltammetry) of 0.868% was found, and at QC2 (Quality Control 2), 100.0 µg/L, a CV of 0.983% was found. The CV of 4.03% was found at the LLOQ (Lower Limit of Quantification) of 0.2 µg/L. Between runs, CV was 11.6% for QC1 and 6.7% for QC2.

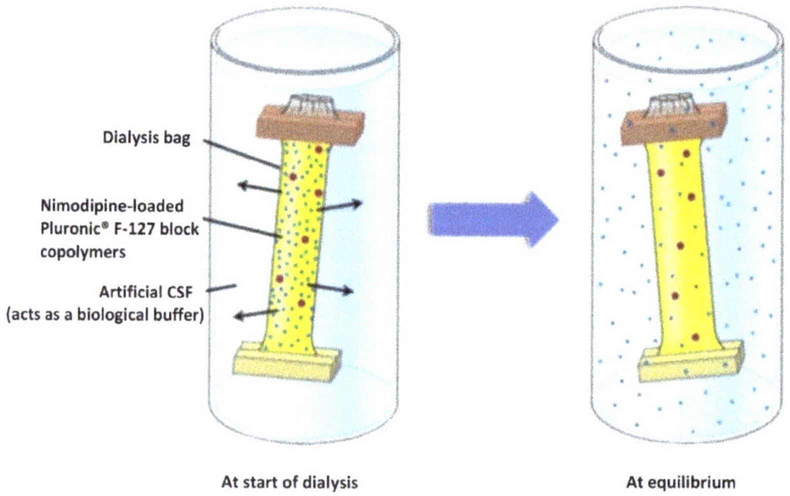

Figure 1. Dialysis bag method with the status at the beginning and after the nimodipine release from the nanodrug.

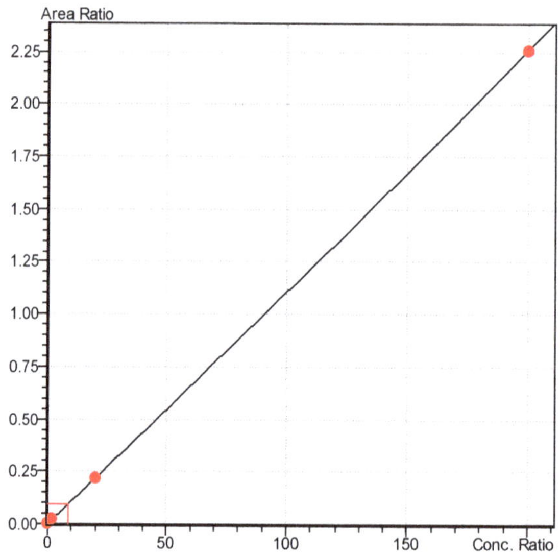

Figure 2. Calibration curve 0.0108x + 0, r = 0.9999693.

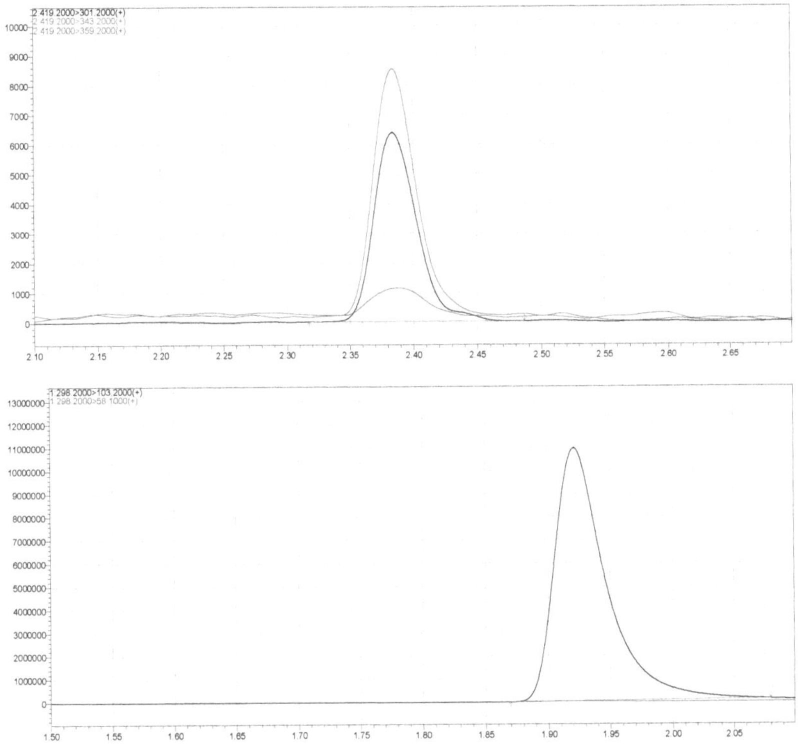

Figure 3. Ion chromatograms of nimodipine (Cal1 0.2 µg/L) and internal Standard D3-trimipramine.

2.5. Ultrasound-Induced Nimodipine Release

For an induced drug release, low frequency ultrasound waves were applied either one or twice using PHYSIOSON-Expert (Physiomed®, Paderborn, Germany). For the experimental setup, two batches of five samples each were sonicated at different intensities. The experimental setup is demonstrated in Figure 4. While the technical variables remained the same (high intensity continuous ultrasound with a frequency of 1 MHz and an intensity of 1.7 W/cm^2), the time variable (t) was modulated: the ultrasound treatment was performed for either 30 or 60 s. As described above, 10 mL of each of the different concentrations of the nimodipine-loaded micelle solution were filled into the dialysis bags and added to 200 mL of artificial CSF. The ultrasound probe, which was previously wetted with ultrasound gel, was positioned on the dialysis bag so that the ultrasound probe touched the surface of the CSF medium in the beaker. The ultrasound treatment was then performed and an aliquot of 300 µL was taken from the dissolution medium at the same predetermined times (0, 5, 15 and 30 min and 2, 4, 24, 48 and 72 h) under static conditions analogous to the measurement of the spontaneous drug release profile described above (36.5 °C for 72 h at 100 rpm). Again, the samples were frozen at minus four degrees Celsius until they were analyzed in a mass spectrometer. The technique used is like that described above (see Section 2.4). As mentioned above, each condition was run five times to determine the mean.

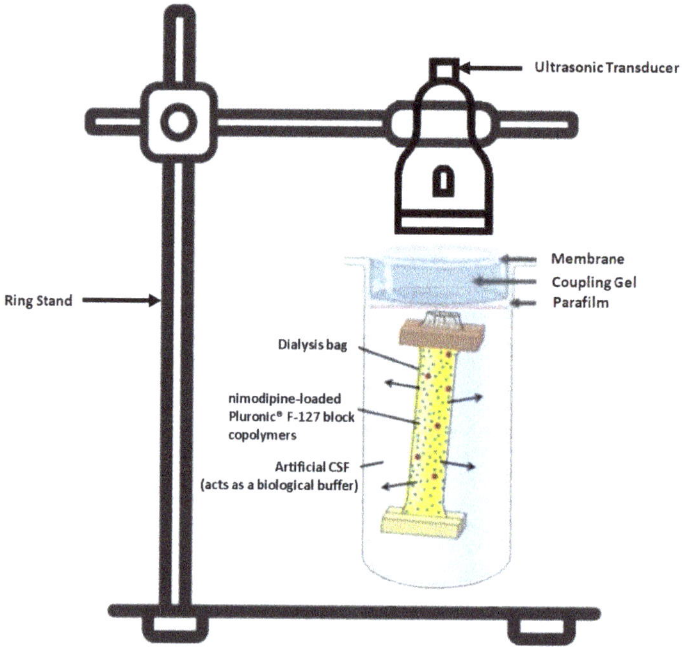

Figure 4. Experimental setup during the ultrasound-induced drug release.

2.6. Statistical Analysis

Statistical analysis was performed using GraphPad Prism (version 9.0, GraphPad Software, San Diego, CA, USA). A p-value of <0.05 was used as the significance level. All data are expressed as mean ± SD or median with 95% confidence interval (CI) and/or interquartile range (IQR). Classical ANOVA analysis was used for subgroup comparisons.

3. Results

3.1. Spontaneous Release Profile of Nimodipine from Nimodipine-Loaded Pluronic® F 127 Block Copolymer

During the first two to four hours, a continuous, slow, and shallow drug release was observed. This was followed by a 6-fold increase in nimodipine concentration after 24 h. A further doubling of the release rate occurred between 48 and 72 h.

3.2. Ultrasound-Induced Drug-Release after Singular vs. Repeated Sonication

A summary of concentrations of nimodipine released spontaneously without external influence (control group), as well as that released after ultrasound application with singular and repeated sonication is given in Table 1.

An increase in the released nimodipine concentration was seen already 30 min after sonication with a potentiation of the effect after repeated sonication. The median nimodipine release without external influence, i.e., concentration of spontaneously released nimodipine after 30 min was 0.24 µg/µL. That increased to 0.60 µg/µL after one sonication, and reached 14.8 µg/µL after repeated sonication, but the difference did not reach statistical significance.

Table 1. Release profile of nimodipine; spontaneous, after one sonication and after repeated sonication.

Experimental Settings	Mean	SD	Median	95% CI	IQR
Control group without sonication					
Control group 2 min	1.439	3.010	0.20	0.2–7.58	0.20–5.40
Control group 15 min	3.588	8.185	0.20	0.19–20.30	0.19–5.40
Control group 30 min	4.867	6.757	0.24	0.2–17.6	0.20–9.12
Control group 2 h	8.547	11.60	2.91	0.2–28.85	0.46–19.11
Control group 4 h	13.35	13.67	10.88	0.2–36.43	1.01–24.42
Control group 24 h	131.6	96.90	118.3	0.2–246.6	51.93–239.6
Control group 48 h	207.7	136.2	219.0	0.2–382.40	104.1–305.7
Control group 72 h	377.7	236.0	355.3	0.2–681.9	228.3–597.1
Treatment group with a singular sonication					
One sonication 2 min	1.243	1.539	0.546	0.24–4.21	0.29–2.24
One sonication 15 min	1.303	2.291	0.454	0.20–5.97	0.21–1.88
One sonication 30 min	1.226	1.687	0.607	0.20–4.63	0.35–1.83
One sonication 2 h	8.296	16.31	1.624	0.20–41.50	0.86–13.18
One sonication 4 h	5.606	9.520	1.822	0.20–24.83	0.61–9.35
One sonication 24 h	115.8	67.53	124.2	0.20–200.4	70.40–164.1
One sonication 48 h	327.5	176.8	360.0	0.43–506.2	220.3–460.2
One sonication 72 h	375.8	270.1	357.2	0.20–754.4	145.5–632.5
Treatment group with repeated sonication					
Repeated sonication 2 min	0.532	0.544	0.27	0.20–1.58	0.20–0.90
Repeated sonication 15 min	1.292	2.414	0.20	0.20–6.20	0.20–2.11
Repeated sonication 30 min	98.72	177.4	14.85	0.51–364.7	3.82–277.5
Repeated sonication 2 h	98.25	204.9	17.48	6.15–516.3	8.10–146.6
Repeated sonication 4 h	168.0	357.1	22.09	0.64–896.1	11.96–262.7
Repeated sonication 24 h	395.6	461.7	204.0	0.65–1226	80.44–780.6
Repeated sonication 48 h	403.7	279.2	422.8	0.54–727.1	166.7–651.9
Repeated sonication 72 h	454.5	334.3	540.3	0.96–736.3	102.5–720.6

SD = standard deviation, CI = confidence interval, IQR = interquartile range.

A direct comparison of the groups with singular sonication and repeated sonication showed a significantly increased early nimodipine release within the first two hours in the group with repeated sonication (median nimodipine concentration 1.62 vs. 17.48 μg/μL, $p = 0.04$). A further trend was seen at 4 h in the group with repeated sonication (median nimodipine concentration 1.82 vs. 22.09 μg/μL, $p = 0.06$) (Figure 5). A comparison of the two groups after 72 h shows no difference in released concentrations (median nimodipine concentrations 357.2 vs. 540.3 μg/μL, $p = 0.60$), indicating that drug release increases early after sonication and returns to baseline in the long term (Figure 6).

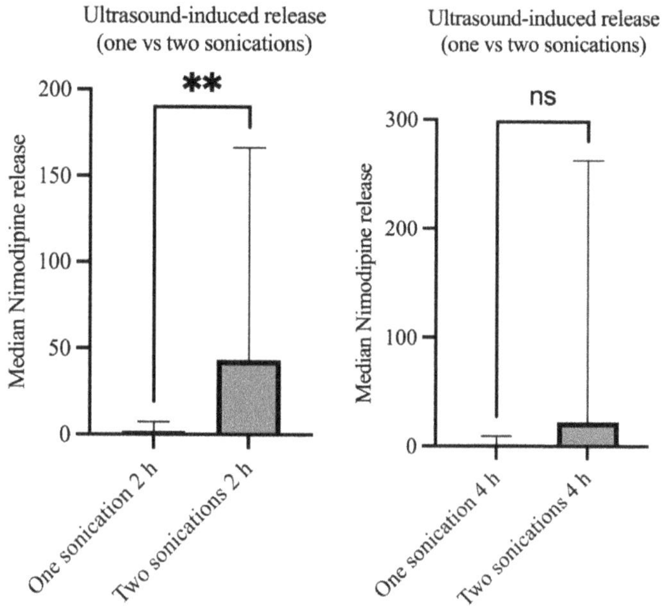

Figure 5. Nimodipine release profile two and four hours after a singular versus repeated sonication showing a significantly increased nimodipine concentration in the group with repeated sonication after two hours, but without a significant difference between the two groups after four hours. "**" states a statistically significant difference. "ns" states non-significant differences.

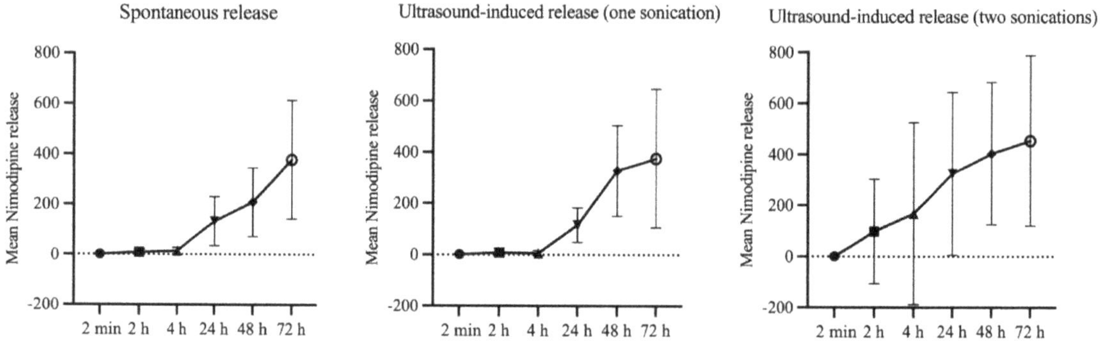

Figure 6. The time course of spontaneous and on-demand nimodipine release profile by singular and repeated sonication over a period of 72 h.

4. Discussion

In this in vitro study, the nimodipine release from a drug-loaded nanocarrier could be successfully enhanced through repeated sonications. These findings proofed the concept of an on-demand drug release by applying ultrasound. A time-dependent increase in nimodipine concentrations was measured within the first two hours after sonication, following a gradual return to baseline again starting four hours after sonication. This allowed a temporary, on-demand increase in nimodipine concentration within the CSF by means of ultrasound, which was a prerequisite for the implementation of this concept in clinical practice. Because previous studies showed that a reversal of angiographic vasospasm does not necessarily result in a better outcome, a neuroprotective effect of nimodipine is deemed to be responsible for the positive impact of nimodipine on the outcome [20–22]. Currently, nimodipine is used in clinical practice with prophylactics (i.e., prevention of cerebral vasospasm) as well as therapeutic interventions (treatment of manifested cerebral vasospasm causing neurological deficits and/or cerebral perfusion deficits). The nimodipine-loaded nanodrug presented in our study with a continuous spontaneous drug release as well as an increased on-demand release through sonication seems to be suitable for both purposes.

4.1. Advantages and Limitations of Systemic Administration Routes for Nimodipine

A meta-analysis conducted by Geraldini et al. in 2022 showed that both oral and intravenous nimodipine were effective in preventing unfavorable outcomes and DCI, but had no influence on mortality [23]. Another meta-analysis published in 2023, which included nine randomized controlled trials, demonstrated no statistically significant difference between intravenous and enteral administration in terms of mortality, DCI, delayed ischemic neurological deficits and outcome [24]. However, the area under the cumulative ranking curve showed a trend for enteral administration to be first, intravenous administration to be second, and placebo to be last in terms of mortality, occurrence of DCI, and poor outcomes [24]. In a more recently published retrospective, multicenter, observational cohort study conducted in 21 hospitals across North America, Mahmoud et al. assessed the extent to which different nimodipine formulations and routes of administration were associated with the safety and efficacy of nimodipine in aSAH [25]. While the administration of nimodipine in liquid form was independently associated with a higher prevalence of diarrhea, the withdrawal of liquid from nimodipine capsules prior to administration was significantly associated with a higher prevalence of nimodipine dose reduction or discontinuation due to hypotension. Crushing the tablets and withdrawing the liquid from the capsules at the bedside before administration were associated with an increased likelihood of DCI [25]. In an observational cohort study, Rass et al. recorded hemodynamic responses in patients with SAH receiving prophylactic nimodipine with either oral or intravenous administration [26]. Hemodynamic responses were assessed within the first hour after the start of nimodipine therapy. It was found that 30% of patients experienced a reduction in blood pressure of more than 10% immediately after the start of nimodipine infusion, with the maximum effect occurring after 15 min [26]. Approximately half of these patients required an immediate increase in norepinephrine, and a further 10% required colloids within one hour of the start of the nimodipine infusion to counteract a further drop in blood pressure [26]. The situation was different with oral nimodipine administration, where significant reductions in blood pressure of >10% occurred later and less frequently—with a consequent increase in the use of noradrenaline. Changes in mean arterial blood pressure (MAP), cerebral perfusion pressure (CPP), cerebral tissue oxygen tension (pbtO$_2$) and cerebral metabolism after oral administration of nimodipine were analyzed in a retrospective study using mixed linear models [27]. Oral administration of nimodipine was shown to reduce MAP, leading to a reduction in cerebral perfusion and oxygenation [27]. However, this study is limited by the small number of cases and the retrospective study design. Furthermore, nimodipine, as a dihydropyridine calcium channel antagonist acts on countless cell types throughout the body and has probably more complex mechanisms of action than simply preventing cerebral vasoconstrictions [28].

4.2. Advantages and Limitation of Local Nimodipine Administration

Advances in the development of alternative administration pathways for nimodipine have reignited interest in refining its potential therapeutic use. A site-specific, sustained-release administration may increase drug concentrations at the site where it is most needed, while avoiding additional adverse effects associated with systemic hypotension. Local drug administration, i.e., pellet-based therapeutics placed around the basal cerebral arteries during aneurysm clipping with continuous release of the calcium antagonist nicardipine, have been shown to be safe [29–31]. Furthermore, local drug administration was associated with less hypotension, led to significantly higher drug concentrations at the target organ, and resulted in a less frequent occurrence of cerebral vasospasm [20,30]. However, pellet-based therapeutics can be used only in surgically treated patients, which limits their use in patients undergoing endovascular coiling to repair ruptured aneurysms [32]. Accordingly, the idea of a new platform for the local administration of nimodipine with delayed release using polymers is maturing. Several studies on the intrathecal administration of calcium channel blockers bound to polymers have already been published [8,18,33,34]. An initial pharmacokinetic evaluation showed that the release of nimodipine after administration consisted of an initial surge followed by a sustained release over 21 days [8].

Based on these encouraging results, the PROMISE (Prolonged Release nimodipine microparticles after Subarachnoid hemorrhage) trial was initially designed in 2015 as a single-center, open-label, non-randomized, dose-escalating Phase I study to evaluate the efficacy, safety and tolerability of the intracisternal administration of EG-1962 (nimodipine in a biodegradable polymer suspended in hyaluronic acid administered as one intraventricular injection that releases nimodipine into the subarachnoid space for at least 21 days) in patients undergoing surgical treatment for aSAH [18]. At the same time, Hänggi et al., who are also the principal investigators and authors of the PROMISE study, initiated the NEWTON study (Nimodipine microparticles to Enhance recovery While reducing Toxicity after subarachnoid hemorrhage) [33]. In contrast to PROMISE, NEWTON is designed as a multicenter, controlled, randomized, open-label, dose-escalation study to evaluate the safety, tolerability, and pharmacokinetics of EG-1962 and nimodipine in patients with aneurysmal SAH, and has already demonstrated efficacy in a Phase 2 study [33]. Across the board, EG-1962 was considered safe and well tolerated. In addition, the group treated with EG-1962 showed a lower rate of DCI—correspondingly, the need for rescue therapy was also lower. Overall, the rate of favorable clinical outcomes was higher in the EG-1962-treated group than in the conventionally treated group [33]. The limitation of these nanodrugs was the lack of ability to externally influence the drug release on demand, which was addressed in our study. With this in vitro study, we were able not only to demonstrate an on-demand increase in drug release through singular sonication, but also to show the possibility of further modifying the drug release by means of repeated sonication, which opens the door for the direct guidance of drug release. In addition to the continuous prophylactic release to prevent vasospasm, we were also able to demonstrate and prove an on-demand release using low-frequency ultrasound, opening up the possibility of on-demand therapeutic intervention in addition to highly effective local prophylaxis.

4.3. Limitations of the Study

As in vitro experiments were conducted, the study does not allow conclusions regarding the effects of the nanodrug in an in vivo scenario. The findings of this experimental study represent the basis for planning and conducting in vivo evaluations of the concept in animal models. Future studies are also needed to shed light on the mechanism involved in ultrasound-mediated drug release from nanodrugs, because this was not the subject of our study and the mechanisms behind it remain unclear. Further experiments are required to answer the question, 'how many sonications are needed to release all of the nimodipine from the nanodrug?' Despite the limitations, the results of our study encourage the further evaluation of the concept in animal models and can be seen as a solid basis for planning future experiments.

5. Conclusions

The data obtained support the successful results of our previously published study of the nanocarrier system of nimodipine-loaded Pluronic® F-127 copolymers in an artificial CSF medium. The experiments presented here confirm a further significant on-demand increase in nimodipine release after repeated sonications. These results support the concept of ultrasound-controlled treatment of cerebral vasospasm by increasing the nimodipine release from a nimodipine-loaded nanodrug on-demand by applying ultrasound.

Further evaluation in animal studies or other in vivo environments is required to further explore this promising concept, the determinants of which have now been tested and proven several times.

Author Contributions: K.D. performed the experiments, contributed to data analysis, and wrote the manuscript draft. S.S. contributed to the methodology of the experiments. M.N. contributed to the supervision of the experiments and critically reviewed the final version of the manuscript. H.L. critically reviewed the final version of the manuscript. F.S. and A.F. contributed to the measurement of nimodipine concentrations and critically reviewed the final version of the manuscript. V.R. contributed to supervision and critically reviewed the final version of the manuscript. V.M. contributed to conceptualization, data analysis and interpretation and supervision and critically reviewed the final version of the manuscript. All authors have read and agreed to the published version of the manuscript.

Funding: The study was funded by a grant awarded to Vesna Malinova by the German Society of Neurosurgery (Stiftung Neurochirurgische Forschung).

Institutional Review Board Statement: Since this is an in vitro study without inclusion of animals or humans, ethics approval was not necessary for this study.

Informed Consent Statement: This is an in vitro experimental study. Therefore, no informed consent was required.

Data Availability Statement: All relevant data and materials are presented in the manuscript.

Conflicts of Interest: The authors declare that they have no known financial interests or personal relationships that could have appeared to influence the work reported in this paper. All authors have seen and approved the final version of the manuscript being submitted.

References

1. Budohoski, K.P.; Guilfoyle, M.; Helmy, A.; Huuskonen, T.; Czosnyka, M.; Kirollos, R.; Menon, D.K.; Pickard, J.D.; Kirkpatrick, P.J. The pathophysiology and treatment of delayed cerebral ischemia following subarachnoid hemorrhage. *J. Neurol. Neurosurg. Psychiatry* **2014**, *85*, 1343–1353. [CrossRef] [PubMed]
2. Flynn, L.; Andrews, P. Advances in the understanding of delayed cerebral ischemia after aneurysmal subarachnoid hemorrhage. *F1000Research* **2015**, *4*, 1200. [CrossRef]
3. Francoeur, C.L.; Mayer, S.A. Management of delayed cerebral ischemia after subarachnoid hemorrhage. *Crit. Care* **2016**, *20*, 277. [CrossRef]
4. Diringer, M.N.; Bleck, T.P.; Claude Hemphill, J., 3rd; Menon, D.; Shutter, L.; Vespa, P.; Bruder, N.; Sander Connolly, E., Jr.; Citerio, G.; Gress, D.; et al. Critical care management of patients following aneurysmal subarachnoid hemorrhage: Recommendations from the Neurocritical Care Society's Multidisciplinary Consensus Conference. *Neurocrit. Care* **2011**, *15*, 211–240. [CrossRef]
5. Dorhout Mees, S.M.; Rinkel, G.J.E.; Feigin, V.L.; Algra, A.; van den Bergh, W.M.; Vermeulen, M.; van Gijn, J. Calcium antagonists for aneurysmal subarachnoid hemorrhage. *Cochrane Database Syst. Rev.* **2007**, *18*, CD000277. [CrossRef]
6. Sandow, N.; Diesing, D.; Sarrafzadeh, A.; Vajkoczy, P.; Wolf, S. Nimodipine dose reductions in the treatment of patients with aneurysmal subarachnoid hemorrhage. *Neurocrit. Care* **2016**, *25*, 29–39. [CrossRef] [PubMed]
7. Hernandez-Duran, S.; Mielke, D.; Rohde, V.; Malinova, V. Does nimodipine interruption due to high catecholamine doses lead to a greater incidence of delayed cerebral ischemia in the setting of aneurysmal subarachnoid hemorrhage? *World Neurosurg.* **2019**, *132*, e834–e840. [CrossRef] [PubMed]
8. Hänggi, D.; Etminan, N.; Steiger, H.J.; Johnson, M.; Peet, M.M.; Tice, T.; Burton, K.; Hudson, B.; Turner, M.; Stella, A.; et al. A side-specific, sustained-release drug delivery system for aneurysmal subarachnoid hemorrhage. *Neurotherapeutics* **2016**, *13*, 439–449. [CrossRef] [PubMed]
9. Mudshinge, S.R.; Deore, A.B.; Patil, S.; Bhalgat, C.M. Nanoparticles: Emerging carriers for drug delivery. *Saudi Pharm.* **2011**, *19*, 129–141. [CrossRef]
10. Mdlovu, N.V.; Juang, R.S.; Weng, M.T.; Lin, K.S. Green synthesis and characterization of silicate nanostructures coated with Pluronic F127/gelatin for triggered drug delivery in tumor microenvironments. *Int. J. Biol. Macromol.* **2023**, *251*, 126337. [CrossRef]
11. Pampaloni, N.P.; Giugliano, M.; Scaini, D.; Ballerini, L.; Rauti, R. Advances in nano neuroscience: From nanomaterials to nanotools. *Front. Neurosci.* **2019**, *12*, 953. [CrossRef] [PubMed]
12. Opris, I.; Lebedev, M.A.; Pulgar, V.M.; Vidu, R.; Enachescu, M.; Casanova, M.F. Editorial: Nanotechnologies in neuroscience and neuroengineering. *Front. Neurosci.* **2020**, *14*, 33. [CrossRef]

13. Hänggi, D.; Etminan, N.; Macdonald, R.L.; Steiger, H.J.; Mayer, S.A.; Aldrich, E.F.; Diringer, M.N.; Hoh, B.L.; Mocco, J.; Strange, P.; et al. NEWTON: Nimodipine microparticles to enhance recovery with reducing toxicity after subarachnoid hemorrhage. *Neurocrit. Care* **2015**, *23*, 274–284. [CrossRef] [PubMed]
14. Chiappetta, D.; Sosnik, A. Poly(ethylene oxide)–poly(propylene oxide) block copolymer micellesas drug delivery agents: Improved hydrosolubility, stability and bioavailability of drugs. *Eur. J. Pharm. Biopharm.* **2007**, *66*, 303–317. [CrossRef] [PubMed]
15. Sun, C.; Wang, J.; Liu, J.; Qui, L.; Zhang, W.; Zhang, L. Liquid proliposomes of nimodipine drug delivery system: Preparation, characterization, and pharmacokinetics. *AAPS Pharm. Sci. Tech.* **2013**, *14*, 332–338. [CrossRef]
16. Etminan, N.; Macdonald, R.L.; Davis, C.; Burton, K.; Steiger, H.J.; Hänggi, D. Intrathecal application of the nimodipine slow-release microparticle system eg-1962 for prevention of delayed cerebral ischemia and improvement of outcome after aneurysmal subarachnoid hemorrhage. *Acta Neurochir. Suppl.* **2015**, *120*, 281–286.
17. Döring, K.; Sperling, S.; Ninkovic, M.; Schroeder, H.; Fischer, A.; Stadelmann, C.; Streit, F.; Binder, L.; Mielke, D.; Rohde, V.; et al. Ultrasound-Induced Release of Nimodipine from Drug-Loaded Block Copolymer Micelles: In Vivo Analysis. *Transl. Stroke Res.* **2022**, *13*, 792–800. [CrossRef] [PubMed]
18. Sotoudegana, F.; Aminib, M.; Faizic, M.; Abofazelia, R. Nimodipine-loaded Pluronic® block copolymer micelles: Preparation, characterization, in-vitro and in-vivo studies. *Iran. J. Pharm. Res.* **2016**, *15*, 641–661.
19. Döring, K.; Sperling, S.; Ninkovic, M.; Gasimov, T.; Stadelmann, C.; Streit, F.; Binder, L.; Rohde, V.; Malinova, V. Ultrasound-induced release of nimodipine from drug-loaded block copolymers: In vitro analysis. *J. Drug Del. Sci. Technol.* **2021**, *66*, 102834. [CrossRef]
20. Bederson, J.B.; Connolly, E.S., Jr.; Batjer, H.H.; Dacey, R.G.; Dion, J.E.; Diringer, M.N.; Duldner, J.E., Jr.; Harbaugh, R.E.; Patel, A.B.; Rosenwasser, R.H.; et al. Guidelines for the management of aneurysmal subarachnoid hemorrhage: A statement for healthcare professionals from a special writing group of the Stroke Council, American Heart Association. *Stroke* **2009**, *40*, 994–1025. [CrossRef]
21. Raabe, A.; Beck, J.; Berkefeld, J.; Deinsberger, W.; Meixensberger, J.; Schmiedek, P.; Seifert, V.; Steinmetz, H.; Unterberg, A.; Vajkoczy, P.; et al. Recommendations for the management of patients with aneurysmal subarachnoid hemorrhage. *Zentralbl. Neurochir.* **2005**, *66*, 79–91. [CrossRef] [PubMed]
22. Vatter, H.; Seifert, V. Vasospams pharmacology. *Acta Neurochir. Suppl.* **2009**, *104*, 115–118.
23. Geraldini, F.; De Cassai, A.; Diana, P.; Correale, C.; Boscolo, A.; Zampirollo, S.; Disaro, L.; Carere, A.; Cacco, N.; Navalesi, P.; et al. A comparison between enteral and intravenoius nimodipine in subarachnoid hemorrhage: A systematic review and network meta-analysis. *Neurocrit. Care* **2022**, *36*, 1071–1079. [CrossRef] [PubMed]
24. Lei, G.; Rao, Z.; Hu, Y. The efficacy of different nimodipine administration route for treating subarachnoid hemorrhage: A network meta-analysis. *Medicine* **2023**, *102*, e34789. [CrossRef]
25. Mahmoud, S.H.; Hefny, F.R.; Panos, N.G.; Delucilla, L.; Ngan, Z.; Perreault, M.M.; Hamilton, L.A.; Rowe, A.S.; Buschur, P.L.; Owusu-Guha, J.; et al. Comparison of nimodipine formulations and administration techniques via enteral feeding tubes in patients with aneurysmal subarachnoid hemorrhage: A multicenter retrospective cohort study. *Pharmacotherapy* **2023**, *43*, 279–290. [CrossRef]
26. Rass, V.; Kindl, P.; Lindner, A.; Kofler, M.; Altmann, K.; Putnina, L.; Ianosi, B.A.; Schiefecker, A.J.; Beer, R.; Pfausler, B.; et al. Blood pressure changes in association with nimodipine therapy in patients with spontaneous subarachnoid hemorrhage. *Neurocrit. Care* **2023**, *39*, 104–115. [CrossRef]
27. Moser, M.; Schwarz, Y.; Herta, J.; Plöchl, W.; Reinprecht, A.; Zeitlinger, M.; Brugger, J.; Ramazanova, D.; Rössler, K.; Hosmann, A. The effect of oral nimodipine on cerebral metabolism and hemodynamic parameters in patients suffering aneurysmal subarachnoid hemorrhage. *J. Neurosurg. Anesthesiol.* **2023**, *36*, 317–325. [CrossRef]
28. Carlson, A.P.; Hänggi, D.; Macdonald, R.L.; Shuttleworth, C.W. Nimodipine reappraised: An old drug with a future. *Curr. Neuropharmacol.* **2020**, *18*, 65–82. [CrossRef]
29. Kerschbaumer, J.; Freyschlag, C.F.; Petr, O.; Adage, T.; Breitenbach, J.J.; Wessels, L.; Wolf, S.; Hecht, N.; Gempt, J.; Wostrack, M.; et al. A randomized, single ascending dose safety, tolerability, and pharmacokinetics study of NicaPlant in aneurysmal subarachnoid hemorrhage patients undergoing clipping. *Brain Spine* **2023**, *3*, 102673. [CrossRef] [PubMed]
30. Kasuya, H.; Onda, H.; Sasahara, A.; Takeshita, M.; Hori, T. Application of nicardipine prolonged-release implants: Analysis of 97 consecutive patients with acute subarachnoid hemorrhage. *Neurosurgery* **2005**, *56*, 895–902. [CrossRef]
31. Vandenbulcke, A.; Messerer, M.; Garvayo Navarro, M.; Peters, D.R.; Starnoni, D.; Giammattei, L.; Ben-Hamouda, N.; Puccinelli, F.; Saliou, G.; Cossu, G.; et al. Cisternal nicardipine for prevention of delayed cerebral ischemia in aneurysmal subarachnoid hemorrhage: A comparative retrospective cohort study. *Acta Neurochir.* **2024**, *166*, 133. [CrossRef] [PubMed]
32. Barth, M.; Pena, P.; Seiz, M.; Thomé, C.; Muench, E.; Weidauer, S.; Hattingen, E.; Kasuya, H.; Schmiedek, P. Feasibility of intraventricular nicardipine prolonged release implants in patients following aneurysmal subarachnoid haemorrhage. *Br. J. Neurosurg.* **2011**, *25*, 677–683. [CrossRef] [PubMed]

33. Hänggi, D.; Etminan, N.; Aldrich, F.; Steiger, H.J.; Mayer, S.A.; Diringer, M.N.; Hoh, B.L.; Mocco, J.; Faleck, H.J.; Loch Macdonald, R.; et al. Randomized, open-label, phase 1/2a study to determine the maximum tolerated dose of intraventricular sustained release nimodipine for subarachnoid hemorrhage (NEWTON [Nimodipine microparticles to enhance recovery while reducing toxicity after subarachnoid hemorrhage]). *Stroke* **2017**, *48*, 145–151.
34. Macdonald, R.L.; Hänggi, D.; Ko, N.U.; Darsaut, T.E.; Carlson, A.P.; Wong, G.K.; Etminan, N.; Mayer, S.A.; Aldrich, E.F.; Diringer, M.N.; et al. NEWTON-2 Cisternal (Nimodipine Microparticles to Enhance Recovery While Reducing Toxicity After Subarachnoid Hemorrhage): A Phase 2, Multicenter, Randomized, Open-Label Safety Study of Intracisternal EG-1962 in Aneurysmal Subarachnoid Hemorrhage. *Neurosurgery* **2020**, *88*, E13–E26. [CrossRef]

brain sciences

MDPI

Article

Management of Anterior Choroidal Artery Aneurysms: A Retrospective Cohort Study

Andrew Falzon [1,*], Shigeta Miyake [2], Tze Phei Kee [3], Hugo Andrade-Barazarte [4,5] and Timo Krings [6,7]

1 Department of Neuroradiology, Atkinson Morley Regional Neuroscience Centre, St George's University Hospital, Tooting, London SW17 0QT, UK
2 Department of Neurosurgery, Yokohama City University School of Medicine, Yokohama 236-004, Japan
3 Department of Neuroradiology, National Neuroscience Institute, Singapore 308433, Singapore
4 Division of Neurosurgery, Toronto Western Hospital, Toronto, ON M5T 2S8, Canada
5 Sprott Department of Surgery, University of Toronto, Toronto, ON M5T 2S8, Canada
6 Division of Neurointerventional Radiology, UMass-Chan Lahey Department of Radiology, Lahey Hospital and Medical Centre—Beth Israel Lahey Health, Burlington, MA 01805, USA
7 TH Chan School of Medicine, UMass Chan Medical School, Worcester, MA 01655, USA
* Correspondence: andrewmfalzon@gmail.com

Abstract: Background: Anterior choroidal artery (AChoA) aneurysms pose a challenge for both endovascular and clipping procedures. The eloquent territory supplied by the parent vessel has limited collateralization and its compromise can lead to significant morbidity. This study aims to analyze the clinical outcomes and procedure-related complications of clipping and endovascular treatment of AChoA aneurysms to aid physician decision making. **Methods:** Thirty-two ruptured and unruptured AChoA aneurysms that underwent catheter angiography at a single neurovascular center between January 2000 and December 2023 were included. Either conservative management, clipping, and/or endovascular treatment were performed. Clinical outcomes and complications were analyzed retrospectively. **Results:** Twenty-four endovascular treatments and seven clipping procedures were included. Of the total 24 endovascular procedures, 46% were primary coiling, 25% were balloon-assisted coiling, 13% were flow diverting stent, 8% were combined balloon-assisted coiling and flow diverting stent, and 8% were combined balloon-assisted and stent-assisted coiling. There was no procedure-related mortality in both groups. No intra- or post-procedural ruptures/re-ruptures occurred during follow-up in both endovascular and clipping cohorts. AChoA territory infarcts occurred in 4% of the endovascular and 29% of the clipping cohorts. Other thromboembolic complications occurred in 4% of the endovascular cohort. The recurrence rate requiring retreatment was 12.5% for the endovascular and 43% for the clipping cohort. A favorable clinical outcome (mRS ≤ 2) was 78% for the endovascular cohort and 67% for the clipping cohort. **Conclusions:** Endovascular and clipping outcomes align with prior studies, with endovascular showing a favorable safety profile. Both approaches are viable, though they present distinct risks and advantages.

Keywords: anterior choroidal artery aneurysm; endovascular; flow diverter stent; balloon-assisted coiling; stent-assisted coiling; clipping

1. Introduction

Anterior choroidal artery (AChoA) aneurysms account for a small proportion of all intracranial aneurysms, comprising 2–5% of the total [1]. The treatment of these aneurysms may pose challenges due to their complex anatomical and hemodynamic characteristics, which are prone to ischemic stroke [2]. Both endovascular and surgical treatment options are possible, each with distinct advantages and disadvantages [3].

More recent advances in endovascular technology and procedural techniques allowed for many cases to be effectively treated this way [4,5]. The efficacy and safety of these two treatment modalities were described previously in relatively small case series due to the low incidence of these aneurysms. A recent meta-analysis of these case series has provided further insight into this rare entity and its treatment; however, many limitations and unknowns remain.

The purpose of this study is to analyze the clinical outcomes and procedure-related complications of endovascular treatment and clipping of the AChoA aneurysms in a single tertiary hospital to help aid future management and improve patient outcome.

2. Materials and Methods

This retrospective cohort study reviewed ruptured and unruptured AChoA aneurysms that underwent assessment with catheter angiography and subsequent conservative management, clipping, or endovascular treatment at a single neurovascular tertiary center between January 2000 and December 2023.

A total of 32 patients were recruited. Nineteen patients underwent primary endovascular treatment. Of these, two patients required endovascular retreatment and one patient required retreatment with clipping. Six patients underwent primary clipping. Of these, three patients required endovascular retreatment. A total of 24 endovascular and 7 clipping procedures were performed.

Twelve patients were initially managed conservatively with modification of risk factors and regular imaging surveillance. Of these, four patients underwent subsequent primary endovascular treatment and one underwent primary clipping. Treatment was not indicated in the remaining seven patients.

The inclusion criteria were: patients with an unruptured or ruptured AChoA aneurysms and (1) pre-treatment digital subtraction angiography; (2) rotational angiography with 3D reconstruction; (3) accessible electronic medical records; and (4) underwent clipping, endovascular treatment, and/or conservative management.

The exclusion criteria were: (1) atypical aneurysms, including dissecting, blister-type, or fusiform; and (2) patients lacking sufficient Digital Imaging and Communications in Medicine (DICOM) data for accurate volume rendering. This ensured more accurate aneurysm characterization.

All clinical data were obtained from a local hospital research database and individual electronic patient records. Hypertension was defined as at least two separate blood pressure measurements recorded in medical records with a systolic blood pressure > 140 mm Hg or a diastolic blood pressure of >90 mm Hg. Smoking was defined as current cigarette smoking at the time of admission with cumulative smoking history of at least five pack years. Family history of aneurysm was defined as having two first degree relatives with a diagnosed intracranial aneurysm.

Data were analyzed using IBM SPSS Statistics 29.0.2.0 for Mac. Continuous variables were demonstrated as mean/median and range. Categorical variables were demonstrated as total numbers and percentages. A STROBE checklist was utilized as a guide throughout.

2.1. Endovascular Procedural Details

All sterile procedures were performed under general anesthesia using a closed system of continuous heparinized saline flush. In total, 22/24 (92%) were performed using right common femoral artery access and 2/24 (8%) were performed using right radial artery access.

Systemic heparinization was administered intravenously with an initial bolus of 100 IU per kg of body weight, and 1000 IU administered every hour after. If radial access was used, a cocktail containing 3000 IU of heparin, 2.5 mg of verapamil, and 150 mcg of nitroglycerin was administered intra-arterially, with additional IV heparin top up. Diagnostic angiography, including rotational angiography with 3D volume rendering, was performed and analyzed to determine the most appropriate endovascular or surgical approach. Endovascular approaches included primary coiling, balloon assisted coiling (BAC), stent assisted coiling (SAC), and flow diverting stent (FDS).

All elective patients were loaded on dual antiplatelet therapy for five days prior to the procedure with Aspirin 81 mg PO OD and Ticagrelor 90 mg PO BD or Clopidogrel 75 mg OD. The choice of antiplatelet therapy was based on operator preference. No platelet function testing was performed. If a flow divertor was implanted, dual antiplatelet therapy was continued for three months. This was converted to single antiplatelet therapy with Aspirin only if follow up surveillance imaging was satisfactory. All acute patients were treated with primary coiling and were not loaded on antiplatelet therapy.

2.2. Clipping Procedural Details

In our approach, the treatment modality would be determined after 3D angiographic evaluation. Endovascular approach would be considered unless an unfavorable outcome was anticipated, therefore requiring clipping.

Three cases were performed through an ipsilateral lateral supra-orbital craniotomy and four cases through an ipsilateral pterional craniotomy. One of these cases was referred with limited intra-operative information. A sub-frontal approach was performed using microsurgical techniques. In all six cases, patency of the AChoA was verified intra-operatively using indocyanine green (ICG) video angiography. Somatosensory and motor evoked potentials (SSEPs and MEPs) were also used to monitor neurological dysfunction intra-operatively.

2.3. Multidisciplinary Approach and Neurovascular Experience

The treatment modality would be determined following angiographic assessment and discussion within a neurovascular board meeting or mini multidisciplinary meeting.

The neurovascular group consists of senior operators, including microvascular neurosurgeons, interventional neuroradiologists, and hybrids. An endovascular approach would typically be considered the preferred first line treatment unless an unfavourable outcome was anticipated, therefore requiring clipping

The institution is a high-volume teaching hospital with approximately 50–65 patients seen in a multidisciplinary neurovascular clinic each week. This includes new referrals and follow-up for microvascular or endovascular procedures. Lead operators include a microvascular neurosurgeon with 15 years out of fellowship and interventional neuroradiologists with 5–20 years out of fellowship. Approximately 70% of treated aneurysms are via endovascular approach, with the remaining being surgical. Exact procedural numbers vary from year to year.

2.4. Post-Procedural Follow-Up

Routine CT or MR angiography follow-up was performed in accordance with local guidelines for all aneurysm patients in our center. Pre- and post-procedural clinical assessments were performed by an interventional neuroradiologist and/or a vascular neurosurgeon. The clinical follow-up was performed through our multidisciplinary outpatient neurovascular clinic. If the patient was lost to follow-up or repatriated to their local institution, the latest clinical outcome available was used.

2.5. Evaluation of Treatment Efficacy, Clinical Outcome, and Complications

All imaging data were reviewed by an interventional neuroradiologist. Treatment efficacy was evaluated using immediate post-procedural modified Raymond Roy classification (mRRC) and by reviewing follow-up imaging data for recurrence, residuum growth, and re-rupture.

Clinical outcome for all patients was evaluated using the modified Rankin scale (mRS) before and after intervention at the last available follow-up. A favorable mRS was defined as $\leq$2. A poor outcome was defined as >2.

For the ruptured cases, the World Federation of Neurological Surgeons grading scale (WFNS) and Hunter and Hess (HH) scale were obtained from medical records. Modified fisher grade was evaluated on the initial non-contrast CT head and interpreted by a blinded neuroradiologist.

Intra-procedural complications were evaluated by reviewing angiographic images and procedure notes. Post-procedural complications were evaluated by reviewing clinic notes and surveillance imaging. The incidence of vasospasm secondary to subarachnoid hemorrhage (SAH) was analyzed as a factor impacting clinical outcome.

3. Results

For the total 32 patients, the mean age was 50, with a range of 20–80 years. There were 5/32 (16%) males and 27/32 (84%) females; 5/32 (16%) patients had hypertension, 14/32 (44%) patients had multiple intracranial aneurysms, and 4/32 (13%) had previous SAH from another aneurysm rupture.

There were 17/32 (53%) ruptured AChoA aneurysms, and 15/32 (47%) were unruptured. For the ruptured aneurysms, the mean PHASES score was 4.5 with a range of 4–7. For the unruptured aneurysms, the mean PHASES score was 4.9 with a range of 4–10 (Table 1).

Table 1. PHASES scores in the endovascular and clipping cohorts with pre-procedural hemorrhage status.

	Ruptured		Unruptured		Total	
PHASES	Endo	Clip	Endo	Clip	Endo	Clip
4	8	3	1	1	9	4
5	3	1	4	0	7	1
6	1	0	0	1	1	1
7	1	0	0	0	1	0
10	0	0	1	0	1	0

Aneurysm size for the entire cohort had a mean of 3.9 mm, with a range of 1.3–11 mm. For the ruptured cohort, the mean size was 4.2 mm with a range of 1.3 to 7 mm. For the unruptured cohort, the mean size was 3.5 mm with a range of 2 to 11 mm.

Aneurysm neck diameter had a mean of 2.4 mm with a range of 1.1–5 mm. For the ruptured patients, the mean neck was 2.6 mm with a range of 1.5 to 3.6 mm, and for the unruptured patients, the mean neck was 2.2 mm with a range of 1.1 to 3.6 mm.

Aspects ratio had a mean of 1.74, with a range of 0.87–3.44. For the ruptured cases, the mean was 1.74 with a range of 0.87 to 3.16 mm. For the unruptured cases, it was 1.60 with a range of 1 to 3.44.

3.1. Conservative Management

Conservative management was indicated in seven patients during the entirety of their follow-up. These aneurysms did not demonstrate an appreciable change in volume or morphology over a median of 31 months of follow-up with an interquartile range of 50.5 months. The average aneurysm size of this group was 2.4 mm, with a median of 2.3 mm and a range of 2–2.6 mm.

3.2. Endovascular and Clipping Cohorts

A total of 25/32 (78%) patients were treated; 12/32 (38%) were initially managed conservatively. Of these, 5/12 (42%) required treatment and 7/12 (58%) did not.

A total of 24 endovascular treatments were performed; 19/24 (79%) were primary endovascular cases, 2/24 (8%) were secondary treatments following primary endovascular treatment, and 3/24 (13%) were secondary treatments following primary clipping (Figure 1).

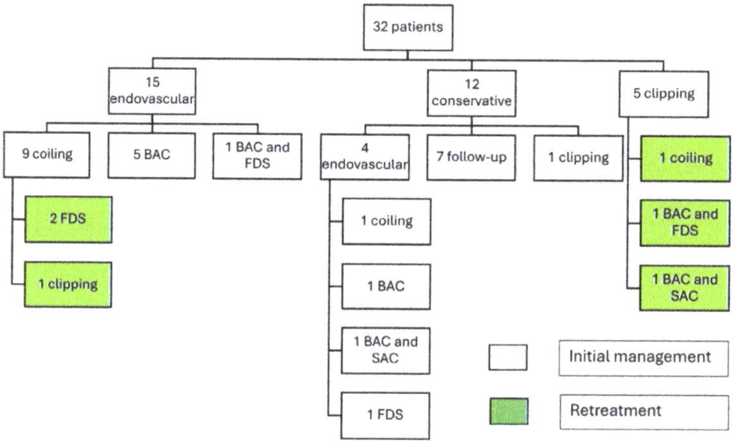

Figure 1. Schematic representation of the conservative, endovascular, and clipping management of each patient. Retreatments are highlighted in green.

Of all 19 primary endovascular cases, 10/19 cases (53%) underwent primary coiling, as a part of the initial management, 6/19 (32%) underwent BAC alone, 1/19 (5%) underwent combined BAC and SAC, 1 case (5%) underwent combined BAC and FDS, and 1 case (5%) underwent FDS.

Of all 5 secondary endovascular cases, 2/5 (40%) were initially treated with primary coiling and retreated with FDS, while 3/5 (60%) were initially treated with primary clipping and retreated with various endovascular techniques, including 1/5 (20%) BAC and FDS, 1/5 (20%) BAC and SAC, and 1/5 (20%) coiling alone.

A total of 7 clipping treatments were performed. Of these, 6/7 (86%) were primary clipping cases and 1/7 (14%) was secondary treatment following primary endovascular treatment.

3.3. Ruptured and Unruptured Cohorts

A total of 21/31 (68%) procedures were for the ruptured aneurysms and 10/31 (32%) were for the unruptured aneurysms. Within the endovascular cohort, 13/24 (54%) patients had a ruptured aneurysm and 11/24 (46%) patients had an unruptured aneurysm. Within the clipping cohort, 5/7 (71%) patients had a ruptured aneurysm and 2/7 (29%) patients had an unruptured aneurysm.

3.4. Procedure Related Complications

The complications of the 24 endovascular cases and 7 clipping cases are discussed below.

3.4.1. Procedure Related Infarction

A total of 4/31 (13%) patients experienced thromboembolic complications, 2 in the endovascular cohort (2/24 = 8.3%) and 2 in the surgical cohort (2/7 = 28.5%). All four patients were ruptured pre-procedure (Table 2).

Table 2. Morphological and clinical details of the four cases that had a procedural related infarct, all of which were treated as acutely ruptured aneurysms.

#	Treatment	ASA Use	AChoA Involvement	Size (mm)	Neck (mm)	Width (mm)	ASPECT Ratio
1	Clip	No	Yes	4.5	3.7	4	1.22
2	Clip	No	Yes	5	2.2	5.9	2.27
3	Coil	No	Yes	2.5	2.4	1.6	1.04
4	BAC	Yes	Yes	3.8	2	2.6	1.90

ASA acetylsalicylic acid; ASPECT Ratio (Dome/Neck); BAC balloon assisted coiling.

Within the endovascular cohort, one patient had an AChoA territory infarct (Figure 1) and the other had a catheter-related PCA (posterior cerebral artery) and MCA (middle cerebral artery) territory infarct. The catheter-related infarct presented with limb hemiparesis after 4 h, which resolved after 1 week.

Within the clipping cohort, both patients had AChoA territory infarcts. The post-procedural mRS were 5 and 3, respectively (Figure 2).

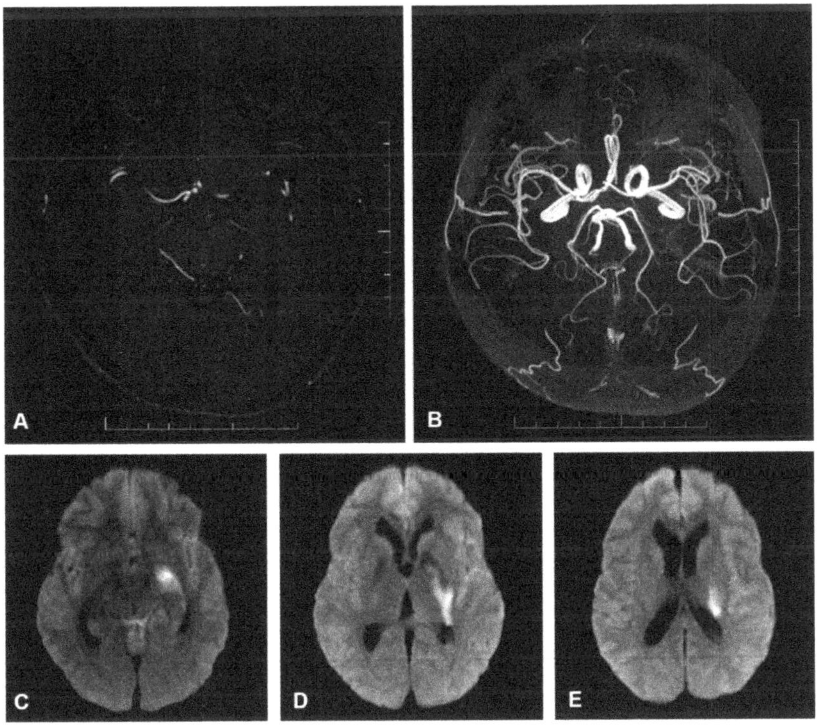

Figure 2. (**A**) axial image of a contrast enhanced MR intracranial angiogram which demonstrates the course of the AChoA. The artery gives rise to multiple perforators as it traverses the carotid, ambient and choroidal cisterns which may supply adjacent eloquent structures including the optic nerve, medial temporal lobe and middle cerebral peduncle. (**B**) axial image of a maximum intensity projection of the same contrast enhanced MR angiogram which demonstrates the path of the AChoA in relation to the anterior and posterior circulation. (**C–E**) B1000 diffusion weighted axial images of the brain arranged caudal to cranial. These panels demonstrate restricted diffusion (hyperintensity) involving the AChoA territory in keeping with acute infarction.There is involvement of the hippocampus/mesiotemporal lobe (**C**), internal limb of the internal capsule encroaching on the lateral thalamus (**D**), and the corona radiate extending towards the caudate tail (**E**).

3.4.2. Recurrence and Retreatment

A total of 6/31 patients (19%) were retreated while 25/31 (81%) did not have a recurrence or need retreatment. Within the endovascular cohort, 3/24 (12.5%) patients required retreatment and 21/24 (87.5%) did not require any further treatment on follow-up (Table 3). Of those requiring retreatment, 2/3 (66%) were ruptured on initial treatment (Figure 1). One patient was initially treated with primary coiling and retreated by flow diverter stent, following recurrence after 5 months. The second patient was initially treated with primary coiling and was retreated with clipping due to recurrence after 3 months. Of these, 1/3 (33%) were unruptured on initial treatment with primary coiling and were retreated with a flow diverting stent (Figure 3).

Table 3. Morphological and clinical details of the six cases that had recurrence requiring retreatment.

#	Initial Bleed	Initial Treatment	Reccurent Treatment	AChoA Involvment	Size (mm)	Neck (mm)	Width (mm)	ASPECT Ratio
1	No	Clip	BAC and FDS	No	4.5	3.6	2.5	1.25
2	Yes	Clip	Coil	Yes	4.5	3.7	4	1.22
3	Yes	Clip	BAC and SAC	Yes	5.6	3.2	4.2	1.75
4	No	Coil	FDS	No	11	3.2	7.5	3.44
5	No	Coil	BAC and SAC	Yes	2.5	2.2	2.8	1.14
6	Yes	Coil	FDS	Yes	4.1	2.3	4	1.78

ASPECT Ratio (Dome/Neck); BAC balloon assisted coiling; FDS Flow diverting stent; SAC stent assisted coiling.

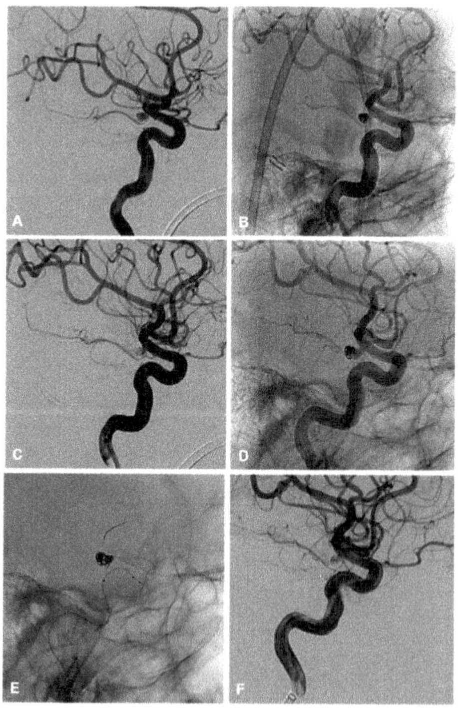

Figure 3. (**A–C**) demonstrate lateral angiographic images from the initial treatment of an unruptured AChoA aneurysm with primary coiling. (**A**) demonstrates a 4 mm smooth and saccular AChoA

aneurysm that incorporates the origin of the AChoA at its neck. (**B**,**C**) are the unsubtracted and subtracted images of the final coil mass demonstrating a mRRC II and patency of the AChoA. (**D**–**F**) demonstrate the lateral angiographic images of the second treatment with coiling and flow diversion following recurrence. (**D**) is the unsubtracted image demonstrating coil compaction with an enlarged neck residuum prior to retreatment. (**E**) demonstrates the unsubtracted image of the final coil mass and flow diverter. (**F**) demonstrates the final subtracted angiographic run post re-treatment with coiling and flow diversion with preserved patency of the AChoA and some filling of the coil interstices. Follow up MRA at 3 months demonstrated complete occlusion of the aneurysm.

Within the clipping cohort, 3/7 (43%) patients required endovascular retreatment and 4/7 (57%) patients did not require any further treatment on follow-up. Of those requiring retreatment, 2/3 (66%) were ruptured on initial treatment with clipping and required endovascular retreatment. One patient was an immediate post-clipping residuum requiring primary coiling and the second patient reoccurred after a year and required a combined balloon and stent-assisted coiling. The third patient requiring retreatment was unruptured on initial treatment with clipping and required endovascular retreatment with BAC and FDS. This recurrence occurred >10 years post-clipping and was identified on routine surveillance for additional unsecured intracranial aneurysms.

3.4.3. Other Complications

In all treatment cases, there were no intra-procedural or post-treatment ruptures or re-ruptures on follow-up. Of these, 1/5 (20%) of the endovascular cases, requiring an intracranial stent or flow diverting stent, had in-stent stenosis on long-term follow-up that was asymptomatic and did not require an angioplasty or re-stenting. None of the treated patients died during hospital admission or due to clipping or endovascular treatment. No delayed surgical complications, such as surgical site infections, were reported.

3.5. *Vasospasm*

A total of 11/17 (65%) patients with a ruptured aneurysm had moderate or severe vasospasm; 9/11 (82%) had a modified fisher scale of 4 and 2/11 (18%) had a scale of 2.

3.6. *Clinical Outcome*

The clinical outcome for all patients was evaluated using the modified Rankin scale before and after intervention at the last available follow-up. Of the 19 patients who underwent primary endovascular treatment (13/19 ruptured), 1 case was lost to follow-up. In total, 14/18 (78%) patients had a good outcome with mRS $\leq$ 2. The median follow-up time was 32 months with an interquartile range of 50.5 months.

Of the 6 patients who underwent primary clipping (5/6 ruptured), 4/6 (67%) had a good outcome with mRS $\leq$ 2. The median follow-up time was 47 months, and the interquartile range was 141 months. With regards to the ruptured cohort, all patients had a preadmission mRS of 0. Within the endovascular cohort, 53% returned to baseline mRS 0 at follow up, 62% had a good outcome with an mRS $\leq$ 2, and 23% had a poor outcome of mRS > 2.

Within the clipping cohort, 50% returned to baseline mRS 0 at follow up and 50% had a poor outcome with an mRS > 2.

3.6.1. Outcome in Patients with a Favorable Hunt and Hess Scale

Of the 19 patients who underwent primary endovascular treatment (1 lost to follow-up), 16/18 (89%) had a HH scale of 0–3. Of these, 12/16 (75%) had a favorable clinical outcome and 4/16 (25%) had a poor outcome. Of the 6 patients who underwent primary clipping, 5/6 (83%) had a HH scale of 0–3. Of these, 4/5 (80%) had a favorable outcome and 1/5 (20%) had a poor outcome (Table 4).

Table 4. Clinical outcome for the endovascular and clipping cohorts based on the presentation Hunter and Hess scale.

	HH 0		HH 1–3		HH 4–5		TOTAL	
MRS	**Endo**	**Clip**	**Endo**	**Clip**	**Endo**	**Clip**	**Endo**	**Clip**
0–2	5	2	7	2	2	0	14	4
>2	1	0	3	1	0	1	4	2

3.6.2. Outcome in Patients with a Favorable WFNS

Of the 13 patients who underwent primary endovascular treatment for rupture, 1 patient was lost to follow-up. Of the 12 remaining patients, 10/12 (83%) had WFNS scale of I–III. Of these, 7/10 (70%) had a favorable clinical outcome and 3/10 (30%) had a poor outcome. Of the 4 patients who underwent clipping for rupture, 3/4 (75%) had WFNS scale of I–III. Of these, 2/3 (67%) had a favorable outcome and 1/3 (33%) had a poor outcome.

4. Discussion

In this section, different aspects of anterior choroidal artery aneurysm treatment, complications, and clinical outcomes were considered. This is an exploratory study with a limited sample size due to the low incidence of AChoA aneurysms. This naturally limits statistical power and precludes subgroup analysis. Allowing for this, we analyze and discuss our results to draw some meaningful conclusions for physicians when managing patients with AChoA aneurysms.

4.1. Anterior Choroidal Artery Anatomy

AChoA arises from the dorsal surface of the ICA (Internal carotid artery) in 98% of cases [4,6]. The cisternal segment traverses the carotid and ambient cisterns, where perforating arteries originate [7]. These perforators supply eloquent structures, including the optic tract, internal capsule (posterior limb, genu, and retrolenticular parts), globus pallidus, caudate tail, lateral thalamus, cerebral peduncle, hippocampus, and amygdala [8,9]. The choroidal segment traverses the choroidal fissure, entering the temporal horn to supply the choroid plexus and anastomose with the choroidal system (Figure 1).

Within our cohort, four procedural related infarcts were documented, all of which were ruptured presentations. These are outlined in Table 2 under Section 3.4.1 (Procedure related infarction). In each case, the origin of the AChoA was incorporated into the neck of the aneurysm, which appears to be a risk factor for both endovascular and surgical approaches. A recent meta-analysis reports a low ischemic complication rate for patients treated with flow diversion as this appears less likely to compromise the parent vessel [10]. In our series, we have not seen ischemic complications in our patients treated with flow diversion. However, this treatment was reserved for elective cases only.

4.2. Follow Up—Impact on Complications and Clinical Outcome

In our study, the median follow up for endovascular cases is 32 months, compared with 47 months for clipping. This is considered a relatively short/medium term follow up for both cohorts and has implications on interpreting complications, including recurrence. The limited follow up and the shorter follow up for endovascular treatment may underestimate the true incidence of recurrence and recurrence requiring retreatment.

4.3. Endovascular Treatment—Complications and Clinical Outcome

In our series, there were no mortalities associated with endovascular treatment. Mortality in endovascular treatment of these aneurysms is often low, with a previously reported 1% mortality rate [2].

An AChoA territory ischemic complication rate of 4% was noticed. We also noticed a 4% catheter related thrombo-embolic infarct that resulted in transient hemiparesis. Our results are comparable to previous studies that reported 4–6.5% AChoA related infarction [2,11–13] and 4–5.4% for other thromboembolic complications [2,3,5].

Patients with ischemic complications presented in the immediate post-procedure period between 0 and 4 h. Other studies reported similar experiences [2,3]. We suggest that close monitoring of neurovitals in this period will help identify the early onset of focal neurology and may prompt management such as GPIIbIIIa inhibitor in select cases.

Our series demonstrated a relatively low recurrence rate for endovascular treatment, with only 3/24 (12.5%) patients requiring retreatment, which is comparable with other studies [5,12–14]. Two of these patients were ruptured, and all patients were initially treated with primary coiling.

One unruptured aneurysm, with a size of 11 mm and neck size of 3.2 mm, underwent primary coiling with mRCC of II. This residuum enlarged after 4 years and was retreated electively with FDS. In medium to large size unruptured AChoA aneurysms, FDS may be considered initially [15–17].

In our series, 78% of endovascular treatments had a good outcome with mRS ≤ 2, which is comparable to other studies [3,10]. This comprises 83% good outcomes for unruptured cases and 75% good outcomes for ruptured cases. The median follow-up time was 32 months, with an interquartile range of 50.5 months.

Our findings corroborate the results of previous studies that demonstrate a favorable safety profile of endovascular approaches for AChoA aneurysm treatment [10,18,19].

4.4. Clipping–Complications and Clinical Outcome

In our series, there were no mortalities associated with clipping. An AChoA territory infarct of 29% is comparable to other studies [20–22]. A 43% retreatment rate was noticed. One recurrence case occurred after more than 10 years of follow-up.

On review of these cases, the mean neck measured 3.5 mm and the origin of the AChoA was incorporated in 66% of cases. These morphological features are thought to be potentially contributing factors to the high recurrence rate seen [18,23].

All recurrences opted for endovascular retreatment with a variety of different endovascular approaches. None of these retreatments required further treatment on follow-up. This preference for endovascular retreatment suggests that the varied armamentarium of endovascular approaches makes it malleable to altered anatomy and possibly less favorable surgical conditions with AChoA aneurysm treatment. This includes the protective micro catheter technique, remodeling with balloons, and reconstructive techniques, using stents and flow diverters. These techniques would be suitable for primary and/or secondary treatment of these aneurysms [3,4,16] (Figure 4).

The demonstration of possible long-term recurrence may also warrant long-term follow-up for this cohort of patients [24]. 3D angiographic evaluation and mimicking the clipping approach allows for better planning and identification of the AChoA location in relationship to the aneurysm dome. This may be helpful, while dissecting the aneurysm neck, for pilot clip placement [25].

Surgical visualization of the aneurysm is often limited as it is within a deep and narrow space lateral to the ICA and in close relation to the skull base. The size and shape of the anterior and posterior clinoid processes, and the close relation to the uncus of the medial temporal lobe, may further complicate visualization, requiring extensive dissection. Retraction of the temporal lobe or uncus may result in rupture of the aneurysm or tearing the AChoA and its perforators. This is further complicated by the limited view of the aneurysm neck, AChoA origin, and its perforators, which are often obscured by the aneurysm and the ICA [4]. AChoA aneurysms lie in close proximity to the optic and oculomotor nerves, which are at risk of injury during dissection [26].

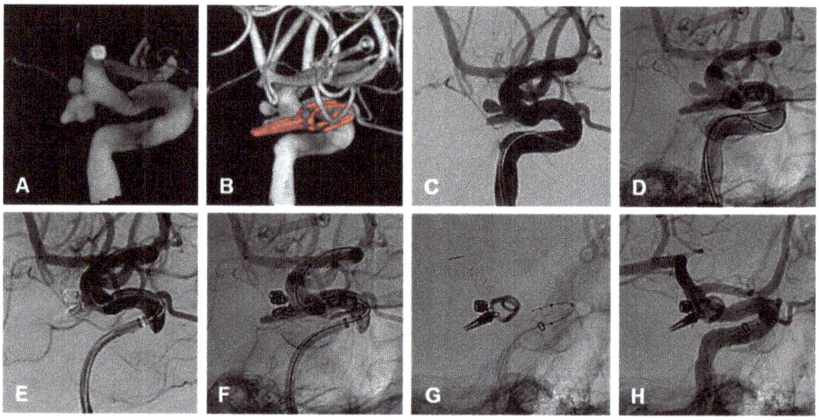

Figure 4. (**A**) demonstrates a 3D shaded surface display of a ruptured irregular AChoA aneurysm with a posteriorly pointing nipple thought to be the rupture point. Note is made of an additional unruptured aneurysm cranial to this. The patient underwent surgical clipping of the ruptured AChoA aneurysm and remodeling of the neck to preserve the AChoA origin. (**B**) The patient developed an enlarging residuum on routine surveillance imaging 52 months after initial treatment. This panel demonstrates a 3D shaded surface display of the clip partly obscuring the recurrence. Note is made of the location of both aneurysm necks, which are posterior to the ICA and not visualized adequately from a sub frontal approach. (**C**,**D**) are unsubtracted and subtracted lateral angiographic images demonstrating the recurrent AChoA aneurysm and the additional untreated and unruptured aneurysm cranial to this. The patient underwent elective re-treatment with balloon assisted coiling of both aneurysms, the results are seen on the subtracted and unsubtracted angiographic images (**E**,**F**). A braided stent was deployed within the ICA, across both aneurysm necks, to promote endothelialization. This is demonstrated on the unsubtracted final angiographic images (**G**,**H**).

Temporary clipping, proximally of the ICA and distally of the A1 and M1, might be required to reduce the pressure within the aneurysm sac and reduce rupture risk of the inherently small and thin-walled aneurysm [6]. This requires a perforator and calcification-free zone for each clip to be placed effectively. These two factors do not complicate endovascular approaches. Excessive manipulation of the ICA during this process may result in rupture of the aneurysm.

Extensive dissection allows for better visualization of final clip placement and allowing for immediate clip repositioning or reconstruction if required [4,23]. In SAH, dissection of the subarachnoid space is more difficult due to acute swelling of the brain or adhesions from a previous SAH [27].

Ensuring that the AChoA territory is not compromised during temporary clipping and confirming patency of the AChoA at the end of the procedure are critical.

Intra-operative assessment using real time neurophysiological monitoring and qualitative measure of flow, with ICG video angiography, are used to help evaluate these [28,29].

Intraoperative neurophysiological monitoring, using MEP and SSEPs, is used to assess potential compromise of the AChoA territory during temporary clipping. Blood flow impairment to the internal capsule and cerebral peduncle, containing the corticospinal tracts, is monitored through MEPs caused by electrical stimulation, often of the hand motor cortex.

It was previously reported that changes in MEPs and SSEPs often lag behind clinical deficits, which may result in false negatives and a poor sensitivity of 33% [22]. In the same study, the use of ICG video angiography improved occlusion rates of aneurysms and clip repositioning, but there was no reduction in AChoA territory infarct. They also describe that 5/6 patients with AChoA territory infarct demonstrated a patent AChoA on immediate post-operative angiograms, suggesting that temporary flow arrest may lead to ischemia. The mean duration of temporary clip occlusion in their series was 5.6 min [22].

In our series, all patients underwent monitoring with MEPs and SSEPs. One of the two patients with AChoA territory procedure-related infarcts had compromised potentials in the upper and lower limbs. SSEPs returned to normal, but MEPs remained at 40% of baseline.

Despite the demanding procedural technicalities, this series demonstrates that a good clinical outcome (67%) with mRS ≤ 2 was achieved in the clipping cohort, which is comparable to other studies [14,20]

4.5. Limitations

This study has several limitations, including its retrospective nature, making it inherently prone to selection bias. The number of endovascular treatments is similar to other small case series but, in the grand scheme of things, represents a relatively small number, thereby affecting the power of the dataset. The small number of clipping-treated aneurysms precludes accurate comparisons between the two treatment arms. The study reviews the experience of a single center, and although there are multiple neurosurgical and endovascular operators, this may limit the generalization of these results. The absence of imaging core lab adjudication for obtaining aneurysm measurements and characteristics means that there is potential variability and bias. To help mitigate this, the measurements were blindly performed by a neuroradiologist twice. Any discrepancies were reviewed by an additional party. All ruptured AChoA that presented to the institution were investigated with catheter angiography and therefore would be captured in our cohort. There may be selection bias for patients with unruptured AChoA who may have only had CTA or MRA imaging and, therefore, are not represented in our study. A well-designed randomized control trial would be the most accurate way of evaluating the efficacy and safety profile of both endovascular and clipping techniques in the treatment of AChoA aneurysms.

5. Conclusions

Clinical outcomes of both clipping and endovascular treatment of AChoA aneurysms look to be comparable. In this study, endovascular treatment demonstrated low recurrence rates and procedure-related thromboembolic complications in keeping with the current literature. Endovascular treatment demonstrated lower recurrence and thromboembolic rates compared to clipping. Both approaches are viable, though they present distinct risks and advantages.

Author Contributions: Conceptualization, A.F. and T.K.; methodology, A.F.; validation, A.F. and T.K.; formal analysis, A.F.; investigation, A.F.; data curation, A.F.; writing—original draft preparation, A.F.; writing—review and editing, A.F., S.M., T.P.K., H.A.-B. and T.K.; visualization, A.F.; supervision, T.K.; project administration, A.F. All authors have read and agreed to the published version of the manuscript.

Funding: This research received no external funding.

Institutional Review Board Statement: The study was conducted in accordance with the Declaration of Helsinki, and approved by the Institutional Ethics Board of UHN (ID: 23-5084) on 2 October 2023.

Informed Consent Statement: Individual patient consent was waived due to the retrospective nature of this study and the non-identifying nature of the data.

Data Availability Statement: Data is unavailable due to ethical and legal restrictions.

Acknowledgments: Ahmed Abdelghafar for assistance with administration, review of clinical charts, technical support, file formatting and editing.

Conflicts of Interest: The authors declare no conflicts of interest.

References

1. Drake, C.G.; Vanderlinden, R.G.; Amacher, A.L. Carotid-choroidal aneurysms. *J. Neurosurg.* **1968**, *29*, 32–36. [CrossRef] [PubMed]
2. Piotin, M.; Mounayer, C.; Spelle, L.; Williams, M.T.; Moret, J. Endovascular treatment of anterior choroidal artery aneurysms. *AJNR Am. J. Neuroradiol.* **2004**, *25*, 314–318. [PubMed]
3. Kim, B.M.; Kim, D.I.; Shin, Y.S.; Chung, E.C.; Kim, D.J.; Suh, S.H.; Kim, S.Y.; Park, S.I.; Choi, C.S.; Won, Y.S. Clinical outcome and ischemic complication after treatment of anterior choroidal artery aneurysm: Comparison between surgical clipping and endovascular coiling. *AJNR Am. J. Neuroradiol.* **2008**, *29*, 286–290. [CrossRef] [PubMed]
4. Lehecka, M.; Dashti, R.; Laakso, A.; van Popta, J.S.; Romani, R.; Navratil, O.; Kivipelto, L.; Kivisaari, R.; Foroughi, M.; Kokuzawa, J.; et al. Microneurosurgical management of anterior choroid artery aneurysms. *World Neurosurg.* **2010**, *73*, 486–499. [CrossRef] [PubMed]
5. Kang, H.S.; Kwon, B.J.; Kwon, O.K.; Jung, C.; Kim, J.E.; Oh, C.W.; Han, M.H. Endovascular coil embolization of anterior choroidal artery aneurysms. Clinical article. *J. Neurosurg.* **2009**, *111*, 963–969. [CrossRef]
6. Kretschmer, T.; Heinen, C.; July, J.; Schmidt, T. Surgery of IC-Anterior Choroidal Aneurysms. In *Neurovascular Surgery*; July, J., Wahjoepramono, E.J., Eds.; Springer: Singapore, 2019; pp. 93–103. [CrossRef]
7. Vogels, V.; Dammers, R.; van Bilsen, M.; Volovici, V. Deep Cerebral Perforators: Anatomical Distribution and Clinical Symptoms: An Overview. *Stroke* **2021**, *52*, e660–e674. [CrossRef] [PubMed]
8. Herman, L.H.; Fernando, O.U.; Gurdjian, E.S. The anterior choroidal artery: An anatomical study of its area of distribution. *Anat. Rec.* **1966**, *154*, 95–101. [CrossRef] [PubMed]
9. Morandi, X.; Brassier, G.; Darnault, P.; Mercier, P.; Scarabin, J.; Duval, J. Microsurgical anatomy of the anterior choroidal artery. *Surg. Radiol. Anat.* **1996**, *18*, 275–280. [CrossRef]
10. Barhouse, P.; Young, M.; Taussky, P.; Pacheco-Barrios, N.; Ogilvy, C.S. Anterior choroidal artery aneurysms: A systematic review and meta-analysis of outcomes and ischemic complications following surgical and endovascular treatment. *J. Neurosurg.* **2024**. *ahead of print*. [CrossRef] [PubMed]
11. Meguro, T.; Kuwahara, K.; Tomita, Y.; Okuma, Y.; Tanabe, T.; Muraoka, K.; Terada, K.; Hirotsune, N.; Nishino, S. Ischemic complications of anterior choroidal artery aneurysm treatment. *No Shinkei Geka* **2014**, *42*, 917–923. [CrossRef]
12. Maeda, T.; Ooigawa, H.; Suzuki, K.; Sato, H.; Iihoshi, S.; Kohyama, S.; Kurita, H. Predictors of Ischemic Complication in Anterior Choroidal Artery Aneurysm Repair. *World Neurosurg.* **2022**, *167*, e157–e164. [CrossRef]
13. Dorfer, C.; Gruber, A.; Standhardt, H.; Bavinzski, G.; Knosp, E. Management of residual and recurrent aneurysms after initial endovascular treatment. *Neurosurgery* **2012**, *70*, 537–553, discussion 553–554. [CrossRef] [PubMed]
14. Roh, H.K.; Jeong, E.O.; Kim, K.H.; Jeong, H.W.; Lee, H.J.; Choi, S.W.; Kim, S.H.; Koh, H.S.; Youm, J.Y.; Kwon, H.J. Treatment results of anterior choroidal artery aneurysms treated mostly with coil embolization: A single-center experience. *J. Cerebrovasc. Endovasc. Neurosurg.* **2022**, *24*, 341–348. [CrossRef]
15. Cagnazzo, F.; Mantilla, D.; Rouchaud, A.; Brinjikji, W.; Lefevre, P.H.; Dargazanli, C.; Gascou, G.; Riquelme, C.; Perrini, P.; Di Carlo, D.; et al. Endovascular Treatment of Very Large and Giant Intracranial Aneurysms: Comparison between Reconstructive and Deconstructive Techniques-A Meta-Analysis. *AJNR Am. J. Neuroradiol.* **2018**, *39*, 852–858. [CrossRef]
16. Bhogal, P.; Ganslandt, O.; Bäzner, H.; Henkes, H.; Aguilar Perez, M. Treatment of Unruptured, Saccular, Anterior Choroidal Artery Aneurysms with Flow Diversion: A Single Centre Experience. *Clin. Neuroradiol.* **2019**, *29*, 459–465. [CrossRef]
17. Brinjikji, W.; Kallmes, D.F.; Cloft, H.J.; Lanzino, G. Patency of the Anterior Choroidal Artery after Flow-Diversion Treatment of Internal Carotid Artery Aneurysms. *AJNR Am. J. Neuroradiol.* **2015**, *36*, 537–541. [CrossRef]
18. Duan, Y.; Qin, X.; An, Q.; Liu, Y.; Li, J.; Chen, G. A New Classification of Anterior Choroidal Artery Aneurysms and Its Clinical Application. *Front. Aging Neurosci.* **2021**, *13*, 596829. [CrossRef] [PubMed]
19. Wang, Y.; Yu, J. Endovascular Treatment and Angiographic Characteristics of Aneurysms at the Origin of the Anterior Choroidal Artery. *Front. Neurol.* **2022**, *13*, 832604. [CrossRef] [PubMed]
20. Friedman, J.A.; Pichelmann, M.A.; Piepgras, D.G.; Atkinson, J.L.; Maher, C.O.; Meyer, F.B.; Hansen, K.K. Ischemic complications of surgery for anterior choroidal artery aneurysms. *J. Neurosurg.* **2001**, *94*, 565–572. [CrossRef]
21. Cho, M.S.; Kim, M.S.; Chang, C.H.; Kim, S.W.; Kim, S.H.; Choi, B.Y. Analysis of Clip-induced Ischemic Complication of Anterior Choroidal Artery Aneurysms. *J. Korean Neurosurg. Soc.* **2008**, *43*, 131–134. [CrossRef] [PubMed]

22. Winkler, E.A.; Lu, A.; Burkhardt, J.K.; Rutledge, W.C.; Yue, J.K.; Birk, H.S.; Alotaibi, N.; Choudhri, O.; Lawton, M.T. Microsurgical Clipping of Anterior Choroidal Artery Aneurysms: A Systematic Approach to Reducing Ischemic Complications in an Experience with 146 Patients. *Oper. Neurosurg.* **2019**, *17*, 413–423. [CrossRef] [PubMed]
23. Aletich, V.A.; Debrun, G.M.; Misra, M.; Charbel, F.; Ausman, J.I. The remodeling technique of balloon-assisted Guglielmi detachable coil placement in wide-necked aneurysms: Experience at the University of Illinois at Chicago. *J. Neurosurg.* **2000**, *93*, 388–396. [CrossRef] [PubMed]
24. Tsutsumi, K.; Ueki, K.; Morita, A.; Usui, M.; Kirino, T. Risk of Aneurysm Recurrence in Patients with Clipped Cerebral Aneurysms: Results of Long-Term Follow-Up Angiography. *Stroke* **2001**, *32*, 1191–1194. [CrossRef] [PubMed]
25. Park, J.; Son, W.; Kim, M.; Shin, I.H. Anterior Choroidal Artery Aneurysm Clipping: Angiographic Diagnostics and Surgical Tactics Focused on Visualizing the Anterior Choroidal Artery Behind the Aneurysm. *World Neurosurg.* **2024**, *187*, e1072–e1082. [CrossRef] [PubMed]
26. Hendricks, B.K.; Spetzler, R.F. Surgical Challenges Associated with Anterior Choroidal Artery Aneurysm Clipping: 2-Dimensional Operative Video. *Oper. Neurosurg.* **2020**, *19*, E289. [CrossRef]
27. Kim, S.Y.; Jeon, H.J.; Kim, S.; Chung, J.; Park, K.Y.; Huh, S.K.; Lee, J.W. Microsurgical clipping of ruptured anterior choroidal artery aneurysms: Incidence of and risk factors for ischemic complications. *Clin. Neurol. Neurosurg.* **2020**, *195*, 105884. [CrossRef] [PubMed]
28. Horton, T.G.; Barnes, M.; Johnson, S.; Kalapos, P.C.; Link, A.; Cockroft, K.M. Feasibility and efficacy of transcranial motor-evoked potential monitoring in neuroendovascular surgery. *AJNR Am. J. Neuroradiol.* **2012**, *33*, 1825–1831. [CrossRef] [PubMed]
29. Raabe, A.; Beck, J.; Gerlach, R.; Zimmermann, M.; Seifert, V. Near-infrared indocyanine green video angiography: A new method for intraoperative assessment of vascular flow. *Neurosurgery* **2003**, *52*, 132–139, discussion 139. [CrossRef] [PubMed]

brain sciences

MDPI

Article

Challenges in the Management of Cavernoma-Related Epilepsy: Seizure Outcomes, Antiseizure Medication Practices, and Access to Intraoperative Technologies in Kazakhstan

Karashash Menlibayeva [1], Chingiz Nurimanov [2,*], Iroda Mammadinova [2], Ainur Turzhanova [3], Serik Akshulakov [2] and Yerbol Makhambetov [2]

1 Department of Population Health Sciences, Faculty of Life Sciences and Medicine, King's College London, London SE1 1UL, UK; karashash.2.menlibayeva@kcl.ac.uk
2 Vascular and Functional Neurosurgery Department, National Centre for Neurosurgery, Astana 010000, Kazakhstan; irodamammadinova@gmail.com (I.M.); yermakh@gmail.com (Y.M.)
3 Department of Research Management, National Centre for Neurosurgery, Astana 010000, Kazakhstan
* Correspondence: chingiz198705@gmail.com

Abstract

Objective: This study aims to analyze the diagnostic patterns of cavernoma-related epilepsy, the management of antiseizure medications, and clinical outcomes following microsurgical treatment in patients with late-diagnosed epilepsy secondary to cavernous malformations in the Central Asian region. Methods: A retrospective cross-sectional study was conducted on 60 patients who underwent microsurgical resection for brain cavernous malformations over a 12-year period (2010–2022) at the National Centre for Neurosurgery, Astana, Kazakhstan. All participants were 18 years or older and presented with seizures. Follow-up evaluations were conducted by neurologists, and seizure outcomes were assessed using the 2017 classification criteria of the International League Against Epilepsy. Results: The mean follow-up period was 83.77 ± 39.81 months. In total, 51.67% of participants demonstrated positive ILAE outcomes, 33.33% had moderate ILAE outcomes, and the remaining 15.00% experienced negative ILAE outcomes. Approximately 47% of patients received antiseizure medication before surgery, primarily as monotherapy with carbamazepine (33%), and administered at a low dose (40%). Early microsurgical resection showed a positive post-surgery seizure outcome. Approximately 67% of patients who experienced seizures within one year prior to surgery showed positive ILAE outcomes, whereas those with a seizure history extending beyond five years were roughly 32% seizure-free ($p = 0.01$). Conclusions. Cavernoma-related epilepsy in Central Asia remains a significant clinical challenge, particularly with respect to diagnostic accuracy and antiseizure medication management. In our cohort, only approximately half of patients achieved favorable seizure control following microsurgical resection. Notably, early surgical intervention within one year of seizure onset was associated with improved outcomes, whereas delayed surgery, restricted availability of intraoperative technologies, and suboptimal antiseizure medication practices were linked to less favorable outcomes. Strengthening diagnostic pathways, antiseizure medication management, and expanding access to advanced surgical technologies are critical steps to improving treatment outcomes in a studied patient population.

Keywords: cerebral cavernous malformations; seizures; ILAE; microsurgical resection; epilepsy

https://doi.org/10.3390/brainsci15090992

1. Introduction

CMs are benign vascular lesions that occur within the brain parenchyma or leptomeninges [1]. Histologically, they are characterized by clusters of dilated vascular caverns lined by endothelium, lacking mature vascular architecture. Although many CMs remain clinically silent, they may present symptomatically, most commonly with intracerebral hemorrhage or seizures [2,3].

Several risk factors are associated with the occurrence of seizures in patients with CMs. These include temporal lobe involvement, cortical location, presence of a hemosiderin rim, patient age, and specific morphological characteristics of the lesion [4–7]. If left untreated, CM-related seizures may evolve into CRE, the management of which involves pharmacological therapy, microsurgical resection, and, in selected cases, stereotactic radiosurgery [8].

The primary treatment for CM-related seizures involves ASMs, with early initiation being critical given the high risk of epilepsy development after a first seizure—estimated at up to 94% within five years [9]. Among therapeutic options, microsurgical resection has demonstrated superior efficacy compared with medication alone or radiosurgery [8,10]. Evidence indicates that resection achieves favorable outcomes even in patients with drug-resistant CRE [11]. Patient-reported outcomes further support its effectiveness, showing significant long-term seizure control and improved quality of life following surgery [12]. Importantly, early intervention, particularly within one year of symptom onset, is associated with the most favorable outcomes [4,13,14]. Patients undergoing surgical resection frequently attain seizure freedom and may discontinue ASM therapy postoperatively [15]. By contrast, delayed surgery and prolonged seizure duration are associated with poorer outcomes, emphasizing the need for early diagnosis and timely surgical management of CRE [16,17].

The diagnosis of CRE requires a multidisciplinary approach involving neuroradiologists, neurologists, and neurosurgeons. MRI and EEG remain essential for identifying epilepsy of structural etiology [18]. Nevertheless, timely diagnosis continues to be a major challenge, particularly in resource-limited settings. Approximately 80% of epilepsy cases occur in low- and middle-income countries, where access to appropriate diagnostic tools and treatment remains limited [19,20]. Furthermore, societal stigma associated with epilepsy often contributes to delays in seeking medical care [21,22], despite existing World Health Organization guidelines aimed at addressing these challenges [23].

In Kazakhstan, the largest upper-middle-income country in Central Asia [24], epilepsy is frequently undiagnosed or diagnosed late, with rising incidence and prevalence observed in the years preceding the COVID-19 pandemic [25]. Data on seizure outcomes following microsurgical resection of CRE in patients with delayed CM diagnosis remain scarce, and information on ASM management patterns in this context is limited. This study therefore aims to analyze the diagnostic pathways, ASM management practices, and seizure outcomes following microsurgical treatment of CRE in patients with late-diagnosed epilepsy secondary to CM in Kazakhstan.

2. Materials and Methods

2.1. Study Design

Retrospective cross-sectional study.

2.2. Participants

A total of 116 medical records of patients who underwent microsurgical resection for CRE were reviewed to assess eligibility. Of these, 56 patients (48.28%) were excluded from the analysis. Nineteen were lost to follow-up despite repeated contact attempts, thirty-one had not experienced preoperative seizures, and six had died, with the cause of death remaining unknown. Notably, four of these deaths occurred in 2020 during the COVID-19 pandemic. The final study cohort consisted of 60 adult patients who underwent microsurgical resection between 2010 and 2022 at the National Centre for Neurosurgery in Astana, Kazakhstan. In this cohort, the primary indication for surgery was drug-resistant epilepsy. A minority of patients presented with preoperative intracerebral hemorrhage, and surgery was performed electively rather than during the acute phase.

2.3. Inclusion and Exclusion Criteria

Adult patients who underwent microsurgical resection for brain CM and presented with CM-related intractable seizures were eligible for inclusion. Only patients who underwent preoperative video-electroencephalographic monitoring to confirm seizure onset localization were included. All patients also underwent preoperative MRI, including T1, T2, and susceptibility-weighted imaging sequences, to characterize the lesion and assess for evidence of hemorrhage.

Patients younger than 18 years, those with incomplete or lost follow-up data, and those with multiple cavernous malformations were excluded to reduce heterogeneity and minimize potential confounding factors influencing seizure outcomes.

2.4. Follow-Up

Neurologists contacted patients by phone and conducted interviews. Follow-up data were subsequently evaluated by an epileptologist and categorized according to the ILAE classifications of epilepsy surgery seizure outcomes. In this study, ILAE classes 1 and 2 were defined as positive outcomes, classes 3 and 4 as moderate outcomes, and classes 5 and 6 as negative outcomes.

During the follow-up period, all patients also underwent postoperative electroencephalographic evaluations. These recordings were reviewed by board-certified epileptologists to detect persistent epileptiform activity and to evaluate the effectiveness of seizure control.

2.5. Variables

Data were collected on participants' demographic and clinical characteristics, CM features, and preoperative as well as postoperative antiseizure medication use. The place of residence was categorized as either a metropolis or a small city. In Kazakhstan, three cities—Astana (the capital), Almaty, and Shymkent—are officially classified as metropolises, each with a population exceeding one million inhabitants. All other towns were grouped as small cities.

The variable "other nationalities" included Russians, Uzbeks, Germans, and Tatars. Seizure types were classified according to the ILAE 2017 Classification of Seizure Types and were further grouped into focal onset, generalized onset, and unknown onset.

Comorbidities were categorized into cardiovascular diseases (arterial hypertension, congestive heart failure, coronary disease, and angina), gastrointestinal disorders (chronic pancreatitis, chronic gastritis, chronic cholecystitis, peptic ulcer, and hepatitis B and C), renal diseases (chronic pyelonephritis, chronic renal disease, malignant neoplasm of the kidney, chronic glomerulonephritis, and nephrolithiasis), respiratory system diseases (chronic bronchitis and pulmonary fibrosis), endocrine system diseases (Huntington's disease, multinodular goiter, immunologic thyroiditis, type 2 diabetes, and cardiometabolic syndrome), and ophthalmological conditions (retinal angiopathy, cataract, astigmatism, and manifest deviation).

Antiseizure medication dosages were categorized according to the maintenance dosage defined in the epilepsy treatment protocol of the Ministry of Health of Kazakhstan. A dosage below the maintenance level was categorized as low, while a dosage above the maintenance level was categorized as high. The following maintenance dose ranges were used: carbamazepine 600–1200 mg/day, sodium valproate 1000–3000 mg/day, valproic acid 1000–3000 mg/day, levetiracetam 1000–3000 mg/day, lamotrigine 100–200 mg/day, oxcarbazepine 900–2400 mg/day, and topiramate 200–400 mg/day [26].

2.6. Statistical Methods

Data were cleaned and coded using Microsoft Excel (version 2411, Microsoft 365). Further statistical analysis was performed in Stata 18.0 SE (StataCorp, College Station, TX, USA). Chi-square and Fisher's exact tests were used, as appropriate, to assess associations between categorical variables. Continuous variables were assessed for normality using the skewness–kurtosis test and visualized using histograms. As the data were not normally distributed, the Kruskal–Wallis test was employed to compare continuous variables across ILAE outcome groups.

3. Results

A total of 60 patients with complete follow-up data were included in the final analysis. The mean follow-up duration was 83.77 ± 39.81 months. The mean age at surgery was 36.98 ± 11.78 years, while the mean age at initial radiographic diagnosis (MRI/CT) was 35.90 ± 11.16 years, and the mean age at first seizure was 32.95 ± 12.22 years.

Most participants were of Kazakhs ethnicity (76.67%) and male (58.33%), with the majority residing in small cities (76.67%). Overall, a tenth of patients reported having a disability, and 15% had experienced a preoperative intracerebral hemorrhage. Headache was the most frequent initial symptom (85.00%), followed by weakness, numbness, or paralysis (38.33%), memory impairment (16.67%), and hearing or vision disturbances with unsteadiness (10.00%).

All patients (100%) presented with seizures. The mean duration of seizures prior to surgery was 48.45 ± 54.65 months, whereas the mean time interval between radiographic diagnosis of CM and surgery was 11.91 ± 31.17 months.

Most participants experienced generalized seizures (40.00%), while 19 patients (31.67%) presented with focal-onset seizures, and 17 patients (28.33%) had seizures of unknown onset. The most prevalent comorbidity was cardiovascular disease (15.00%), including arterial hypertension, congestive heart failure, coronary artery disease, and angina.

Regarding seizure location, approximately one-third of CMs were discovered in the frontal lobe, 28.33% in the temporal lobe, one-fifth in the parietal lobe, 12.00% in deep brain structures, and 5.00% in the occipital lobe. Laterality analysis showed that 53.33% of lesions were located in the left hemisphere.

The demographic and clinical characteristics of the cohort are summarized in Table 1.

Table 1. Baseline demographic and clinical characteristics of 60 patients.

Variable	n (%)
No. of patients	60 (100)
Mean follow up time (months) ± SD	83.77 ± 39.81
Age (years) at the time of surgery	
Mean ± SD	36.98 ± 11.78
16–30	24 (40.00)
31–40	14 (23.33)
41 and older	22 (36.67)

Table 1. *Cont.*

Variable	n (%)
Age (years) at first radiographic diagnosis (MRI/CT) of CM	
Mean ± SD	35.90 ± 11.16
16–30	26 (43.33)
31–40	14 (23.33)
41 and older	20 (33.33)
Age (years) when the initial seizure occurs	
Mean ± SD	32.95 ± 12.22
16–30	27 (45.00)
31–40	19 (31.67)
41 and older	14 (23.33)
Gender	
Female	25 (41.67)
Male	35 (58.33)
Nationality	
Kazakh	46 (76.67)
Other	14 (23.33)
City type	
Metropolises	14 (23.33)
Small cities	46 (76.67)
Disability	
Yes	6 (10.00)
No	54 (90.00)
Time since radiographic diagnosis (months)	
Mean ± SD	11.91 ± 31.17
<1 year	54 (90.00)
1–5 year	1 (1.67)
>5 years	5 (8.33)
Time since initial presenting seizure (months)	
Mean ± SD	48.45 ± 54.65
<1 year	27 (45.00)
1–5 year	14 (23.33)
>5 years	19 (31.67)
Type of seizure	
Focal onset	19 (31.67)
Generalized onset	24 (40.00)
Unknown onset	17 (28.33)
Preoperative hemorrhage	
Yes	9 (15.00)
No	51 (85.00)

Table 1. *Cont.*

Variable	n (%)
Initial presenting symptoms	
Headaches	51 (85.00)
Hearing or vision changes	6 (10.00)
Weakness, numbness, or paralysis	23 (38.33)
Memory deficits	10 (16.67)
Unsteadiness	6 (10.00)
Comorbidities	
Cardiovascular system diseases	9 (15.00)
Gastrointestinal system diseases	5 (8.33)
Renal system diseases	3 (5.00)
Respiratory system diseases	1. (1.67)
Endocrine system diseases	3 (5.00)
Ophthalmological condition	2 (3.33)
Location of the cavernous malformation	
Deep brain structures	7 (11.67)
Frontal lobe	21 (35.00)
Occipital lobe	3 (5.00)
Parietal lobe	12 (20.00)
Temporal lobe	17 (28.33)
Location of the cavernous malformation (side)	
Left	32 (53.33)
Right	28 (46.67)

Table 2 summarizes the preoperative (Preop) and postoperative (Postop) use of antiseizure medications (ASMs), including dosage patterns. More than half of participants (53.33%) did not receive any ASM prior to surgery. Among those treated, carbamazepine was the most frequently prescribed agent, both before and after resection. Overall, prescribed dosages tended to be at the lower end of the recommended therapeutic range.

The relationship between patients' antiseizure medication (ASM) use and their ILAE seizure outcomes is presented in Table 3.

Among the 60 patients, 28 (46.67%) received ASM therapy prior to surgery, and 25 of this continued treatment postoperatively. Among those who continued ASM, 56% achieved positive ILAE outcomes at long-term follow-up. By contrast, 32 patients (53.33%) did not receive medication before surgery, with half of them initiating treatment postoperatively. Among those, 56.25% achieved positive long-term outcomes. However, the differences between groups were not statistically significant. The role of preoperative ASM therapy is further analyzed and presented in Table 4.

Table 2. Preoperative and postoperative data on ASM and ILAE outcomes.

Variable	Preop, n (%)	Postop, n (%)
Treatment with ASM		
Yes	28 (46.67)	41 (68.33)
No	32 (53.33)	19 (31.67)
Medication Name		
Carbamazepine	20 (33.33)	31 (51.67)
Lamotrigine	2 (3.33)	1 (1.67)
Topiramate	1 (1.67)	1 (1.67)
Valproic acid	5 (8.33)	8 (13.33)
None	32 (53.33)	19 (31.67)
Medication Dosage		
Initial dose	24 (40.00)	38 (63.33)
Maintenance dose	4 (6.67)	3 (5.00)
None	32 (53.33)	19 (31.67)

Table 3. Impact of medication behavior on ILAE outcomes.

Variable, n (%)	Negative ILAE Outcomes	Moderate ILAE Outcomes	Positive ILAE Outcomes	All
No. of patients	9 (15.00)	20 (33.33)	31 (51.67)	60 (100)
Patients who took medication before surgery and continued after surgery	8 (32.00)	3 (12.00)	14 (56.00)	25 (41.67)
Patients who took medication before surgery and discontinued after surgery	1 (33.33)	1 (33.33)	1 (33.33)	3 (5.00)
Patients who did not take medication before surgery and did not start after surgery	7 (43.75)	2 (12.50)	7 (43.75)	16 (26.67)
Patients who did not take medication before surgery and started after surgery	4 (25.00)	3 (18.75)	9 (56.25)	16 (26.67)

Table 4. Preoperative ASM management on ILAE outcomes.

Variable, n (%)	Negative ILAE Outcomes	Moderate ILAE Outcomes	Positive ILAE Outcomes	All
The number of patients who received preop ASM	9 (32.14)	4 (14.29)	15 (53.57)	28 (100)
Preop ASM name				
Carbamazepine	7 (35.00)	2 (10.00)	11 (55.00)	20 (71.43)
Lamotrigine	0	1 (50.00)	1 (50.00)	2 (7.14)
Topiramate	1 (100.00)	0	0	1 (3.57)
Valproic acid	1 (20.00)	1 (20.00)	3 (60.00)	5 (17.86)
Preop ASM dosage				
Initial dose	9 (37.50)	4 (16.67)	11 (45.83)	24 (85.71)
Maintenance dose	0	0	4 (100)	4 (14.29)

Among patients who received ASMs prior to surgery (N = 28), treatment with carbamazepine at initial dosing levels was associated with higher rate of favorable ILAE outcomes, with 53.57% achieving seizure control.

The seizure outcomes following microsurgical resection of CM in the entire cohort of 60 patients are summarized in Table 5. The mean follow-up duration was 83.77 ± 39.81 months (range, 14–169 months). At the final follow-up, 51.67% of patients achieved favorable outcomes, 33.33% had moderate outcomes, and the remaining 15.00% experienced negative ILAE outcomes.

Table 5. Seizure outcomes after surgical resection of CM in 60 patients.

Variable, n (%)	Negative ILAE Outcomes	Moderate ILAE Outcomes	Positive ILAE Outcomes	All
No. of patients	9 (15.00)	20 (33.33)	31 (51.67)	60 (100)
Mean follow-up time (months) ± SD	93.11 ± 27.87	83.25 ± 40.22	81.39 ± 43.04	83.77 ± 39.81
Age (years) at the time of surgery, mean ± SD	37.44 ± 10.72	33.65 ± 8.08	39.00 ± 13.75	36.98 ± 11.78
Age (years) at the time of initial seizures, mean ± SD	34.54 ± 11.68	28.02 ± 10.13	35.66 ± 12.94	32.95 ± 12.22
Age (years) at the time of radiographic diagnosis (MRI/CT) of CM, mean ± SD	37.11 ± 10.88	32.90 ± 8.19	37.48 ±12.72	35.90 ± 11.16
Gender				
Female	3 (12.00)	11 (44.00)	11 (44.00)	25 (41.67)
Male	6 (17.14)	9 (25.71)	20 (57.14)	35 (58.33)
Type of seizure				
Focal onset	2 (10.53)	10 (52.63)	7 (36.84)	19 (31.67)
Generalized onset	4 (16.67)	6 (25.00)	14 (58.33)	24 (40.00)
Unknown onset	3 (17.65)	4 (23.53)	10 (58.82)	17 (28.33)
Preoperative hemorrhage				
Yes	2 (28.57)	2 (28.57)	3 (42.86)	7 (11.67)
No	7 (13.21)	18 (33.96)	28 (52.83)	53 (88.33)
Treatment with ASM (preop)				
Yes	4 (14.29)	9 (32.14)	15 (53.57)	28 (46.67)
No	5 (15.62)	11 (34.38)	16 (50.00)	32 (53.33)
Preop ASM dosage				
Low	4 (16.67)	9 (37.50)	11 (45.83)	24 (40.00)
Maintenance	0	0	4 (100.00)	4 (6.67)
None	5 (15.62)	11 (34.38)	16 (50.00)	32 (53.33)
Location of the cavernous malformation				
Deep brain structures	1 (14.29)	4 (57.14)	2 (28.57)	7 (11.67)
Frontal lobe	3 (14.29)	5 (23.81)	13 (61.90)	21 (35.00)
Occipital lobe	0	0	3 (100)	3 (5.00)
Parietal lobe	1 (8.33)	5 (41.67)	6 (50.00)	12 (20.00)
Temporal lobe	9 (15.00)	20 (33.33)	31 (51.67)	17 (28.33)

Table 5. *Cont.*

Variable, n (%)	Negative ILAE Outcomes	Moderate ILAE Outcomes	Positive ILAE Outcomes	All
Location of the cavernous malformation (side)				
Left	3 (9.38)	11 (34.38)	18 (56.25)	32 (53.33)
Right	6 (21.43)	9 (32.14)	13 (46.43)	28 (46.67)
Time since initial presenting seizure *				
<1 year	**3 (11.11)**	**6 (22.22)**	**18 (66.67)**	**27 (45.00)**
1–5 year	**5 (35.71)**	**2 (14.29)**	**7 (50.00)**	**14 (23.33)**
>5 years	**1 (5.26)**	**12 (63.16)**	**6 (31.58)**	**19 (31.67) (* $p = 0.01$)**
Time since radiographic diagnosis				
<1 year	9 (16.67)	18 (33.33)	27 (50.00)	54 (90.00)
1–5 year	0	0	1 (100)	1 (1.67)
>5 years	0	2 (40.00)	3 (60.00)	5 (8.33)

Bold indicates statistically significant (* $p = 0.01$).

The mean age at surgery was 37 years, with the youngest subgroup observed among patients with moderate ILAE outcomes (33.65 $\pm$ 8.08 years). Among patients with a history of intracerebral hemorrhage, 71.43% achieved moderate or favorable outcomes, compared with 86.8% of those without hemorrhage. CMs located in deep brain structures were predominantly associated with moderate outcomes (57.14%), whereas lesions in other brain regions more frequently resulted in favorable outcomes.

The only statistically significant association was found for seizure duration prior to surgery. Approximately 67% of patients who underwent surgery within one year of seizure onset achieved favorable outcomes, whereas only 32% of those with a seizure history extending five years attained favorable outcomes.

4. Discussion

This study evaluated diagnostic patterns of CREs, the management of ASMs, and postoperative seizure outcomes in patients with late-diagnosed epilepsy secondary to cerebral CM in a Kazakhstani cohort. Overall, 51.67% of patients achieved favorable long-term outcomes (ILAE classes 1–2) after surgery, with a mean follow-up of approximately seven years. These results were less favorable compared to prior studies, which have reported seizure freedom rates of about 70% following CM resection [17,27].

A deeper understanding of the mechanisms of epileptogenesis in CM is critical for interpreting surgical outcomes. Although CMs themselves are not intrinsically epileptogenic, epilepsy arises through two primary mechanisms: (1) local epileptogenesis of the surrounding tissue and (2) secondary epileptogenesis in remote brain regions [28]. Cortical excitability surrounding CMs, driven by reactive gliosis, hemosiderin deposits, and architectural disturbances, plays a key role in the development of CRE [29]. In addition, secondary epileptogenesis in distant brain areas underscores the intricate network changes and synaptic alterations that perpetuate seizure activity, particularly within the limbic system. A comprehensive understanding of these processes will inform more targeted therapeutic strategies aimed at improving seizure control in patients with CMs [28].

Studies from other countries provide valuable context for interpreting our findings on CRE. Microsurgical resection remains the most effective treatment for seizure control, particularly for lesions in the temporal and frontal lobes, achieving higher rates of epilepsy control compared to radiosurgery, although neurosurgery may carry a slightly higher risk of permanent morbidity [8,17].

Emerging minimally invasive techniques, such as laser interstitial thermal therapy (LITT), have shown promise for seizure control and prevention of symptomatic progression or hemorrhage in selected patients [30]. For patients with lesions considered unsuitable for surgery due to location or other risk factors, stereotactic radiosurgery offers an alternative, providing meaningful reductions in bleeding and seizure frequency with relatively low adverse effects [31].

Advanced surgical techniques, such as 3.0 Tesla MRI with an epilepsy-specific protocol, intraoperative electrocorticography, modern navigation systems, and cortical mapping, are critical for achieving seizure freedom after surgery [32,33]. Because the number and localization of lesions strongly influence post-surgery outcomes [8], these innovations, together with the expertise of trained epileptologists, have substantially improved surgical outcomes by enabling more precise identification and resection of epileptogenic tissue [34–36].

In the present cohort, the limited availability of advanced intraoperative technologies—introduced at our center only in 2021—likely contributed to suboptimal resection accuracy and the relatively modest seizure-free rate observed (51.67%). The absence of intraoperative MRI or CT, which can delineate the hemosiderin rim and facilitate more complete lesion removal, further limited surgical efficacy. These limitations represented significant barriers to optimal epilepsy surgery outcomes in Kazakhstan until recently. Looking ahead, we plan to conduct a comparative study assessing seizure outcomes in CM patients operated on with intraoperative EEG and MRI versus those treated without these tools.

Lesion location is a critical determinant of both the choice of intervention and the likelihood of favorable surgical outcomes. Temporal CMs, particularly those in the mesiotemporal lobe, are strongly associated with the development of CRE, as this region represents the most epileptogenic zone [37]. For CMs located in the frontal and temporal lobes, microsurgical resection generally offers superior seizure control compared with radiosurgery. By contrast, radiosurgery has demonstrated greater effectiveness in managing CMs situated in the parietal and occipital lobes [38]. In the present cohort, however, no differences were observed between the CM location and the post-surgery seizure outcome.

Another key factor associated with positive post-surgery seizure freedom is the duration of epilepsy prior to surgery [14]. In this study, the interval between the initial presenting seizure and surgery demonstrated a statistically significant association with postoperative ILAE outcomes. Prolonged seizure duration before surgery was associated with poorer outcomes, whereas patients whose first seizure occurred within one year prior to surgery achieved substantially better results, with approximately 67% achieving seizure freedom (ILAE classes 1–2).

These findings were consistent with prior studies. Early surgical intervention has been shown to be effective in multiple settings, including a cohort from Sheffield [39] and large-volume cerebrovascular centers [14,40]. However, those studies largely evaluated outcomes of microsurgery following the initial seizure without explicitly considering the timing of CM diagnosis as the underlying etiology. In the present cohort, delayed surgical intervention was primarily attributable to late diagnosis of CM rather than to clinical decision making alone. These results reinforce existing evidence supporting early microsurgical intervention for seizure control in CRE, while also highlighting the importance of timely and accurate diagnosis of CM to optimize surgical outcomes.

In the analyzed cohort, a substantial delay was observed between the onset of initial seizures and the confirmation of a diagnosis of CM and associated epilepsy using diagnostic tools such as MRI, CT, or EEG. The number of patients who underwent microsurgery within one year after radiographic confirmation of CRE was approximately twice that of patients who pursued surgical intervention after the initial seizure (54 vs. 27). The reasons for this delay remain unclear but may be related to limited access to primary care services or to the strong stigma associated with epilepsy [41,42]. As reported by Guo and colleagues, patients with epilepsy often conceal their condition and withdraw from social interactions [41]. This behavior appears to be particularly common in Asian countries [43,44], where self-perception of the diagnosis and coping mechanisms exert greater influence on psychosocial adjustment than the clinical manifestations of epilepsy themselves [45]. Moreover, negative societal attitudes toward marriage, parenthood, and employment are more prevalent in culturally homogeneous societies [46,47]. By contrast, public perceptions in Western countries are generally more favorable [48,49], with only about 10% of respondents expressing negative attitudes toward people with epilepsy [50], and these views have remained relatively stable for nearly two decades [51]. In the studied Kazakhstani cohort, epilepsy-related stigma may have contributed to diagnostic delays, late surgical intervention, and, consequently, less favorable postoperative outcomes.

Another critical aspect concerns the management of ASMs in Kazakhstan. Inappropriate prescribing practices remain a significant challenge, with monotherapy being the most common strategy [52]. Suboptimal medication selection and underdosing likely contribute to inadequate seizure control both before and after surgery [53]. In this study cohort, only 46.67% of patients with CRE received ASM therapy, most commonly low-dose carbamazepine monotherapy. Similar findings were reported by Guekht and colleagues, who observed that nearly one-quarter of individuals with epilepsy were not receiving pharmacological treatment and that prescribed regimens were frequently suboptimal [54]. This predominance of low-dose monotherapy in our cohort raises concerns regarding limited adherence to treatment protocols, inappropriate prescribing practices, and possible restrictions in ASM availability within the country.

4.1. Limitations

This study has several limitations. First, its retrospective design constrained the scope and accuracy of data collection. Reliance on self-reported outcomes may have introduced self-selection and survivorship bias.

Second, the proportion of patients lost to follow-up may have influenced the results. Several context-specific factors likely contributed to this attrition, including inadequate medical record management, underdeveloped digital medical record infrastructure resulting in loss of contact information, and cultural attitudes toward health disclosure. In some cases, patients expressed reluctance or skepticism in responding to health-related questions, even when contacted by their treating physicians.

Third, the relatively small sample size may have limited the statistical power of the study and reduced the generalizability of the findings. Finally, the lack of clinical data regarding the resection of hemosiderin-stained areas restricted the analysis. The absence of intraoperative imaging and navigation systems impeded consistent identification and documentation of these regions, thereby preventing a thorough evaluation of their association with CRE.

4.2. Future Directions

Further research is warranted to investigate the patterns of diagnosis and management of patients presenting with seizures, as well as the practices of physicians in prescribing diagnostic tests following an initial seizure episode. Additionally, a survey studying attitudes toward epilepsy, as well as self-stigma among patients, are needed to better understand barriers to timely care. Studies evaluating patterns of ASM prescribing and administration would also provide valuable insights into current treatment gaps. Moreover, a comparative analysis of postoperative seizure outcomes in patients with CRE before and after the implementation of intraoperative tools is essential, alongside efforts to address persistent limitations in early diagnosis and treatment approaches.

5. Conclusions

Seizure control following microsurgical resection of CRE in Kazakhstan was limited, with favorable outcomes achieved in only half of patients. Early surgery within one year of seizure onset was associated with improved outcomes, whereas delayed surgery, restricted access to intraoperative resources, and suboptimal ASM management were associated with less favorable outcomes. Strengthening diagnostic pathways, optimizing ASM management, and advancing surgical technology are essential steps toward improving outcomes in this patient population.

Author Contributions: Conceptualization, K.M. and C.N.; methodology, K.M.; validation, I.M. and A.T.; formal analysis, C.N.; investigation, I.M.; resources, I.M.; data curation, K.M., C.N. and I.M.; writing—original draft preparation, K.M., I.M. and A.T.; writing—review and editing, K.M., C.N. and S.A.; supervision, Y.M.; project administration, S.A. All authors have read and agreed to the published version of the manuscript.

Funding: This research received no external funding.

Institutional Review Board Statement: The study was conducted in accordance with the Declaration of Helsinki and approved by the National Centre for Neurosurgery's bioethics committee (protocol code 4, dated 11 November 2022).

Informed Consent Statement: Not applicable, as this study was conducted retrospectively using existing medical records without direct patient involvement. All data were de-identified to ensure patient confidentiality, and the study was approved by the institutional ethics committee.

Data Availability Statement: The data presented in this study are available from the corresponding author upon reasonable request. De-identified data may be shared with qualified researchers to ensure the protection of patient confidentiality.

Conflicts of Interest: The authors declare no conflicts of interest.

Abbreviations

CM	Cavernous malformations
CRE	CM-related epilepsy
ASM	Antiseizure medication
MRI	Magnetic Resonance Imaging
EEG	Electroencephalogram
ILAE	International League Against Epilepsy
CT	Computed Tomography

References

1. Smith, E.R.; Scott, R.M. Cavernous Malformations. *Neurosurg. Clin. N. Am.* **2010**, *21*, 483–490. [CrossRef]
2. Rosenow, F.; Alonso-Vanegas, M.A.; Baumgartner, C.; Blümcke, I.; Carreño, M.; Gizewski, E.R.; Hamer, H.M.; Knake, S.; Kahane, P.; Lüders, H.O.; et al. Cavernoma-Related Epilepsy: Review and Recommendations for Management—Report of the Surgical Task Force of the ILAE Commission on Therapeutic Strategies. *Epilepsia* **2013**, *54*, 2025–2035. [CrossRef]
3. Alalfi, M.O.; Lanzino, G.; Flemming, K.D. Clinical Presentation, Hemorrhage Risk, and Outcome in Patients with Familial Cavernous Malformations: A Pragmatic Prospective Analysis of 75 Patients. *J. Neurosurg.* **2023**, *139*, 1018–1024. [CrossRef] [PubMed]

4. Huang, C.; Chen, M.-W.; Si, Y.; Li, J.-M.; Zhou, D. Factors Associated with Epileptic Seizure of Cavernous Malformations in the Central Nervous System in West China. *Pak. J. Med. Sci.* **2013**, *29*, 1116–1121. [CrossRef]
5. Zhang, P.; Zhang, H.; Shi, C.; Zhou, J.; Dong, J.; Liang, M.; Li, R.; Cheng, J.; Chen, Y.; Yuan, J.; et al. Clinical Characteristics and Risk Factors of Cerebral Cavernous Malformation-Related Epilepsy. *Epilepsy Behav.* **2023**, *139*, 109064. [CrossRef] [PubMed]
6. Menzler, K.; Chen, X.; Thiel, P.; Iwinska-Zelder, J.; Miller, D.; Reuss, A.; Hamer, H.M.; Reis, J.; Pagenstecher, A.; Knake, S.; et al. Epileptogenicity of Cavernomas Depends on (Archi-) Cortical Localization. *Neurosurgery* **2010**, *67*, 918–924. [CrossRef] [PubMed]
7. Narita, M.; Miyairi, Y.; Motobayashi, M.; Chiba, A.; Inaba, Y. Incidence of Cerebral Cavernous Malformation-Related Epilepsy in Children: A Single Center Survey. *Cureus* **2023**, *15*, e38178. [CrossRef]
8. Gao, X.; Yue, K.; Sun, J.; Cao, Y.; Zhao, B.; Zhang, H.; Dai, S.; Zhang, L.; Luo, P.; Jiang, X. Treatment of Cerebral Cavernous Malformations Presenting with Seizures: A Systematic Review and Meta-Analysis. *Front. Neurol.* **2020**, *11*. [CrossRef]
9. Josephson, C.B.; Leach, J.-P.; Duncan, R.; Roberts, R.C.; Counsell, C.E.; Al-Shahi Salman, R. Seizure Risk from Cavernous or Arteriovenous Malformations. *Neurology* **2011**, *76*, 1548–1554. [CrossRef]
10. Santos, A.N.; Rauschenbach, L.; Riess, C.; Georgiades, I.; Fiçilar, B.; Gallardo, E.G.; Quesada, C.M.; Li, Y.; Tippelt, S.; Dohna-Schwake, C.; et al. Outcome after Conservative or Surgical Treatment for New-Onset Epilepsy in Children with Cerebral Cavernous Malformation. *Seizure* **2023**, *111*, 23–29. [CrossRef]
11. Schuss, P.; Marx, J.; Borger, V.; Brandecker, S.; Güresir, Á.; Hadjiathanasiou, A.; Hamed, M.; Schneider, M.; Surges, R.; Vatter, H.; et al. Cavernoma-Related Epilepsy in Cavernous Malformations Located within the Temporal Lobe: Surgical Management and Seizure Outcome. *Neurosurg. Focus.* **2020**, *48*, E6. [CrossRef]
12. Van Gompel, J.J.; Marsh, W.R.; Meyer, F.B.; Worrell, G.A. Patient-Assessed Satisfaction and Outcome after Microsurgical Resection of Cavernomas Causing Epilepsy. *Neurosurg. Focus* **2010**, *29*, E16. [CrossRef]
13. Kapadia, M.; Walwema, M.; Smith, T.R.; Bellinski, I.; Batjer, H.; Getch, C.; Rosenow, J.M.; Bendok, B.R.; Schuele, S.U. Seizure Outcome in Patients with Cavernous Malformation after Early Surgery. *Epilepsy Behav.* **2021**, *115*, 107662. [CrossRef]
14. Nico, E.; Adereti, C.O.; Hackett, A.M.; Bianconi, A.; Naik, A.; Eberle, A.T.; Cifre Serra, P.J.; Koester, S.W.; Malnik, S.L.; Fox, B.M.; et al. Assessing the Relationship between Surgical Timing and Postoperative Seizure Outcomes in Cavernoma-Related Epilepsy: A Single-Institution Retrospective Analysis of 63 Patients with a Review of the Literature. *Brain Sci.* **2024**, *14*, 494. [CrossRef]
15. Dammann, P.; Wrede, K.; Jabbarli, R.; Neuschulte, S.; Menzler, K.; Zhu, Y.; Özkan, N.; Müller, O.; Forsting, M.; Rosenow, F.; et al. Outcome after Conservative Management or Surgical Treatment for New-Onset Epilepsy in Cerebral Cavernous Malformation. *J. Neurosurg.* **2017**, *126*, 1303–1311. [CrossRef]
16. von der Brelie, C.; Kuczaty, S.; von Lehe, M. Surgical Management and Long-Term Outcome of Pediatric Patients with Different Subtypes of Epilepsy Associated with Cerebral Cavernous Malformations. *J. Neurosurg. Pediatr.* **2014**, *13*, 699–705. [CrossRef]
17. Shoubash, L.; Nowak, S.; Greisert, S.; Al Menabbawy, A.; Rathmann, E.; von Podewils, F.; Fleck, S.; Schroeder, H.H.W. Cavernoma-Related Epilepsy: Postoperative Epilepsy Outcome and Analysis of the Predictive Factors, Case Series. *World Neurosurg.* **2023**, *172*, e499–e507. [CrossRef] [PubMed]
18. Cerebral Angioma. Available online: https://www.epilepsydiagnosis.org/aetiology/cerebral-angioma-genetics.html (accessed on 14 November 2024).
19. Epilepsy: A Public Health Imperative. Available online: https://www.who.int/publications/i/item/epilepsy-a-public-health-imperative (accessed on 14 November 2024).
20. Bankole, N.D.A.; Dokponou, Y.C.H.; Koning, R.D.; Dalle, D.U.; Kesici, Ö.; Egu, C.; Ikwuegbuenyi, C.; Adegboyega, G.; Ooi, S.Z.Y.; Dada, O.E.; et al. Epilepsy Care and Outcome in Low- and Middle-Income Countries: A Scoping Review. *J. Neurosci. Rural. Pract.* **2024**, *15*, 8. [CrossRef] [PubMed]
21. Pellinen, J. Treatment Gaps in Epilepsy. *Front. Epidemiol.* **2022**, *2*, 976039. [CrossRef]
22. Kuehn, B. Fighting Epilepsy Stigma. *JAMA* **2019**, *322*, 603. [CrossRef] [PubMed]
23. Katchanov, J.; Birbeck, G.L. Epilepsy Care Guidelines for Low- and Middle- Income Countries: From WHO Mental Health GAP to National Programs. *BMC Med.* **2012**, *10*, 107. [CrossRef]
24. World Bank Country and Lending Groups—World Bank Data Help Desk. Available online: https://datahelpdesk.worldbank.org/knowledgebase/articles/906519-world-bank-country-and-lending-groups (accessed on 14 November 2024).
25. Akhmedullin, R.; Kozhobekova, B.; Gusmanov, A.; Aimyshev, T.; Utebekov, Z.; Kyrgyzbay, G.; Shpekov, A.; Gaipov, A. Epilepsy Trends in Kazakhstan: A Retrospective Longitudinal Study Using Data from Unified National Electronic Health System 2014–2020. *Seizure Eur. J. Epilepsy* **2024**, *122*, 58–63. [CrossRef]
26. Эпилепсия у Детей и Взрослых > Клинические Протоколы МЗ РК—2016 (Казахстан) > MedElement. Available online: https://diseases.medelement.com/disease/%D1%8D%D0%BF%D0%B8%D0%BB%D0%B5%D0%BF%D1%81%D0%B8%D1%8F-%D1%83-%D0%B4%D0%B5%D1%82%D0%B5%D0%B9-%D0%B8-%D0%B2%D0%B7%D1%80%D0%BE%D1%81%D0%BB%D1%8B%D1%85/14753 (accessed on 27 March 2024).
27. Cossu, M.; Raneri, F.; Casaceli, G.; Gozzo, F.; Pelliccia, V.; Lo Russo, G. Surgical Treatment of Cavernoma-Related Epilepsy. *J. Neurosurg. Sci.* **2015**, *59*, 237–253.

28. Jehi, L.E.; Palmini, A.; Aryal, U.; Coras, R.; Paglioli, E. Cerebral Cavernous Malformations in the Setting of Focal Epilepsies: Pathological Findings, Clinical Characteristics, and Surgical Treatment Principles. *Acta Neuropathol.* **2014**, *128*, 55–65. [CrossRef] [PubMed]
29. Rajeswarie, R.; Aravinda, H.; Arivazhagan, A.; Bevinahalli, N.N.; Rao, M.B.; Mahadevan, A. Evaluating the Role of Perilesional Tissue in Pathobiology of Epileptogenesis of Vascular Malformations of the Central Nervous System. *J. Epilepsy Res.* **2022**, *12*, 53–61. [CrossRef]
30. Jimenez, A.E.; Geist, E.G.; Connolly, E.S.; McKhann, G.M.; Youngerman, B.E. Laser Interstitial Thermal Therapy for Cavernous Malformations: A Meta-Analysis of Individual Patient-Level Data. *J. Neurosurg.* **2025**, *142*, 1014–1024. [CrossRef]
31. Berber, T.; Celik, S.E.; Aksaray, F.; Yoney, A.; Harmanci, K.; Tambas, M.; Yılmaz, B.D.; Numanoglu, C.; Yolcu, A.; Açan, H.İ.; et al. Radiosurgery Effects and Adverse Effects in Symptomatic Eloquent Brain-Located Cavernomas. *J. Radiat. Res.* **2023**, *64*, 133–141. [CrossRef]
32. Yang, T.; Hakimian, S.; Schwartz, T.H. Intraoperative ElectroCorticoGraphy (ECog): Indications, Techniques, and Utility in Epilepsy Surgery. *Epileptic Disord.* **2014**, *16*, 271–279. [CrossRef] [PubMed]
33. Vakani, R.; Nair, D.R. Electrocorticography and Functional Mapping. *Handb. Clin. Neurol.* **2019**, *160*, 313–327. [CrossRef] [PubMed]
34. He, K.; Alriashy, M.H.S.; Fan, Z.; Qiao, N.; Liao, Y.; An, Q.; Xu, B.; Song, J.; Zhang, X.; Zhu, W.; et al. Cavernoma-Associated Epilepsy Within the Mesial Temporal Lobe: Surgical Management and Seizure Outcome. *World Neurosurg.* **2022**, *160*, e464–e470. [CrossRef]
35. Phal, P.M.; Usmanov, A.; Nesbit, G.M.; Anderson, J.C.; Spencer, D.; Wang, P.; Helwig, J.A.; Roberts, C.; Hamilton, B.E. Qualitative Comparison of 3-T and 1.5-T MRI in the Evaluation of Epilepsy. *AJR Am. J. Roentgenol.* **2008**, *191*, 890–895. [CrossRef]
36. Prat-Acín, R.; Galeano-Senabre, I.; López-Ruiz, P.; García-Sánchez, D.; Ayuso-Sacido, A.; Espert-Tortajada, R. Intraoperative Brain Mapping during Awake Surgery in Symptomatic Supratentorial Cavernomas. *Neurocirugía* **2021**, *32*, 217–223. [CrossRef] [PubMed]
37. Shih, Y.-C.; Chou, C.-C.; Peng, S.-J.; Yu, H.-Y.; Hsu, S.P.C.; Lin, C.-F.; Lee, C.-C.; Yang, H.-C.; Chen, Y.-C.; Kwan, S.-Y.; et al. Clinical Characteristics and Long-Term Outcome of Cerebral Cavernous Malformations-Related Epilepsy. *Epilepsia* **2022**, *63*, 2056–2067. [CrossRef]
38. Tuleasca, C.; Peciu-Florianu, I.; Strachowski, O.; Derre, B.; Vannod-Michel, Q.; Reyns, N. How to Combine the Use of Intraoperative Magnetic Resonance Imaging (MRI) and Awake Craniotomy for Microsurgical Resection of Hemorrhagic Cavernous Malformation in Eloquent Area: A Case Report. *J. Med. Case Rep.* **2023**, *17*, 160. [CrossRef] [PubMed]
39. Alexander, R.; Kirsty, H.; Imron, H.; Saminderjit, K.; Shungu, U.; Dev, B.; Varduhi, C. Cavernoma Related Epilepsy—A Sheffield Cohort. *J. Neurol. Neurosurg. Psychiatry* **2023**, *94*, A40–A41. [CrossRef]
40. Dziedzic, T.A.; Koczyk, K.; Nowak, A.; Maj, E.; Marchel, A. Long-Term Management of Seizures after Surgical Treatment of Supratentorial Cavernous Malformations: A Retrospective Single Centre Study. *J. Korean Neurosurg. Soc.* **2022**, *65*, 415–421. [CrossRef]
41. Guo, W.; Wu, J.; Wang, W.; Guan, B.; Snape, D.; Baker, G.A.; Jacoby, A. The Stigma of People with Epilepsy Is Demonstrated at the Internalized, Interpersonal and Institutional Level in a Specific Socio-Cultural Context: Findings from an Ethnographic Study in Rural China. *Epilepsy Behav.* **2012**, *25*, 282–288. [CrossRef]
42. Tian, N.; Kobau, R.; Zack, M.M.; Greenlund, K.J. Barriers to and Disparities in Access to Health Care Among Adults Aged ≥18 Years with Epilepsy—United States, 2015 and 2017. *MMWR Morb. Mortal. Wkly. Rep.* **2022**, *71*, 697–702. [CrossRef]
43. Demirci, S.; Dönmez, C.M.; Gündoğar, D.; Baydar, C.L. Public Awareness of, Attitudes toward, and Understanding of Epilepsy in Isparta, Turkey. *Epilepsy Behav.* **2007**, *11*, 427–433. [CrossRef]
44. Lai, C.W.; Huang, X.S.; Lai, Y.H.; Zhang, Z.Q.; Liu, G.J.; Yang, M.Z. Survey of Public Awareness, Understanding, and Attitudes toward Epilepsy in Henan Province, China. *Epilepsia* **1990**, *31*, 182–187. [CrossRef]
45. Lau, V.W.; Lee, T.M.; Ng, P.K.; Wong, V.C. Psychosocial Adjustment of People with Epilepsy in Hong Kong. *Epilepsia* **2001**, *42*, 1169–1175. [CrossRef] [PubMed]
46. Choi-Kwon, S.; Park, K.A.; Lee, H.J.; Park, M.S.; Lee, C.H.; Cheon, S.E.; Youn, M.H.; Lee, S.K.; Chung, C.-K. Familiarity with, Knowledge of, and Attitudes toward Epilepsy in Residents of Seoul, South Korea. *Acta Neurol. Scand.* **2004**, *110*, 39–45. [CrossRef]
47. AlHarbi, F.A.; Alomari, M.S.; Ghaddaf, A.A.; Abdulhamid, A.S.; Alsharef, J.F.; Makkawi, S. Public Awareness and Attitudes toward Epilepsy in Saudi Arabia: A Systematic Review and Meta-Analysis. *Epilepsy Behav.* **2021**, *124*, 108314. [CrossRef] [PubMed]
48. Diamantopoulos, N.; Kaleyias, J.; Tzoufi, M.; Kotsalis, C. A Survey of Public Awareness, Understanding, and Attitudes toward Epilepsy in Greece. *Epilepsia* **2006**, *47*, 2154–2164. [CrossRef]
49. Jensen, R.; Dam, M. Public Attitudes toward Epilepsy in Denmark. *Epilepsia* **1992**, *33*, 459–463. [CrossRef]

50. Spatt, J.; Bauer, G.; Baumgartner, C.; Feucht, M.; Graf, M.; Mamoli, B.; Trinka, E.; Austrian Section of the International League Against Epilepsy. Predictors for Negative Attitudes toward Subjects with Epilepsy: A Representative Survey in the General Public in Austria. *Epilepsia* **2005**, *46*, 736–742. [CrossRef]
51. Gosavi, T.D.; Wang, S.; See, S.J.; Ng, J.; Lim, S.H. Revisiting the Public Awareness, Attitudes, and Understanding towards Epilepsy among Singapore Residents. *Epilepsy Behav.* **2018**, *89*, 143–147. [CrossRef]
52. Jacob, L.; Kerimbaeva, Z.; Kalyapin, A.; Kostev, K. Prescription Patterns of Antiepileptic Drugs in Kazakhstan in 2018: A Retrospective Study of 57,959 Patients. *Epilepsy Behav.* **2019**, *99*, 106445. [CrossRef] [PubMed]
53. Lee, J.W.; Dworetzky, B. Rational Polytherapy with Antiepileptic Drugs. *Pharmaceuticals* **2010**, *3*, 2362–2379. [CrossRef]
54. Guekht, A.; Zharkinbekova, N.; Shpak, A.; Hauser, W.A. Epilepsy and Treatment Gap in Urban and Rural Areas of the Southern Kazakhstan in Adults. *Epilepsy Behav.* **2017**, *67*, 98–104. [CrossRef]

brain sciences

Article

Clinical Presentations and Treatment Approaches in a Retrospective Analysis of 128 Intracranial Arteriovenous Malformation Cases

Corneliu Toader [1,2], Mugurel Petrinel Radoi [1,2,*], Milena-Monica Ilie [1], Razvan-Adrian Covache-Busuioc [1], Vlad Buica [1], Luca-Andrei Glavan [1], Christian-Adelin Covlea [1], Antonio Daniel Corlatescu [1], Horia-Petre Costin [1], Carla Crivoi [3] and Leon Danaila [1,2,4]

1 Department of Neurosurgery, "Carol Davila" University of Medicine and Pharmacy, 020021 Bucharest, Romania; corneliu.toader@umfcd.ro (C.T.); milena-monica.ilie0720@stud.umfcd.ro (M.-M.I.); razvan-adrian.covache-busuioc0720@stud.umfcd.ro (R.-A.C.-B.); vlad.buica0720@stud.umfcd.ro (V.B.); luca-andrei.glavan0720@stud.umfcd.ro (L.-A.G.); christian-adelin.covlea0720@stud.umfcd.ro (C.-A.C.); antonio.corlatescu0920@stud.umfcd.ro (A.D.C.); horia-petre.costin0720@stud.umfcd.ro (H.-P.C.); acad.leondanaila@gmail.com (L.D.)

2 Department of Vascular Neurosurgery, National Institute of Neurology and Neurovascular Diseases, 077160 Bucharest, Romania

3 Faculty of Mathematics and Computer Science, University of Bucharest, 010014 Bucharest, Romania; crivoicarla02@gmail.com

4 Romanian Academy, Medical Sciences Section, 010071 Bucharest, Romania

* Correspondence: petrinel.radoi@umfcd.ro

Abstract: Background: Intracranial AVMs are a highly heterogeneous group of lesions that, while not very common, can pose significant risks. The therapeutic management of AVMs is complicated by ambiguous guidelines, particularly regarding which Spetzler–Martin grades should dictate specific treatment options. This study analyzed the clinical presentations and treatment approaches of 128 brain AVM cases managed between 2014 and 2022 at the National Institute of Neurology and Neurovascular Diseases in Bucharest, Romania. Methods: A retrospective analysis was conducted on patient demographics, clinical symptoms, Spetzler–Martin categorization, nidus localization, therapeutic management, and outcomes. Statistical analysis was performed using Python 3.10. Results: In our cohort of patients, the median age was 45 years, with a slight male predominance (67 males, 61 females). At admission, 51.5% presented with elevated blood pressure. The majority of patients had a Spetzler–Martin score of 2 (37.5%), followed by scores of 3 (31.3%) and 1 (20.3%). Treatment strategies included microsurgical resection in 32% of cases, conservative management in 31.2%, Gamma Knife radiosurgery in 22.6%, and endovascular embolization in 13.3%. Notably, open surgery was predominantly chosen for Grade II AVMs. The functional outcomes were favorable, with 69.5% achieving a good recovery score on the Glasgow Outcome Scale. Only four in-hospital deaths occurred, all in patients who underwent open surgery, and no deaths were recorded during the two-year follow-up. Conclusions: AVMs within the same Spetzler–Martin grade display considerable complexity, necessitating personalized treatment strategies. Our findings highlight the limitations of open surgery for Grade I cases but affirm its effectiveness for Grade II AVMs.

Keywords: arteriovenous malformation; Spetzler–Martin grading system; surgery; radiosurgery; endovascular embolization

1. Introduction

Intracranial arteriovenous malformations (AVMs) are congenital cerebrovascular anomalies characterized by direct, high-pressure connections between arteries and veins without intermediary capillaries, forming a nidus of dysplastic vessels [1]. This structural deficiency allows blood to flow directly from arteries to veins, leading to vessel dilation and tortuosity, significantly increasing the risk of hemorrhage and neurological impairment [2]. Although AVMs can occur throughout the body, intracranial AVMs are particularly concerning due to their heightened bleeding risk.

The true prevalence of brain AVMs (bAVMs) remains uncertain, largely because many cases are asymptomatic. Postmortem analyses suggest a prevalence between 5 and 613 cases per 100,000, while epidemiological studies estimate an incidence of 1.12 to 1.42 per 100,000, with hemorrhage as the first presenting symptom in 38–68% of cases [3,4]. Advances in MRI technology have increased the detection of unruptured AVMs, while the incidence of ruptured cases remains stable [2]. Most symptomatic patients are diagnosed between the ages of 20 and 50, with no significant gender differences in prevalence [2,5]. There is not a significant difference in incidence between males and females [1]. Hemorrhage occurs in approximately 65% of cases, most commonly in parenchymal regions (82%), followed by intraventricular and subarachnoid sites [5–7]. Risk factors for rupture include frontal lobe location, deep venous drainage, deep nidus location, and associated aneurysms [8–11]. Pregnancy as a risk factor is debated, with mixed evidence on increased rupture risk [5,12,13]. Other common symptoms include seizures, headaches, and neurological deficits [5].

The etiology of bAVMs is poorly understood, though likely congenital. Deficient capillary formation during fetal development may play a role [2]. Syndromic associations, such as hereditary hemorrhagic telangiectasia (Rendu–Weber–Osler syndrome), Cobb syndrome, and cerebrofacial arteriovenous metameric syndromes, suggest a genetic component in some cases [4,14,15]. Abnormal angiogenesis, vasculogenesis, and inflammation, mediated by factors such as VEGF, angiopoietin-2, TGF-β, and MMPs, are implicated in AVM development [10,16–18].

Grading systems assess AVM morbidity and mortality risk, with the Spetzler–Martin scale being a primary tool, evaluating nidus size, location eloquence, and venous drainage type. Eloquent areas include sensorimotor, language, and visual cortices, as well as deep brain structures like the hypothalamus, thalamus, and brainstem. The Lawton–Young scale and Spetzler–Ponce classification further refine risk and outcome prediction [4,10].

Treatment strategies for bAVMs include microsurgical resection, endovascular embolization, and stereotactic radiosurgery, especially Gamma Knife radiosurgery. When surgical risks are high, conservative management focuses on symptom control and hemorrhage prevention through antiepileptic drugs (AEDs), monitoring, and lifestyle adjustments [19]. For inoperable AVMs, alternative therapies such as Botox injections for refractory migraine management have shown symptom relief [20].

The management of unruptured AVMs remains debated. The ARUBA trial (2014) suggested medical management as preferable for unruptured AVMs over surgical interventions, though critiques highlight limitations such as early termination, selection bias, and broad inclusion criteria [11,21,22]. Despite these limitations, the ARUBA trial has influenced a trend toward conservative management in unruptured cases [23].

While significant data on AVMs exist globally, particularly from high-resource healthcare settings, regional data from Romania remain scarce due to limited national statistics and centralized reporting. This study offers novel insights into AVM cases in Romania by providing a comprehensive assessment of patient demographics, clinical presentations, and treatment strategies based on nidus location and Spetzler–Martin grading. Given the constraints and unique aspects of the Romanian healthcare system, our findings may inform localized treatment protocols, guide healthcare policy, and support the better allocation of resources for multidisciplinary AVM management [24].

2. Materials and Methods

This study presents a retrospective unicentric analysis of 128 cases of cerebral AVMs treated at the Department of Neurosurgery, National Institute of Neurology and Neurovascular Diseases in Bucharest, Romania, between 2014 and 2022. Patients were subjected to one of four management approaches: microsurgical resection, Gamma Knife radiosurgery, endovascular embolization, or conservative treatment as determined by the medical team.

A comprehensive analysis was conducted, focusing on specific variables throughout the preoperative, intraoperative, and postoperative stages of patient medical management. Particular attention was given to factors such as bleeding, presence of arterial hypertension, seizures, location of the nidus, Spetzler–Martin score, and hemorrhage. Additionally, postoperative complications were discussed, and the number of reoperations was noted.

The research adhered to the main principles of the Declaration of Helsinki and received approval from the Ethics Committee of the National Institute of Neurology and Neurovascular Diseases in Bucharest, Romania (Approval No. [7230]). Clinical data, including age, sex, Glasgow Coma Scale score, bleeding, and treatment, were extracted from relevant patient files. All data processing was conducted in compliance with the current General Data Protection Regulation (GDPR), and informed consent was obtained from all patients included in this study.

Statistical analysis and figure plotting were performed using Python version 3.10, developed by the Python Software Foundation (9450 SW Gemini Dr., ECM# 90772, Beaverton, OR 97008, USA). The analysis utilized Python libraries such as pandas, numpy, seaborn, and matplotlib.

3. Results

3.1. Patient Demographics and Comorbidities

3.1.1. Age and Sex

A dataset comprising 128 intracranial AVM cases treated between 2010 and 2022 was collected from the National Institute of Neurology and Neurovascular Diseases in Romania. We analyzed (Figure 1) the demographic characteristics of patients diagnosed with AVMs, focusing on age and gender distribution. Among the patients, 67 were male and 61 were female. The median age at diagnosis was 45 years, and the mean age was 44.5 years. The highest prevalence was observed in the 40–50 age group, which accounted for 29.6% of the total cases.

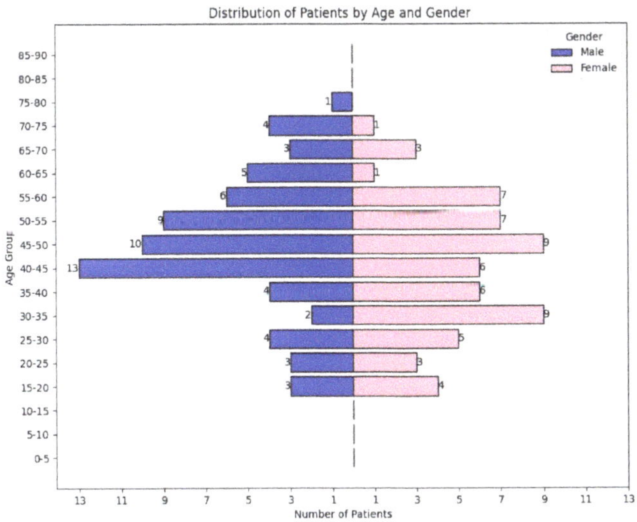

Figure 1. Distribution of patients with intracranial AVM by age and gender.

3.1.2. Arterial Hypertension at Admission Time

Arterial blood pressure was measured at the time of admission for all patients. Of these, 51.5% (n = 66) had systolic and diastolic pressures exceeding 140/90 mmHg. Specifically, 27.3% (n = 35) had stage 1 hypertension, 21.1% (n = 27) had stage 2 hypertension, and 3.1% (n = 4) experienced a hypertensive crisis (Figure 2).

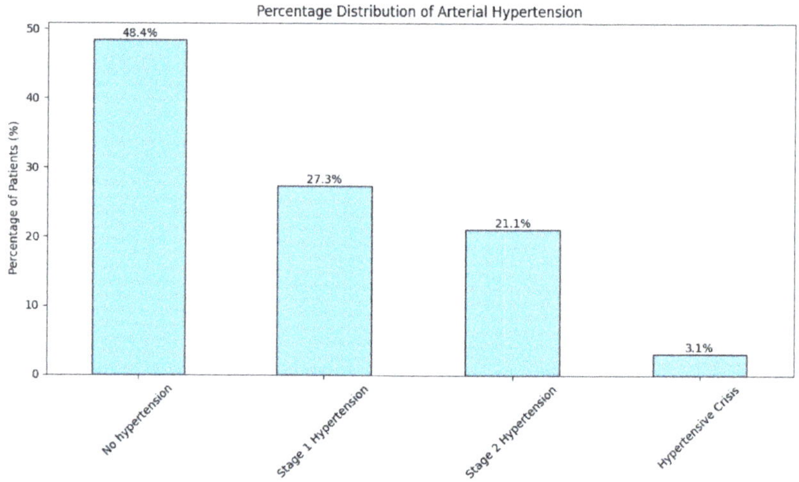

Figure 2. Assessment of arterial hypertension of intracranial AVM patients.

3.2. *Presentation*

3.2.1. Glasgow Coma Scores

At presentation, the mental state of the patients was assessed using the Glasgow Coma Scale. The majority of patients, 75.8% (n = 97), had minor brain injuries with scores of 13 or higher. Specifically, 49.2% (n = 63) had a score of 15, 14.1% (n = 18) had a score of 14, and 12.5% (n = 16) had a score of 13 (Figure 3).

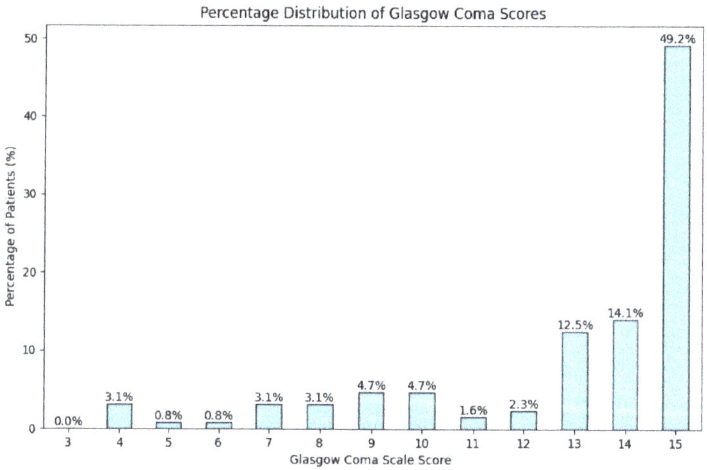

Figure 3. Distribution of patients by Glasgow Coma Scale.

3.2.2. Headaches, Nausea and Vomiting

A total of 51.6% (n = 66) of patients presented with headaches, characterized by persistent and severe headaches, while 32.8% (n = 42) experienced episodes of vomiting prior to admission.

3.2.3. Comitial Seizures

A history of epilepsy was present in 32.2% (n = 41) of the patients, either under focal or generalized seizures (Figure 4).

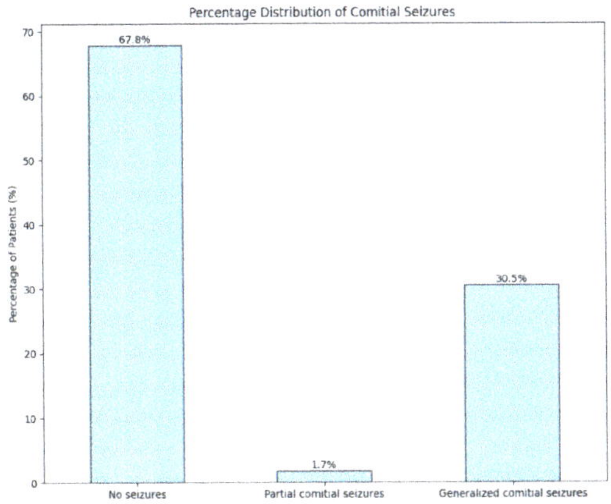

Figure 4. Percentage distribution of comitial seizures in intracranial AVM patients.

3.2.4. Spetzler–Martin Scores

Among the patients, 20.3% (n = 26) had a score of 1, indicating a nidus smaller than 3 cm, a non-eloquent location, and venous drainage into the superficial system. The majority of patients had a score of 2, accounting for 37.5% (n = 48), while 31.3% (n = 40) had a score of 3. Scores of 4 and 5 were less common, with 7.8% (n = 10) and 3.1% (n = 4) of patients, respectively (Figure 5).

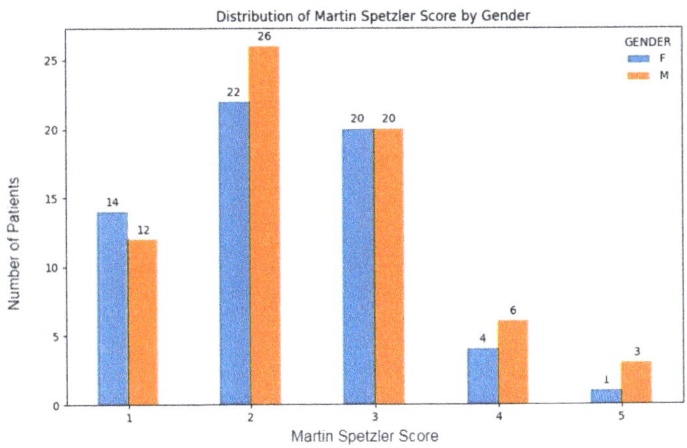

Figure 5. Distribution of Spetzler–Martin score by gender in intracranial AVM patients.

3.3. Rupture Status Resulting in Intracranial Hemorrhage

In this patient cohort, 63.3% (n = 81) of patients presented with unruptured AVMs, while 36.7% (n = 47) of patients had ruptured AVMs, resulting in intracranial hemorrhage. Of those with ruptures, 20.3% (n = 26) of patients experienced subarachnoid hemorrhage. The ruptured cases were assessed according to the RAGS classification (Figure 6), with distributions as follows: 56.7% of ruptured AVMs were scored as RAGS 1, indicating minimal rupture risk, followed by 27.6% as RAGS 2, 14.2% as RAGS 3, and 3.5% as RAGS 4. This grading reflects the extent and severity of hemorrhagic events, aiding in clinical stratification and management decisions for patients with ruptured AVMs.

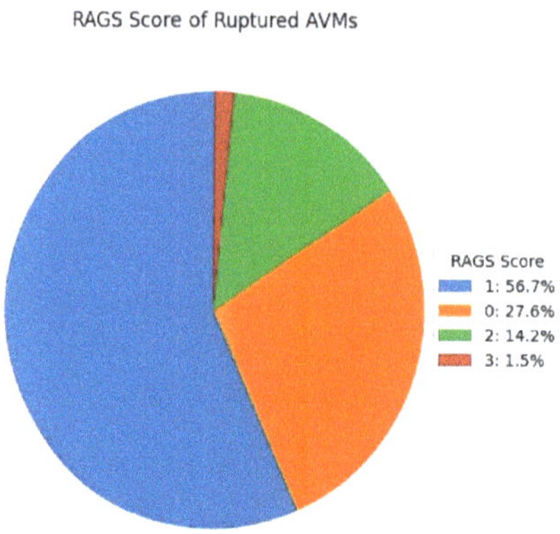

Figure 6. Percentage distribution of patients with intracranial AVM by RAGS.

3.4. Cases Management

This study identified five distinct treatment options for patients with intracranial AVMs, distributed according to the Spetzler–Martin score (Figure 7) and the nidus localization (Figure 8). Microsurgical AVM resection was chosen for 32% of patients (n = 41), while conservative treatment was selected for 31.2% (n = 40). Gamma Knife radiosurgery was used for 22.6% (n = 29), and endovascular embolization was applied to 13.3% (n = 17). A combination of endovascular embolization and Gamma Knife radiosurgery was used for 0.8% (n = 1).

Figure 7 illustrates a marked preference for open surgery in the treatment of Grade II intracranial AVMs.

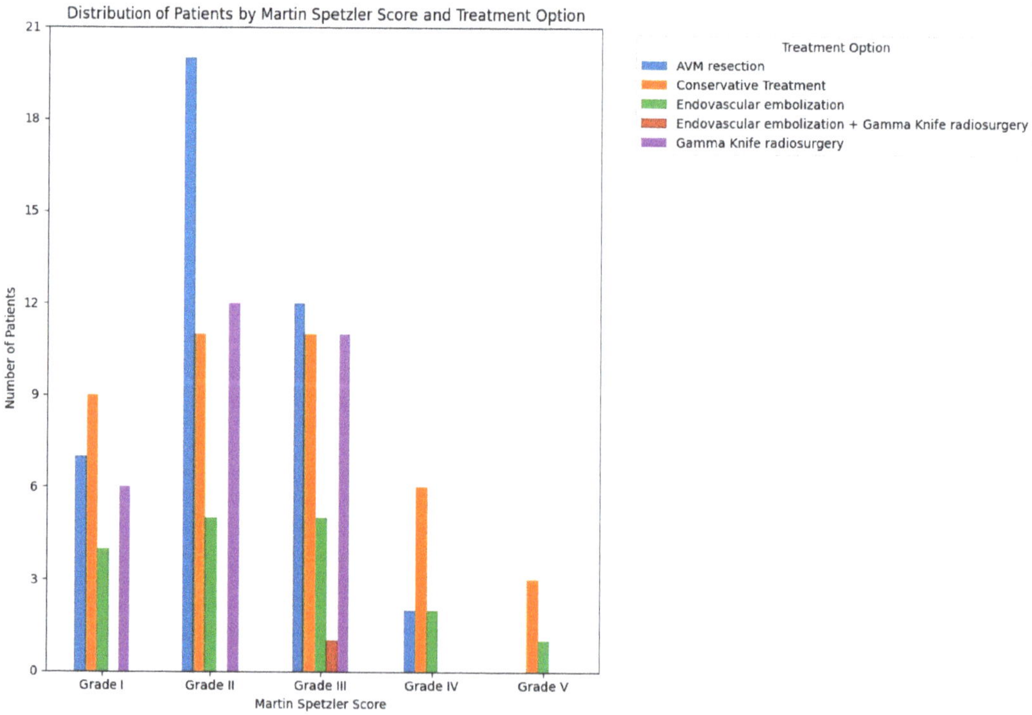

Figure 7. Distribution of patients with intracranial AVM by treatment and Spetzler–Martin score.

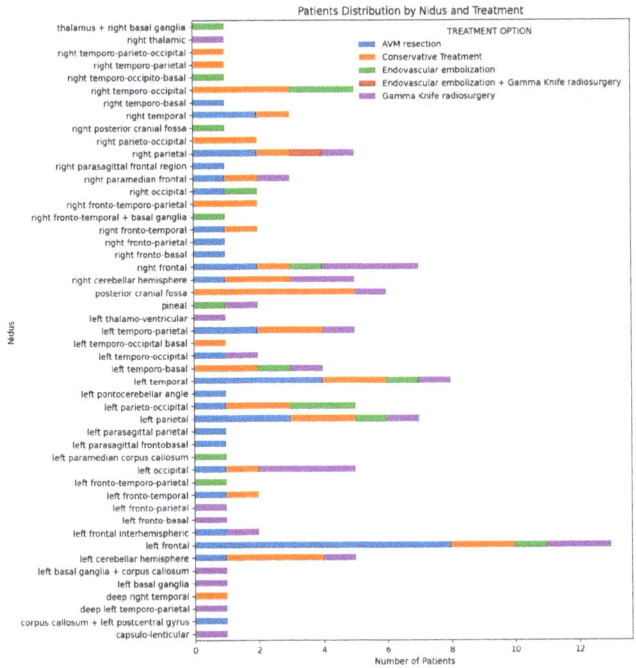

Figure 8. Distribution of nidus locations and treatment options in AVM patients.

3.5. Short-Term Outcomes

Functional outcomes were assessed before hospital discharge. According to the Glasgow Outcome Scale (Figure 9), the majority of patients (69.5%, n = 89) achieved a score of 5, indicating good recovery. A smaller percentage, 24.2% (n = 31), had a score of 4, reflecting moderate disability. Scores of 1 and 3 were observed in 3.1% (n = 4) of patients each, indicating death or persistent disabilities. No patients received a score of 2. Only four in-hospital deaths were reported, all occurring in patients who underwent open surgery. All patients were followed-up for a minimum of two years, with some patients receiving extended follow-up based on clinical need and availability.

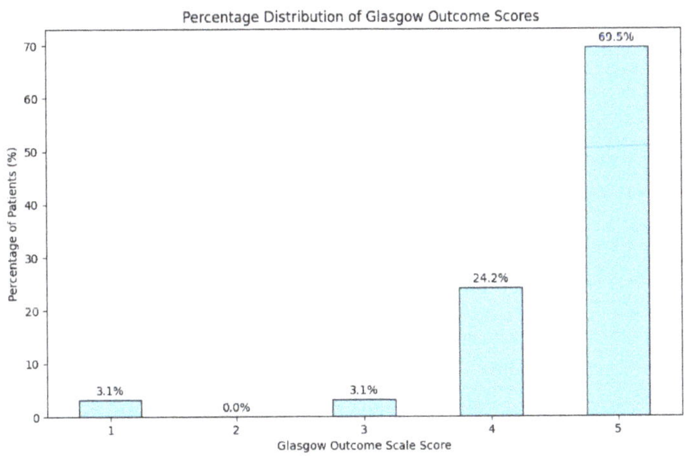

Figure 9. Distribution of Glasgow Outcome Scores in patients with intracranial AVM.

This approach ensured consistent post-treatment monitoring and allowed for the comprehensive assessment of long-term outcomes across the cohort.

4. Discussion

The literature (Table 1) exposes a diverse range of findings regarding AVM treatment outcomes across various patient populations. Studies have examined numerous facets of AVM management, including patient demographics, Spetzler–Martin grading, treatment modalities, and key clinical outcomes. Collectively, these studies shed light on important patterns and challenges in AVM treatment, offering valuable insights for contemporary clinical practice.

Table 1. Literature review table that analyzes significant studies about AVM and treatment outcomes.

Study	Population (n)	Male-to-Female Ratio	Spetzler–Martin Grades Included	Variables Assessed, Similarly to Our Study	Treatment Method	Key Findings
Von Der Brelie et al. [25]	293 (out of which 103 presented with epilepsy and had follow-up)	59 males/ 44 females	I–III	Seizure outcomes, hemorrhage, treatment type	Microsurgery	Favorable seizure outcomes post-surgery; seizure control improved in AVM patients post-resection
De Castro-Afonso et al. [26]	203 (117 unruptured AVMs—86 ruptured AVMs)	108 males/ 95 females	I–IV	Venous drainage, nidus size, AVM rupture	Microsurgery, EVT	Larger draining veins linked to higher hemorrhage risk; supports aggressive treatment for high-risk AVMs
Nesvick et al. [27]	352	150 males/ 202 females	I–III	Obliteration rates, biological effective dose (BED)	Stereotactic radiosurgery	BED > 133 Gy predicts high obliteration rates post-SRS; recommended dose adjustments for AVM obliteration
Steiner et al. [28]	247	132 males/ 115 females	I–IV	Treatment outcomes, angiographic obliteration	Gamma Knife radiosurgery	High obliteration rates with SRS; few adverse events, supporting radiosurgery for specific AVM grades
Heros et al. [29]	153	83 males/ 70 females	I–V	Surgical outcomes, hemorrhage, neurological deficits	Surgical resection	Surgical resection beneficial for Grades I-III, less so for IV-V; conservative management recommended for higher grades
Redekop et al. [30]	97 patients with AVM and intranidal aneurysm	52 males/ 45 females	I–III	Aneurysm presence, hemorrhage risk	EVT, micro-surgery	Intranidal aneurysms increase hemorrhage risk; surgical intervention recommended for associated aneurysms
Mast et al. [31]	281	133 males/ 148 females	I–IV	Initial hemorrhage, re-bleed risk	EVT, resection, SRS	Initial hemorrhage predicts higher re-bleed risk; suggests monitoring high-risk AVMs post-initial bleed
Al Shahi et al. [32]	92	49 males/ 43 females	I–IV	Detection rates, public health impact	Not specified	Provides baseline AVM detection rates; calls for resource allocation for AVM management

Table 1. *Cont.*

Study	Population (n)	Male-to-Female Ratio	Spetzler–Martin Grades Included	Variables Assessed, Similarly to Our Study	Treatment Method	Key Findings
Maruyama et al. [33]	500	287 males/ 213 females	I–IV	Hemorrhage risk post-SRS	Gamma Knife radiosurgery	SRS reduces hemorrhage risk; highlights latency period where hemorrhage risk remains until obliteration

Although the exact mechanism by which epilepsy occurs in patients with AVMs is not fully understood, several risk factors have been identified that increase the likelihood of seizures. These include younger age, temporal lobe location, cortical involvement, and a nidus diameter exceeding 3 cm [34]. In our cohort, we observed that out of 41 patients with AVMs located in or involving the temporal region, 17 experienced epileptic seizures. These seizures were either focal or progressed to generalized seizures, supporting the association between temporal lobe AVMs and increased seizure incidence. All patients experiencing seizures were prescribed oral AEDs at discharge to maintain effective seizure control and manage their condition in the long term.

The ARUBA trial did not evaluate surgical outcomes for patients with Grade I or II AVMs, who are considered optimal candidates for surgery [35]. This limitation reduces the trial's ability to provide comprehensive recommendations. Therefore, we aim to address treatment option controversies and present our own findings to offer a more inclusive perspective.

In contrast to the ARUBA trial findings, a study by Potts et al. concluded that surgery remains the "gold standard" treatment for most low-grade AVMs. This study emphasized using endovascular embolization as a preoperative adjunct. High surgical cure rates and excellent functional outcomes in patients with both ruptured and unruptured AVMs support a strong preference for surgical intervention, offering the best cure rate, lowest risk profile, and greatest protection against hemorrhage for low-grade AVMs [36]. A prospective study by Baharvahdat et al. demonstrated that endovascular treatment (EVT) was highly effective for low-grade AVMs classified as Spetzler–Martin I–II. This study reported a high rate of complete exclusion with a low complication rate of 5%. EVT was recommended as the first-line treatment for both ruptured and unruptured low-grade AVMs located in deep or eloquent regions, where the risks of open surgery are significant [37]. Out of 48 patients with Spetzler–Martin Grade II AVMs, 20 (41.6%) underwent microsurgical resection, supporting Potts's assertion that open surgery is the gold standard for low-grade AVMs. Conversely, among 26 Grade I AVMs, 9 received conservative treatment and only 7 underwent microsurgical resection, indicating a decline in the preference for open surgery in these cases and supporting ARUBA's claims. Our findings suggest that while open surgery may be the gold standard for Grade II AVMs, it is not necessarily the optimal solution for all Grade I AVMs.

In line with Lawton's proposal to further classify Grade III AVMs into subtypes such as S1V1E1, S2V1E0, S2V0E1, and S3V0E0, our cohort also reflects the heterogeneous nature of these AVMs [38]. The data show no clear preference for treatment options among patients with Grade III AVMs, as similar numbers underwent AVM resection, Gamma Knife therapy, and conservative treatment. This diversity in treatment approaches underscores the complexity and variability within Grade III AVMs, supporting the idea of further subclassification to better tailor treatment strategies [38]. Notably, conservative treatment is typically recommended for high-grade AVMs, highlighting the nuanced decision-making required for Grade III cases.

Stereotactic radiosurgery (SRS) achieves a 70–80% obliteration rate for bAVMs. Recognizing that the effects of SRS are delayed, the annual hemorrhage rate during the latency period between radiation and complete nidus obliteration following Gamma Knife radiosurgery (GKRS) was found to be 1.4%, which is lower than the general rate of 2–4% [32,39]. In our cohort, GKRS was selected exclusively for Grade I to III AVMs when open surgery was unequivocally declined due to patient comorbidities, patient refusal, or when the AVM was located in a deep area that made surgical access challenging (such as basal ganglia or corpus callosum). The case of the single patient who underwent EVT followed by SRS further supports the recommendations for multimodal approaches in managing Grade III and IV AVMs [35,40]. Aside from Grade V AVMs in older patients, there is no established consensus on conservative management, particularly in light of critiques following the ARUBA study [35]. In our patient cohort, the use of medications such as AEDs, analgesics, and antihypertensive drugs for hemorrhagic stroke control, combined with regular monitoring during follow-ups, resulted in no deaths over the strict two-year follow-up period. This outcome was observed in patients who received only conservative management, meaning that they did not undergo any of the aforementioned procedures.

5. Conclusions

Our study reveals previously unrecognized distinctions within Spetzler–Martin Grade II AVMs, uncovering that nuanced patient and AVM characteristics—such as lesion depth, vascular complexity, and the presence of hypertension—significantly direct optimal treatment pathways. Contrary to generalized protocols, our data suggest that microsurgery provides superior outcomes for Grade II AVMs in eloquent regions, whereas GKRS proves particularly effective for deep-seated AVMs in hypertensive patients, where traditional risk models might discourage intervention. Furthermore, we identified that EVT is most beneficial in non-eloquent, less complex vascular structures, demonstrating that tailored treatment approaches guided by these newly elucidated factors can substantially improve patient outcomes. These findings challenge existing paradigms, advocating for a refined treatment framework that integrates detailed anatomical and comorbidity profiles to enhance therapeutic precision and reduce risks associated with AVM management.

Author Contributions: Conceptualization, C.T. and L.D.; data curation, C.T., M.-M.I., C.-A.C. and H.-P.C.; formal analysis, M.P.R.; investigation, C.T. and A.D.C.; methodology, M.P.R. and A.D.C.; resources, R.-A.C.-B. and V.B.; software, L.-A.G. and C.C.; supervision, C.T. and L.D.; validation, M.P.R.; visualization, H.-P.C. and C.C.; writing—original draft, M.-M.I. and V.B.; writing—review and editing, R.-A.C.-B., L.-A.G., C.-A.C. and L.D. All authors have read and agreed to the published version of the manuscript.

Funding: Publication of this paper was supported by the University of Medicine and Pharmacy Carol Davila, through the institutional program Publish not Perish.

Institutional Review Board Statement: No applicable.

Informed Consent Statement: Not applicable.

Data Availability Statement: The data that support the findings of this study are available from the corresponding author upon reasonable request. The data are not publicly available due to privacy and ethical restrictions.

Conflicts of Interest: The authors declare no conflicts of interest.

References

1. Bokhari, M.R.; Bokhari, S.R.A. Arteriovenous Malformation of the Brain. In *StatPearls*; StatPearls Publishing: Treasure Island, FL, USA, 2024. Available online: http://www.ncbi.nlm.nih.gov/books/NBK430744/ (accessed on 10 August 2024).
2. Lawton, M.T.; Rutledge, W.C.; Kim, H.; Stapf, C.; Whitehead, K.J.; Li, D.Y.; Krings, T.; terBrugge, K.; Kondziolka, D.; Morgan, M.K.; et al. Brain arteriovenous malformations. *Nat. Rev. Dis. Primer* **2015**, *1*, 15008. [CrossRef] [PubMed]
3. Berman, M.F.; Sciacca, R.R.; Pile-Spellman, J.; Stapf, C.; Connolly, E.S.; Mohr, J.P.; Young, W.L. The Epidemiology of Brain Arteriovenous Malformations. *Neurosurgery* **2000**, *47*, 389–397. [CrossRef] [PubMed]
4. Ozpinar, A.; Mendez, G.; Abla, A.A. Epidemiology, genetics, pathophysiology, and prognostic classifications of cerebral arteriovenous malformations. In *Handbook of Clinical Neurology*; Elsevier: Amsterdam, The Netherlands, 2017; Volume 143, pp. 5–13, ISBN 978-0-444-63640-9.
5. Naranbhai, N.; Pérez, R. Management of Brain Arteriovenous Malformations: A Review. *Cureus* **2023**. [CrossRef] [PubMed]

6. Morgan, M.; Sekhon, L.; Rahman, Z.; Dandie, G. Morbidity of Intracranial Hemorrhage in Patients with Cerebral Arteriovenous Malformation. *Stroke* **1998**, *29*, 2001–2003. [CrossRef]
7. Sato, S.; Kodama, N.; Sasaki, T.; Matsumoto, M.; Ishikawa, T. Perinidal Dilated Capillary Networks in Cerebral Arteriovenous Malformations. *Neurosurgery* **2004**, *54*, 163–170. [CrossRef]
8. Stapf, C.; Mast, H.; Sciacca, R.R.; Choi, J.H.; Khaw, A.V.; Connolly, E.S.; Pile-Spellman, J.; Mohr, J.P. Predictors of hemorrhage in patients with untreated brain arteriovenous malformation. *Neurology* **2006**, *66*, 1350–1355. [CrossRef]
9. Khaw, A.V.; Mohr, J.P.; Sciacca, R.R.; Schumacher, H.C.; Hartmann, A.; Pile-Spellman, J.; Mast, H.; Stapf, C. Association of Infratentorial Brain Arteriovenous Malformations with Hemorrhage at Initial Presentation. *Stroke* **2004**, *35*, 660–663. [CrossRef]
10. Kim, H.; Al-Shahi Salman, R.; McCulloch, C.E.; Stapf, C.; Young, W.L. For the MARS Coinvestigators Untreated brain arteriovenous malformation: Patient-level meta-analysis of hemorrhage predictors. *Neurology* **2014**, *83*, 590–597. [CrossRef]
11. Mohr, J.P.; Parides, M.K.; Stapf, C.; Moquete, E.; Moy, C.S.; Overbey, J.R.; Salman, R.A.-S.; Vicaut, E.; Young, W.L.; Houdart, E.; et al. Medical management with or without interventional therapy for unruptured brain arteriovenous malformations (ARUBA): A multicentre, non-blinded, randomised trial. *Lancet* **2014**, *383*, 614–621. [CrossRef]
12. Bateman, B.T.; Schumacher, H.C.; Bushnell, C.D.; Pile-Spellman, J.; Simpson, L.L.; Sacco, R.L.; Berman, M.F. Intracerebral hemorrhage in pregnancy: Frequency, risk factors, and outcome. *Neurology* **2006**, *67*, 424–429. [CrossRef]
13. Gross, B.A.; Du, R. Hemorrhage from Arteriovenous Malformations During Pregnancy. *Neurosurgery* **2012**, *71*, 349–356. [CrossRef] [PubMed]
14. Putman, C.M.; Chaloupka, J.C.; Fulbright, R.K.; Awad, I.A.; White, R.I.; Fayad, P.B. Exceptional multiplicity of cerebral arteriovenous malformations associated with hereditary hemorrhagic telangiectasia (Osler-Weber-Rendu syndrome). *AJNR Am. J. Neuroradiol.* **1996**, *17*, 1733–1742. [PubMed]
15. Bhattacharya, J.J.; Luo, C.B.; Suh, D.C.; Alvarez, H.; Rodesch, G.; Lasjaunias, P. Wyburn-Mason or Bonnet-Dechaume-Blanc as Cerebrofacial Arteriovenous Metameric Syndromes (CAMS): A New Concept and a New Classification. *Interv. Neuroradiol.* **2001**, *7*, 5–17. [CrossRef] [PubMed]
16. Sturiale, C.L.; Puca, A.; Sebastiani, P.; Gatto, I.; Albanese, A.; Di Rocco, C.; Maira, G.; Pola, R. Single nucleotide polymorphisms associated with sporadic brain arteriovenous malformations: Where do we stand? *Brain* **2013**, *136*, 665–681. [CrossRef] [PubMed]
17. Starke, R.M.; Komotar, R.J.; Hwang, B.Y.; Hahn, D.K.; Otten, M.L.; Hickman, Z.L.; Garrett, M.C.; Sisti, M.B.; Lavine, S.D.; Meyers, P.M.; et al. Systemic Expression of Matrix Metalloproteinase-9 in Patients With Cerebral Arteriovenous Malformations. *Neurosurgery* **2010**, *66*, 343–348. [CrossRef]
18. Moftakhar, P.; Hauptman, J.S.; Malkasian, D.; Martin, N.A. Cerebral arteriovenous malformations. Part 2: Physiology. *Neurosurg. Focus* **2009**, *26*, E11. [CrossRef]
19. Al-Shahi Salman, R.; White, P.M.; Counsell, C.E.; Du Plessis, J.; Van Beijnum, J.; Josephson, C.B.; Wilkinson, T.; Wedderburn, C.J.; Chandy, Z.; St. George, E.J.; et al. Outcome After Conservative Management or Intervention for Unruptured Brain Arteriovenous Malformations. *JAMA* **2014**, *311*, 1661. [CrossRef]
20. Mezaal, M.; Abdulelah, M.M.; Mehanna, R.A. Dramatic Effect of Botox Injection in Disabling Chronic Migraine Secondary to Inoperable Cerebral Arteriovenous Malformation. *Cureus* **2024**, *16*, e53326. [CrossRef]
21. Mohr, J.P.; Hartmann, A.; Kim, H.; Pile-Spellman, J.; Stapf, C. Viewpoints on the ARUBA Trial. *Am. J. Neuroradiol.* **2015**, *36*, 615–617. [CrossRef]
22. Bambakidis, N.C.; Cockroft, K.M.; Hirsch, J.A.; Connolly, E.S.; Amin-Hanjani, S.; Meyers, P.M.; Friedlander, R.M. The Case Against A Randomized Trial of Unruptured Brain Arteriovenous Malformations: Misinterpretation of a Flawed Study. *Stroke* **2014**, *45*, 2808–2810. [CrossRef]
23. Wahood, W.; Alexander, A.Y.; Doherty, R.J.; Bhandarkar, A.; Lanzino, G.; Bydon, M.; Brinjikji, W. Elective intervention for unruptured cranial arteriovenous malformations in relation to ARUBA trial: A National Inpatient Sample study. *Acta Neurochir.* **2021**, *163*, 2489–2495. [CrossRef] [PubMed]
24. Ding, D. Pathobiology of Cerebral Arteriovenous Malformations: Correlating Genetic Polymorphisms to Clinical Presentation and Nidus Angioarchitecture. *Cerebrovasc. Dis.* **2014**, *38*, 75. [CrossRef] [PubMed]
25. Von Der Brelie, C.; Simon, M.; Esche, J.; Schramm, J.; Boström, A. Seizure Outcomes in Patients with Surgically Treated Cerebral Arteriovenous Malformations. *Neurosurgery* **2015**, *77*, 762–768. [CrossRef] [PubMed]
26. De Castro-Afonso, L.H.; Vanzim, J.R.; Trivelato, F.P.; Rezende, M.T.; Ulhôa, A.C.; Chodraui-Filho, S.F.; De Abreu Mattos, L.G.; Mounayer, C.; Nakiri, G.S.; Colli, B.O.; et al. Association between draining vein diameters and intracranial arteriovenous malformation hemorrhage: A multicentric retrospective study. *Neuroradiology* **2020**, *62*, 1497–1505. [CrossRef]
27. Nesvick, C.L.; Graffeo, C.S.; Brown, P.D.; Link, M.J.; Stafford, S.L.; Foote, R.L.; Laack, N.N.; Pollock, B.E. The Role of Biological Effective Dose in Predicting Obliteration After Stereotactic Radiosurgery of Cerebral Arteriovenous Malformations. *Mayo Clin. Proc.* **2021**, *96*, 1157–1164. [CrossRef]
28. Steiner, L.; Lindquist, C.; Adler, J.R.; Torner, J.C.; Alves, W.; Steiner, M. Clinical outcome of radiosurgery for cerebral arteriovenous malformations. *J. Neurosurg.* **1992**, *77*, 1–8. [CrossRef]
29. Heros, R.C.; Korosue, K.; Diebold, P.M. Surgical Excision of Cerebral Arteriovenous Malformations: Late Results. *Neurosurgery* **1990**, *26*, 570–578. [CrossRef]
30. Redekop, G.; TerBrugge, K.; Montanera, W.; Willinsky, R. Arterial aneurysms associated with cerebral arteriovenous malformations: Classification, incidence, and risk of hemorrhage. *J. Neurosurg.* **1998**, *89*, 539–546. [CrossRef]

31. Mast, H.; Young, W.L.; Koennecke, H.-C.; Sciacca, R.R.; Osipov, A.; Pile-Spellman, J.; Hacein-Bey, L.; Duong, H.; Stein, B.M.; Mohr, J. Risk of spontaneous haemorrhage after diagnosis of cerebral arteriovenous malformation. *Lancet* **1997**, *350*, 1065–1068. [CrossRef]
32. Al-Shahi, R.; Bhattacharya, J.J.; Currie, D.G.; Papanastassiou, V.; Ritchie, V.; Roberts, R.C.; Sellar, R.J.; Warlow, C.P. Prospective, Population-Based Detection of Intracranial Vascular Malformations in Adults: The Scottish Intracranial Vascular Malformation Study (SIVMS). *Stroke* **2003**, *34*, 1163–1169. [CrossRef]
33. Maruyama, K.; Kawahara, N.; Shin, M.; Tago, M.; Kishimoto, J.; Kurita, H.; Kawamoto, S.; Morita, A.; Kirino, T. The Risk of Hemorrhage after Radiosurgery for Cerebral Arteriovenous Malformations. *N. Engl. J. Med.* **2005**, *352*, 146–153. [CrossRef] [PubMed]
34. Derdeyn, C.P.; Zipfel, G.J.; Albuquerque, F.C.; Cooke, D.L.; Feldmann, E.; Sheehan, J.P.; Torner, J.C. Management of Brain Arteriovenous Malformations: A Scientific Statement for Healthcare Professionals from the American Heart Association/American Stroke Association. *Stroke* **2017**, *48*, 8. [CrossRef] [PubMed]
35. Kato, Y.; Dong, V.; Chaddad, F.; Takizawa, K.; Izumo, T.; Fukuda, H.; Hara, T.; Kikuta, K.; Nakai, Y.; Endo, T.; et al. Expert consensus on the management of brain arteriovenous malformations. *Asian J. Neurosurg.* **2019**, *14*, 1074–1081. [CrossRef]
36. Potts, M.B.; Lau, D.; Abla, A.A.; Kim, H.; Young, W.L.; Lawton, M.T. Current surgical results with low-grade brain arteriovenous malformations. *J. Neurosurg.* **2015**, *122*, 912–920. [CrossRef]
37. Baharvahdat, H.; Blanc, R.; Fahed, R.; Smajda, S.; Ciccio, G.; Desilles, J.-P.; Redjem, H.; Escalard, S.; Mazighi, M.; Chauvet, D.; et al. Endovascular Treatment for Low-Grade (Spetzler-Martin I–II) Brain Arteriovenous Malformations. *Am. J. Neuroradiol.* **2019**, *40*, 668–672. [CrossRef]
38. Lawton, M.T. Spetzler-Martin Grade III Arteriovenous Malformations: Surgical Results and a Modification of the Grading Scale. *Neurosurgery* **2003**, *52*, 740–749. [CrossRef]
39. China, M.; Vastani, A.; Hill, C.S.; Tancu, C.; Grover, P.J. Gamma Knife radiosurgery for cerebral arteriovenous malformations: A systematic review and meta-analysis. *Neurosurg. Rev.* **2022**, *45*, 1987–2004. [CrossRef]
40. Toader, C.; Covache-Busuioc, R.-A.; Bratu, B.-G.; Glavan, L.A.; Corlatescu, A.D.; Ciurea, A.V. Case Study of a Complex Neurovascular Disorder: Choroidal Arteriovenous Malformation. *Medicina* **2024**, *60*, 302. [CrossRef]

brain sciences

Review

Prevention and Management of Spinal Cord Ischemia After Aortic Surgery: An Umbrella Review

Alexandros G. Brotis [1,*], Adamantios Kalogeras [2], Metaxia Bareka [3], Eleni Arnaoutoglou [3], Kostas Spanos [4], Miltiadis Matsagkas [4] and Kostas N. Fountas [5]

1 Department of Neurosurgery and Medical, Faculty of Medicine, School of Thessaly Health Sciences, University of Thessaly, 41500 Larissa, Greece
2 Department of Neurosurgery, University Hospital of Larissa, 41500 Larissa, Greece; kalogadam@gmail.com
3 Department of Anaesthesiology, Medical Faculty of Medicine, School of Thessaly Health Sciences, University of Thessaly, 41500 Larissa, Greece; barekametaxia@hotmail.com (M.B.); earnaout@gmail.com (E.A.)
4 Department of Vascular Surgery, Medical Faculty of Medicine, School of Thessaly Health Sciences, University of Thessaly, 41500 Larissa, Greece; spanos.kon@gmail.com (K.S.) mimats@uth.gr (M.M.)
5 Department of Neurosurgery, Medical Faculty of Medicine, School of Thessaly Health Sciences, University of Thessaly, 41500 Larissa, Greece; fountas@uth.gr
* Correspondence: amprotis@med.uth.gr

Abstract: Background/Objectives: Spinal cord injury is a devastating complication of aortic surgery, with significant morbidity and mortality. This review aimed to summarize the current literature on preventing and managing spinal cord ischemia after open and endovascular aortic repair. **Methods**: We conducted a comprehensive review of PubMed, Scopus, and the Web of Science, focusing on systematic reviews and meta-analyses of the pathophysiology, risk factors, and strategies for mitigating the risk of spinal cord injury after aortic repair. We assessed the quality of the reporting for the eligible studies using the AMSTAR-2 tool and evaluated the strength of the evidence using the GRADE approach. Due to the absence of homogeneous clinical data, the evidence was synthesized in a narrative form. **Results:** Spinal cord ischemia can occur after both open and endovascular aortic repair, with a higher incidence reported in more extensive thoraco-abdominal aortic aneurysm repairs. The underlying pathogenesis is largely understudied. Several preventive strategies have been partially investigated, including cerebrospinal fluid drainage, hypothermia, and distal aortic perfusion. While the employment of neuromonitoring has been established in spine surgery, its efficacy in aortic repair remains uncertain due to confounding factors like hypothermia, anesthesia medications, and cardiopulmonary bypass. The prompt management of spinal cord complications is crucial to optimizing outcomes. No clear treatment algorithm has been universally adopted. **Conclusions:** Spinal cord ischemia remains a major challenge in aortic surgery, with a significant impact on patient outcomes. Further research is needed to elucidate the relevant pathophysiology and develop more effective intraoperative monitoring and management strategies.

Keywords: spinal cord ischemia; aortic surgery; incidence; risk factors; prevention; early detection; treatment; prognosis; umbrella review

1. Introduction

Spinal cord ischemia (SCI) is a devastating complication, which can occur after aortic surgery, resulting in permanent paralysis and significant patient morbidity [1–3]. Multiple factors, including the extent of aortic disease, the duration of circulatory arrest, and the techniques of cerebral and spinal cord protection, have been implicated in the development of this complication [4–6].

Although the literature on the management of SCI, including optimal perfusion and temperature strategies, is extensive, it remains a subject of ongoing debate [4–6]. Significant variations exist regarding the actual complication's incidence and predisposing risk factors across published studies. The existing knowledge on the early prediction of ischemia is also limited. There is an ongoing debate regarding the benefit of preventive measures such as cerebrospinal fluid drainage (CSFD), along with their potential complications [7,8]. Presently, there is no widely agreed-upon treatment for SCI [9].

To address this gap, we performed an umbrella review of the available evidence to provide an overview of the current state of knowledge and identify areas for future research. This study aims to provide a comprehensive overview of the current knowledge regarding SCI following aortic surgery based on systematic reviews and meta-analyses. The primary objectives are to summarize the incidence risk factors (Q1), pathogenesis (Q2), methods for early diagnosis (Q3), and management strategies, including preventive measures (Q4) and the potential complications associated with CSFD (Q5), as well as the treatment (Q6) and prognosis (Q7) of this devastating complication (Table 1). We will also discuss potential sources of heterogeneity across studies and make recommendations for future research directions.

Table 1. The research questions summarized in the PICOT format.

Research Question	Patient	Intervention	Comparator	Outcome	Time
Q1	Patients undergoing aortic surgery	Risk factors related to SCI following surgery	None or standard aortic surgery	Incidence and risk factors for SCI	ANY
Q2	Patients experiencing SCI post-aortic surgery	Mechanisms leading to SCI	Standard aortic surgery patients without SC	Understanding of pathogenesis in SCI after surgery	ANY
Q3	Patients at risk for SCI post-aortic surgery	Early diagnostic methods	Standard diagnostic methods or no early diagnostic approach	Diagnostic accuracy, timeliness, and effectiveness in detecting SC	Intraoperative and early postoperative periods
Q4	Patients undergoing aortic surgery at risk for SCI	Preventive interventions	Standard care without specific preventive measures	Incidence of SCI, early detection, and neurological outcomes	Intraoperative period, early post surgery
Q5	Patients undergoing aortic surgery at risk for SCI	Presence of complications linked to CSFD	No CSFD or standard care	Incidence of complications linked to CSFD	Early and late postoperative periods

Table 1. *Cont.*

Research Question	Patient	Intervention	Comparator	Outcome	Time
Q6	Patients with SCI post-aortic surgery	Treatment options	No treatment or standard management protocols	Recovery of neurological function and reduction in SCI severity	Immediate postoperative to long-term follow-up
Q7	Patients with SCI following aortic surgery	Factors influencing prognosis	No SCI or standard aortic surgery without complication	Functional recovery, quality of life, mortality rates	Short-term to long-term follow-up

This review will be of interest to vascular and cardiothoracic surgeons, neurologists, and neurosurgeons, as well as anesthesiologists and critical care physicians involved in managing patients undergoing aortic surgery.

2. Materials and Methods

2.1. Study Design

This umbrella review provides a comprehensive overview of available systematic reviews and meta-analyses on SCI following aortic surgery. The study was conducted and reported in alignment with the Preferred Reporting Items for Systematic Reviews and Meta-Analyses (PRISMA) guidelines. This secondary research synthesis did not require ethical approval, as it did not involve direct patient involvement. Additionally, this project was conducted without external funding.

2.2. Information Sources

From inception to December 2024, two review authors (A.B. and A.K.) systematically searched several electronic databases, including PubMed, Scopus, and Web of Science, for relevant systematic reviews and meta-analyses. We also searched the reference lists of included studies for potential additional references. Additionally, the authors searched for gray literature, such as conference proceedings and unpublished studies, to minimize the risk of publication bias.

2.3. Search Strategy

The search strategy combined keywords related to SCI, aortic surgery, and the study design (systematic reviews and meta-analyses). The full search strategy was ("spinal cord ischemia" OR "neurological deficits" OR "spinal cord injury" OR paraplegia OR paraparesis) AND ("endovascular aortic repair" OR "abdominal aortic surgery" OR "aortic aneurysm") AND "(management" OR "treatment" OR "hypothermia" OR "cerebrospinal fluid drainage" OR "intercostal artery reimplantation"), with modifications according to the database requirements.

2.4. Study Selection

Two review authors (A.B. and A.K.) independently screened the titles and abstracts of identified studies, retrieving full-text articles for further assessment. Studies were included if they met the following criteria: (1) systematic review or meta-analysis; (2) focused on SCI following aortic surgery; (3) reported at least one of the following parameters: incidence, risk factors, early diagnosis, prevention, treatment, or prognosis; and (4) written in English. Narrative reviews, expert opinions in languages other than English, and individual primary studies were excluded. The authors used the Rayyan web application for collaborative reviews during the screening process [10]. In case of disagreement, the authors consulted a senior author (K.N.F.) (Figure 1).

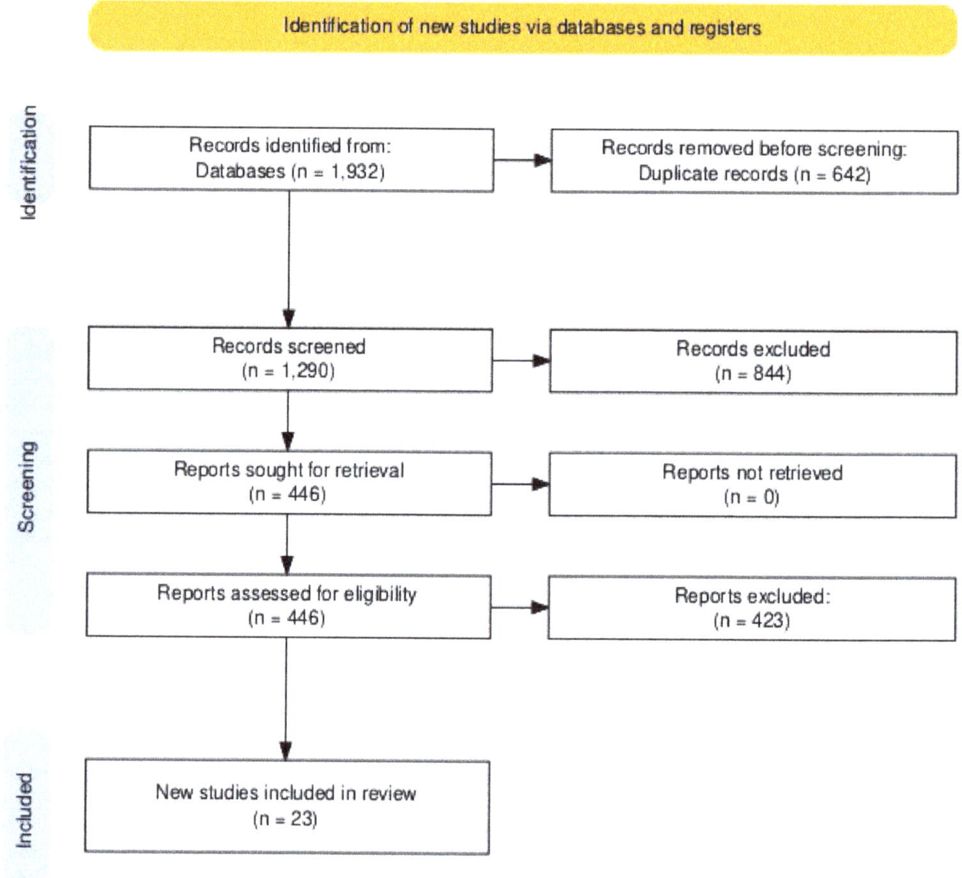

Figure 1. Prisma flow chart of our literature search.

2.5. Data Extraction

Two review authors (A.B. and A.K.) independently extracted relevant data using a pre-designed data extraction form from the included studies. The extracted data included study characteristics (authors, year of publication, study design, number of included studies, and total number of patients), details on the population, intervention or exposure, comparison, and outcomes. We additionally extracted the author's search keywords, databases, eligibility criteria, and quality assessment methods.

2.6. Data Synthesis

For qualitative data, the evidence synthesis for this umbrella review will be presented in a narrative format, providing a comprehensive overview of the key findings from the included systematic reviews and meta-analyses. The narrative synthesis will summarize the incidence, risk factors, diagnostic methods, management strategies, and prognosis of SCI following aortic surgery. Relevant data, such as pooled estimates, will be presented in table format to aid in the interpretation of the results. The narrative review will also discuss potential sources of heterogeneity across the included studies and will highlight areas for future research to address the existing knowledge gaps in this field. For quantitative data, where appropriate, we conducted umbrella meta-analyses using the "metaumbrella" package for R version 4.3.3 to provide pooled estimates of the incidence of SCI, the effectiveness of specific management strategies, and the risk associated with various risk factors. The "metaumbrella" package allows for the synthesis of multiple meta-analyses, enabling us to provide a comprehensive overview of the quantitative evidence on this topic. This approach will help identify patterns and sources of heterogeneity across the included studies.

2.7. Quality Appraisal

Two review authors (A.B. and A.K.) appraised the gathered literature using AMSTAR-2 [11,12]. The quality appraisal of the literature using AMSTAR-2 involved a rigorous assessment of systematic reviews based on 16 key domains. These domains cover crucial aspects of review methodology, including protocol registration, search strategy comprehensiveness, risk of bias assessment, and methods of data extraction [11,12]. Seven of these domains were designated as "critical", carrying greater weight in the overall appraisal. AMSTAR 2 does not generate a numerical score, but provides an overall rating of "high", "moderate", "low", or "critically low" based on the number of "no" responses for each domain. This rating reflects the methodological rigor and trustworthiness of the reviewed systematic reviews, aiding in the identification of high-quality evidence for clinical decision-making and research [11,12]. The results were visualized using amstar2Vis [11,12].

The overall quality of the output evidence was assessed according to GRADE recommendations [13]. The GRADE system is a widely used framework for evaluating the certainty of evidence in systematic reviews and meta-analyses [13]. It assesses the certainty of evidence on a scale from high to very low, based on factors such as risk of bias, inconsistency, indirectness, imprecision, and publication bias [13].

3. Results

3.1. Literature Search

The systematic literature search yielded a total of 1932 records. After removing duplicates, 1290 unique citations were screened. Of these, 121 full-text articles were assessed for eligibility, and 23 systematic reviews and meta-analyses were included in the final synthesis.

3.2. Study Characteristics

The included studies were published between 2004 and 2024 (Table 2). Sixteen employed quantitative meta-analysis, while six were qualitative in nature. The most frequently utilized databases were PubMed Ovid, Cochrane Library, ClinicalTrials.gov, Embase, Scopus, CINAHL, and Embase. The study population comprised patients undergoing open aortic surgery with EVAR and TEVAR for thoraco-abdominal aortic aneurysms (TAAA) or dissections. The most common prophylactic measure was CSFD.

Table 2. Basic characteristics of the twenty-three eligible studies.

Authors	SD	Databases	Period	Patients	Intervention	Comparator	Outcomes	Moderators	Quality Assessment	Studies (Patients)	Study Question (s)
Cina (2004) [8]	MA	Ovid software	Until June 2002	Patients requiring TAAA repair	Prophylactic CSFD	No prophylactic CSFD	SCI and complications	Subgroup analysis for study design	Jadad three-item scale	8 (1143)	Q1, Q4
Wong (2012) [14]	MA	PubMed, the Cochrane Library, and Conference abstracts	2000–2011	Patients undergoing TEVAR	Prophylactic CSFD	No prophylactic CSFD	SCI	(-)	Downs and Black checklist	46 (4936)	Q1, Q5
Tanaka (2016) [15]	MA	MEDLINE, the Cochrane Central Register, EMBASE, CINAHAL, and the Japanese Central Review of Medicine	Until September 1st 2015	Patients requiring TAAA repair	TAAA surgery with MEPs	(-)	Sensitivity and specificity for detecting SCI	Anesthesia, and surgery details as moderators for MEPs accuracy; subgroup for several cut-off values	QUADAS-2	19 (-)	Q3
Khan (2016) [5]	MA	Clinicaltrials.gov, Cochrane Library, PubMed/MEDLINE, and Scopus	Until August 2015	Patients requiring TAAA repair	CSFD	W/O or selective CSFD	SCI	Early vs. late SCI	Jadad and NOS	10 (2013)	Q1, Q4, Q5
Li (2017) [11]	MA	PubMed, EMBASE, Cochrane Library, Web of Science, and ScienceDirect	(-)	Patients with TBAD requiring surgery	TEVAR	OS, BMT	30-day/in-hospital mortality and morbidity, including paraplegia	(-)		16 (10,307)	Q1

Table 2. *Cont.*

Authors	SD	Databases	Period	Patients	Intervention	Comparator	Outcomes	Moderators	Quality Assessment	Studies (Patients)	Study Question (s)
Moulakakis (2018) [1]	SR	PubMed and Scopus	Until December 2017	Patients with infrarenal AAA	Elective endovascular repair	(-)	SCI, including its incidence, risk factors, clinical presentation, and outcomes	Patient characteristics, procedural factors, and anatomical variations		18 (25)	Q1, Q7
Harky (2019) [16]	SR	PubMed, MEDLINE, EMBASE, Google Scholar, SCOPUS, and Cochrane	(-)	Patients requiring TAAA repair	(-)	(-)	SCI	(-)	(-)	15 (265)	Q3
Rocha (2020) [4]	MA	MEDLINE and EMBASE	January 2006 to March 201	Patients with thoracic aortic pathology	Open repair	Endovascular repair	In-hospital or 30-day mortality and morbidity, including SCI	Permanent vs. overall	Checklist	71 (-)	Q1, Q2
Malloy (2020) [17]	SR	PubMed/MEDLINE, Scopus, Ovid, Cochrane, and EMBASE	1 January 2016 to 17 December 2018	Patients with aortic aneurysm requiring repair	TEVAR	(-)	SCI (overall vs. temporary)	Various CSF protocols	Joanna Briggs Institute checklist	8 (859)	Q1, Q4, Q5
Batubara (2022) [18]	MA	PubMed, Ovid Medline, and Cochrane	NR	Patients undergoing Thoracic EVAR	With LSAR	W/O LSAR	Ischemia, stroke, and SCI	(-)	NOS	22 (11,386)	Q4

Table 2. *Cont.*

Authors	SD	Databases	Period	Patients	Intervention	Comparator	Outcomes	Moderators	Quality Assessment	Studies (Patients)	Study Question (s)
Zhang (2022) [19]	MA	MEDLINE, EMBASE, and Cochrane	Until 1 April 2020	Patients undergoing TEVAR	Prophylactic CSFD	W/O or selective prophylactic CSFD	SCI, CSFD-related complications	Pathology (aneurysm vs. dissection); hybrid procedures	Downs and Black score	34 (3561)	Q1, Q4, Q5
Pini (2022) [20]	MA	PubMed, EMBASE, and Cochrane Database	Until 1 February 2021	Patients with TAAA	Endovascular repair	(-)	SCI	(1) TAAA extension; (2) overall vs. permanent SCI; (3) use of CSFD; (4) prophylactic vs. symptomatic; (5) staged vs. nonstaged approach	NOS	27 (2333)	Q1, Q4, Q6
Lella (2022) [9]	SR	Cochrane and PubMed	2012 to 2021	Patients with DTA and TAAA	Open or endovascular repair	(-)	SCI	Type and extent of aortic pathology, operative technique, SCI protection or mitigation strategies, and rates of overall and permanent SCI	NR	41 (-)	Q1, Q4, Q6

Table 2. *Cont.*

Authors	SD	Databases	Period	Patients	Intervention	Comparator	Outcomes	Moderators	Quality Assessment	Studies (Patients)	Study Question (s)
Cheng-Hao (2023) [21]	MA	Scopus, EMBASE, Medline, and Cochrane and Evidence-Based Medicine Reviews	Until September 2022	Patients undergoing TEVAR	Routine CSFD	Selective CSFD and no CSFD	SCI (any vs. permanent vs. transient) rate, complication rates, and operative outcomes	Immediate vs. delayed; transient vs. permanent; aneurysm vs. dissection; emergency vs. elective	Modified Institute of Health Economics scale	40 (4973)	Q1, Q4, Q5
Frankort (2023) [7]	MA	MEDLINE, EMBASE, and CINAHL	Until November 2022	Patients undergoing TEVAR	Prophylactic CSFD	W/O prophylactic CSFD	SCI (early onset of late), complications, and mortality	Risk of bias	NOS/GRADE	28 (4814)	Q1, Q4, Q5, Q7
Muston (2023) [3]	MA	EMBASE, PubMed, Scopus	Until 3 January 2023		Open group	Endovascular (TEVAR and F/B EVAR), and hybrid groups	SCI (permanent, in-hospital)	(-)	CNIHE tool	20 (924)	Q1, Q4
Spinella (2023) [22]	MA	PubMed/MEDLINE	Until November 2020	Patients with TAAA	Type A: single step	Type B: staged with reperfusion branches; Type C: staged with positioning of the thoracic component	SCI (transient and permanent)	Age, extent of the aneurysm, the diameter of the aneurysm, and the use of CSFD	(-)	53 (3095)	Q1, Q4

Table 2. *Cont.*

Authors	SD	Databases	Period	Patients	Intervention	Comparator	Outcomes	Moderators	Quality Assessment	Studies (Patients)	Study Question (s)
Sef (2023) [23]	SR	PubMed, EMBASE via Ovid, Cochrane library, and Clinical Trials Gov	Until December 2022	Patients undergoing open TAAA repair	Neuromonitoring methods MEPs, SSEPs, NIRS, and TCD		Mortality, SCI, and neurologic deficit	(-)	NOS	27 (3130)	Q1. Q2, Q3
Alzghari (2024) [2]	MA	Ovid MEDLINE, Ovid EMBASE, and the Cochrane Library	Until September 2022	Patients with DTA and TAAA	Open or endovascular repair	(-)	SCI, temporary SCI, operative mortality, long-term mortality, postoperative stroke, and CSFD-related complications	Subgroup analyses and multivariate analyses for a multitude of factors	NOS	239 (61,962)	Q1, Q4, Q5, Q7
Leone (2024) [24]	MA	MEDLINE, EMBASE, and Scopus	2000–2023	Patients undergoing F/B-EVAR	CSFD	(-)	CSFD-related mortality and morbidity	(-)	NOS	6 (730)	Q4, Q5
Zheng (2024) [6]	MA	PubMed, EMBASE, Web of Science, and Cochrane Library	Up to May 2023	Patients undergoing TEVAR (elective or emergency) for TBAD	Routine prophylactic CSFD	Selective prophylactic CSFD, W/O prophylactic CSFD	Permanent SCI, temporary SCI, CSFD-related complications, and 30-day mortality	With or W/O CSFD	Downs and Black score	34 (2749)	Q1, Q4, Q5

Table 2. *Cont.*

Authors	SD	Databases	Period	Patients	Intervention	Comparator	Outcomes	Moderators	Quality Assessment	Studies (Patients)	Study Question (s)
Thet (2024) [25]	SR	PubMed, MEDLINE via Ovid, EMBASE, Scopus, and Cochrane CENTRAL	1998–2024	Patients with TAAA	TEVAR or F/B-EVAR	(-)	SCI and early mortality	Permanent vs. transient, neuromonitoring (MEPs, SSEPs, NIRS)	NOS	11 (1069)	Q1, Q3, Q4
Soliman (2024) [26]	SR	PubMed, Scopus, and Google Scholar	1995–2022	Experimental animals or patients undergoing TAAA repair	Detection and monitoring of SCI using various monitoring techniques	(-)	SCI, SC-blood flow	(-)	NR	59 (-)	Q3

BMT, best medica treatment; CSF, cerebrospinal fluid; CSFD, cerebrospinal fluid drain; CT, computed tomography; CNIHE, Canadian National Institute of Health Economics; DTA, descending thoracic aorta; F/B-EVAR, fenestrated or branched endovascular repair; GRADE, Grading of Recommendations Assessment, Development and Evaluation; LSAR, left subclavian artery revascularization; MA, meta-analysis; MEPs, motor-evoked potentials; MICACE, minimally invasive segmental artery embolization; MRI, magnetic resonance imaging; NIRS, near-infrared spectroscopy; NOS, Newcastle Ottawa scale; OS, open surgery; SC, spinal cord; SCI, spinal cord ischemia; SD, study design; SR, systematic review; SSEPs, somatosensory evoked potentials; QUADAS-2, Quality Assessment of Diagnostic Accuracy Studies—2; TAAA, thoracoabdominal aortic aneurysm; TASP, temporary aneurysm sac perfusion; TBAD, Type B aortic dissection; TCD, transcranial Doppler; TEVAR, thoracic endovascular aortic repair; US, ultrasound; W/O, without.

3.3. Incidence and Risk Factors (Q1)

Twelve studies have examined the incidence of SCI as a primary or secondary focus (Table 3), six of which comprised the primary question. However, the included studies exhibited significant heterogeneity in their techniques, case selection, and outcome measures, leading to a wide range of reported incidences, from as low as 0% to as high as 33%.

The overall incidence of SCI after surgical and endovascular aortic repair is about 10% and 3.5%, respectively [3,4,7,9,14,19–21] (Table 4). However, permanent deficit remains in approximately 3.3%, while late events are rare and limited to less than 2% of the cases [3,4,7,9,14,19–21,23,25].

A systematic review and meta-analysis by Rocha et al. found a higher overall incidence of SCI following endovascular TAAA repair (13.5%) compared to open repair (7.4%) [4]. Yet, the occurrence of permanent spinal cord injury was comparable, with a combined incidence of 5.2% for endovascular and 4.4% for open repair [4].

According to a systematic review by Lella et al. (2022), the incidence of SCI varies depending on the type of aortic repair. For endovascular descending thoracic aortic repair, the overall SCI rates ranged from 0% to 10.6%, with permanent SCI ranging from 0% to 5.1% [9]. For endovascular thoraco-abdominal aortic repair, the overall SCI rates ranged from 0% to 35%, with permanent SCI ranging from 2% to 20.5% [9]. In the case of open thoraco-abdominal aortic repair, one study reported a permanent SCI rate of 1.1%, while the overall SCI rates were described as being within the 0–35% range, although not explicitly stated [9].

The study by Pini et al. reported an overall pooled incidence of SCI of 11% after endovascular TAAA repair [20]. However, the incidence varied based on the extent of the TAAA repair, with extent IV repairs having a pooled rate of 6%, while repairs involving extents I–III and V had a higher rate of 13% [20]. Although there was a trend towards lower SCI rates in staged procedures, the difference was not statistically significant [20]. Additionally, the study explored other potential risk factors, such as age and aneurysm diameter, but did not find consistent associations with SCI [20].

Muston et al. examined SCI as a primary outcome in staged TAAA repairs, comparing open, endovascular, and hybrid approaches [3]. They found an overall pooled SCI incidence of 5.4% across all staged repairs [3]. While there was a trend towards lower SCI rates with the hybrid approach (3.2%) compared to open (1.4%) and endovascular (9.8%), these differences were not statistically significant [3]. The study highlighted the challenges in comparing SCI rates due to variations in reporting across studies and emphasized the need for standardized reporting in future research [3].

According to a meta-analysis by Alzghari et al., the pooled incidence of permanent spinal cord injury was 3.3% [2]. This incidence varied based on the surgical approach, with 4% for open repairs and 2.9% for endovascular repairs [2]. Additionally, the permanent SCI rate differed by the location of the aneurysm, being 2.0% for descending thoracic aneurysm repair and 4.7% for TAAA repair [2]. The permanent SCI rate also varied with the extent of the TAAA, ranging from 3.8% for Crawford extent I to 13.4% for extent II, 7.1% for extent III, 2.3% for extent IV, and 6.7% for extent V [2].

Separately, a meta-analysis by Zheng et al. in 2024 reported a pooled estimated risk for permanent SCI after TEVAR of 2.0%, based on 22 studies with 1479 patients [6]. The pooled estimated risk for temporary SCI was 1.0% based on 24 studies with 2048 patients [6].

The incidence of delayed SCI after aortic surgery was examined indirectly by two eligible studies, only as a secondary question. In a systematic review by Sef et al., the reported incidence of delayed SCI varied considerably, ranging from as low as 1% to as high as 12% across the included studies [23]. This variation likely reflects differences in patient populations, surgical techniques, and definitions of delayed SCI used across the included studies [23]. This systematic review underscored the challenges in determining a precise incidence due to these inconsistencies [23]. In a meta-analysis, Chen et al. investigated the relationship between prophylactic CSFD and SCI during thoracic and thoraco-abdominal endovascular aortic repair [21]. They reported incidences of 1.3% for immediate SCI, defined as the presence of paraplegia at the emergence of anesthesia, and 1.9% for delayed SCI, although the definition of delayed SCI was not clearly specified [21].

3.4. Pathogenesis (Q2)

Only the systematic review by Sef et al. discussed in depth the potential mechanisms underlying SCI after aortic surgery [23]. The proposed mechanism of neurologic injury following TA repair involves the disruption of the spinal cord's blood supply at some point, leading to hypoxia [23]. Spinal cord edema and microthrombi development can further reduce perfusion pressure [23]. Existing evidence indicates that the spinal cord relies extensively on a collateral network, often as much as on any nominal vessel, allowing for sufficient blood flow even in the face of ischemia [23]. In addition, experimental data show that spinal cord perfusion pressure drops after segmental artery sacrifice, which gradually recovers over time, however [23].

3.5. Early Diagnosis (Q3)

Five studies examined the role of various diagnostic modalities in the early detection of SCI. The systematic review by Sef et al. (2023) explored the use of perioperative neuromonitoring during open TAAA repair [23]. The authors analyzed studies investigating different neuromonitoring methods, such as motor-evoked potentials (MEPs), somatosensory evoked potentials (SSEPs), and near-infrared spectroscopy (NIRS), to assess their ability to predict and prevent SCI [23]. MEPs emerged as the most commonly used and studied modality, demonstrating reasonable sensitivity and specificity for detecting SCI [23]. While SSEPs and NIRS were also investigated, the evidence supporting their use was less robust, with limitations in sensitivity and specificity [23]. The review suggested that a multimodal approach, combining different neuromonitoring techniques, might offer the best chance of detecting SCI [23].

Tanaka et al. conducted a systematic review and meta-analysis to establish the effectiveness of MEPs in predicting SCI during open surgical repair of thoracic and TAAAs [15]. MEPs had an estimated 77% pooled sensitivity in identifying cases of SCI, and a 95% pooled specificity in accurately ruling out the condition [23]. The diagnostic odds ratio was 30, indicating a strong association between MEPs changes and SCI. However, the authors noted substantial heterogeneity among the included studies, while the study's methodological quality was moderate [23]. The authors concluded that MEPs constitute a valuable tool for predicting SCI during open TAAA repair, but its sensitivity may be limited [23].

The systematic review by Harky et al. investigated the potential of CSF biomarkers in predicting SCI after TAAA repair, including S-100β, neuron-specific enolase, lactate, glial fibrillary acidic protein A, Tau, heat shock proteins 70 and 27 (HSP70, HSP27), and pro-inflammatory cytokines [16]. The review found that, while several biomarkers showed potential, there is a lack of high-quality studies with consistent findings, suggesting limited evidence. Furthermore, commonly measured markers like lactate, S-100β, NSE, and Tau did not reliably correlate with SCI occurrence, indicating an inconsistent correlation with SCI [16]. However, their review identified GFAP, HSP70, HSP27, and IL-8 as promising parameters, as they showed significant increases in SCI patients, warranting further investigation [16].

Thet et al.'s review documented the current evidence on neuromonitoring during endovascular repair of descending thoracic aortic and TAAAs [25]. The review found that somatosensory-evoked potentials and motor-evoked potentials are the most frequently employed neuromonitoring techniques, offering reasonable sensitivity for identifying critical spinal cord injury [25]. The review also discussed other methods, such as near-infrared spectroscopy, but the evidence supporting their use is less established [25]. The review highlighted that neuromonitoring is particularly valuable in high-risk patients, enabling timely intervention to prevent or mitigate SCI [25].

Soliman et al. covered both established methods like motor-evoked potentials (MEPs) and somatosensory-evoked potentials (SSEPs), as well as newer modalities such as near-infrared spectroscopy (NIRS), computed tomography (CT), magnetic resonance imaging (MRI), and CSF biomarkers [26]. Although the perioperative use of MEPs and SSEPs is limited due to the lack of an established protocol, NIRS appears to offer the continuous, non-invasive monitoring of spinal cord oxygenation [26]. However, the effectiveness of NIRS is constrained by its shallow penetration depth and susceptibility to artifacts [26]. Similarly, CT and MRI offer detailed anatomy, but still, they are expensive, time-consuming, and lack real-time continuous recording [26]. Diffusion-weighted MRI shows promise for early SCI detection but cannot be used intraoperatively [26]. CSF and serum biomarkers have uncertain clinical utility [26]. The authors concluded that a multimodal approach combining various neuromonitoring modalities could be the most effective for postoperative SCI monitoring [26].

3.6. Prevention (Q4)

The review by Cina et al. showed that CSFD significantly reduces the risk of paraplegia after open aortic repair, with an absolute risk reduction of 10 [8]. With the use of prophylactic CSFD, one case of paraplegia is prevented for every 10 patients treated [8]. The review suggests that maintaining CSF pressure below 10 mmHg may be crucial for the effectiveness of CSFD in preventing paraplegia [8]. In conclusion, the review affirms that CSFD is an effective method for preventing paraplegia, while emphasizing the importance of careful patient selection and meticulous CSFD management to minimize potential complications [8].

Wong et al. analyzed strategies for preventing spinal cord injury in thoracic endovascular aortic repair [14]. The review focused on CSFD and discussed its potential utility, particularly for high-risk patients [14]. The optimal CSF pressure target during drainage, below 10 mmHg, was also discussed. Other strategies used in open surgical repair, such as maintaining spinal cord perfusion pressure and minimizing aortic occlusion duration, were briefly mentioned, but their applicability and effectiveness in TEVAR were not extensively explored [14].

Khan et al. demonstrated that CSFD significantly reduced the risk of SCI following TAAA repair [5]. The pooled analysis showed a nearly 50% reduction in SCI with CSFD [5]. The protective effect was more pronounced for early SCI but not statistically significant for late SCI [5]. The study concluded that CSFD could be an effective strategy, cautioned about potential complications, and emphasized the need for careful drain management [5]. However, the optimal drainage parameters and patient selection criteria were not adequately defined [5].

Batubara et al. discussed spinal cord ischemia prevention in the context of left subclavian artery revascularization during thoracic endovascular aortic repair [18]. The authors showed that LSA revascularization is associated with a statistically significant reduction in the risk of several ischemic complications [18]. Specifically, LSA revascularization significantly lowers the risk of stroke (OR 0.41), spinal cord ischemia (0.34), and left arm ischemia

(0.22) [18]. However, the optimal revascularization techniques and patient selection criteria still warrant further investigation [18].

The role of prophylactic CSFD in preventing SCI after thoracic endovascular aortic repair was also examined by Zhang et al. [19]. Their review compared the use of prophylactic CSFD (placed before any signs of SCI) versus selective CSFD (inserted only after SCI symptoms appear) [19]. The use or not of prophylactic CSFD did not significantly affect the overall incidence of spinal cord injury ($p = 0.51$) in both the aortic aneurysm ($p = 0.76$) and aortic dissection subgroups ($p = 0.70$) [19]. However, the authors also acknowledge the limitations of the available evidence, including the utilized studies' heterogeneity and the potential for publication bias [19].

Pini et al. found that the pooled SCI rate was lower for staged procedures compared to non-staged procedures (9% vs. 18%, respectively; $p = 0.02$), without significant difference in SCI rates between procedures staged over 1 month apart and those staged under 1 month apart [20]. While the staged approach showed a benefit in reducing SCI, the review also reported an inter-stage mortality rate of 1.6%, highlighting the potential risks associated with the staged approach [20]. In addition, the authors reported a similar pooled SCI rate of approximately 10% for both prophylactic and symptomatic CSFD, suggesting that prophylactic CSFD might not have offered a significant advantage in preventing SCI after TAAA-ER [20]. Finally, the authors commented that factors beyond hemodynamic changes, such as atheroembolization from a "shaggy aorta," could also have contributed to SCI, and that focusing solely on CSFD might not have addressed all potential causes of SCI [20].

Chen et al. (2023) directly compared SCI rates in patients undergoing thoracic endovascular aortic repair with and without prophylactic CSFD [21]. The meta-analysis found no statistically significant difference in SCI rates between patients who received prophylactic CSFD and those who did not (OR 1.34, 95% CI 0.88–2.04, $p = 0.17$). These findings suggest that routine prophylactic CSFD may not offer a substantial benefit in reducing SCI risk for all TEVAR patients [21]. The study found no statistically significant difference in either transient or permanent SCI rates between the CSFD and non-CSFD groups [21]. The review also conducted subgroup analyses based on factors such as the type of aortic pathology and the CSFD strategy employed, yet these analyses likewise failed to reveal any significant differences in SCI rates [21].

Similarly, Frankort et al. incorporated twenty-eight observational, retrospective studies into their meta-analysis, involving a total of 4814 patients [7]. No significant reduction in spinal cord injury (SCI) was observed with the use of cerebrospinal fluid (CSF) drainage (OR 0.67, 95% CI 0.29–1.55, $p = 0.35$) [7]. The authors concluded that the placement of pre-operative CSF drainage did not correlate with a positive outcome in terms of SCI rates during endovascular repairs of thoraco-abdominal aortic aneurysms and descending thoracic aortic aneurysms (DTAA), but given the low quality of evidence, a definitive recommendation for the pre-operative use of CSF drainage placement could not be established [7].

According to Spinella et al.'s analysis of 53 studies involving 3095 patients, both the staged approach with reperfusion branches and the staged sequential approach with positioning of the thoracic component alternatives were associated with lower SCI risk, with type latter showing greater reduction, though less pronounced in older patients [22]. Additionally, the absence of cerebrospinal fluid, larger aortic diameter, and smaller aneurysm extent were associated with lower SCI risk [22]. Thus, a staged endovascular treatment, based on the patient's anatomy and endovascular repair feasibility criteria, may provide significant advantages over single-step treatment in lowering the risk of spinal cord injury, irrespective of the reperfusion method employed [22].

Alzghari et al. discussed a couple of strategies for preventing SCI in the context of aortic repair, focusing on the use of prophylactic CSFD [2]. They suggested that CSFD can lower SCI rates after open TAAA repair, with less clear evidence of its effectiveness in TEVAR [2]. Additionally, the review states that maintaining adequate spinal cord perfusion is crucial for preventing SCI without delving into strategies to maintain mean arterial pressure within a specific target range and avoid hypotension. Finally, their study emphasizes the complexity of SCI prevention after aortic repair and the need for a multi-faceted approach [2].

Muston et al. discussed protective measures to reduce the risk of SCI during TAAA repair [3]. The authors state that most studies utilized spinal cord protection methods beyond induced hypothermia and rewarming, such as staging operations to allow spinal vasculature repair, and CSFD to lower pressure around the spinal cord [3]. Temporary aneurysm sac perfusion (TASP) was also used to maintain blood flow during surgery, while minimally invasive segmental spinal artery coil embolization (MISSACE) was less frequently employed [3].

Leone et al. summarized the complications associated with CSFD. At the same time, the authors recorded important details in the adopted CSFD protocols, depicting the heterogeneity in the clinical use of CSFD for SCI protection [24]. According to their review, the drains were placed using either anatomical landmarks or fluoroscopy guidance [24]. In most cases, the type of drain was not specified, but in two studies, the authors used Liquogard. Drains targeted either a specific pressure (10–12 mmHg) or a fixed CSF-flow rate (5–10 mL/h) [24]. In some studies, the drain was intermittently opened for 15 min every hour, allowing for a maximal CSF drainage of 20 mL [24].

Table 3. Incidence of spinal cord ischemia in the gathered studies.

Authors	Studies (Patients)	Overall	Transient	Permanent	Early	Late
Cina (2004) [8]	8 (1143)	33%	(-)	(-)		
Wong (2012) [14]	46 (4936)	3.47% (95% CI, 1.98–5.37%)				
Tanaka (2016) [15]	19 (-)	0 to 16.7%				
Khan (2016) [5]	10 (2013)	(-)				
Li (2017) [11]	16 (10,307)	0 to 50%				
Moulakakis (2018) [1]	18 (25)	1% (range: 0–8%)				
Harky (2019) [16]	15 (265)	(-)				
Rocha (2020) [4]	71 (-)	Endovascular: 13.5% (95% CI, 10.5–16.7%); Open: 7.4% (95% CI, 6.2–8.7%, $p < 0.01$)		Endovascular: 5.2% (95% CI, 3.8–6.7%); Open: 4.4% [95% CI, 3.3–5.6%, $p = 0.39$]		

Table 3. *Cont.*

Authors	Studies (Patients)	Overall	Transient	Permanent	Early	Late
Malloy (2020) [17]	8 (859)	0–17%		0–2%		
Batubara (2022) [18]	22(11,386)	2.5% (*n* = 283, R = 11,065)				
Zhang (2022) [19]	34 (3561)	Endovascular for aortic: 3.49% (95% CI, 0.23–6.76%); Endovascular for dissection: 3.20% (95% CI, 0.00–7.20%)				
Pini (2022) [20]	27 (2333)	Endovascular: 11% (95%CI, 8–15%)				
Lella (2022) [9]	41 (-)	Overall: 0–16%; Endovascular 0–35%; Open: 3.1–33.5%		Endovascular: 2–20.5%; Open: 1.11%		
Cheng-Hao (2023) [21]	40 (4973)	TEVAR: 3.5% (95% CI: 2.6–4.4%)			1.3% (95% CI: 0.7–1.8%)	1.9% (95% CI: 1.2–2.5%
Frankort (2023) [7]	28 (4814)	Endovascular: 5%, (95% CI 0–14%)				
Muston (2023) [3]	20 (924)	Overall: 5.4% (95%CI 5.1–5.8%); Open: 1.4% (95% CI, 1.3–1.5%); Hybrid: 3.2% (95% CI, 2.8–3.6%); Endovascular: 9.8% (95% CI, 9.2–10.1%)				
Sef (2023) [23]	27 (3130)				0% to 17.0%	1.3% to 12.0%
Alzghari (2024) [2]	239 (61,962)			Overall: 3.3% (95%CI 2.9–3.8%); Open 4.0% (95% CI, 3.3–4.8%); Endovascular: 2.9% (95% CI, 2.4–3.5%)		
Zheng (2024) [6]	34 (2749)		1.0% (95% CI, 0.00–1.0%)	2.0% (95% CI, 1.0–2.0)		
Thet (2024) [25]	11 (1069)	3.8 to 17.3%		2.7 to 5.8%		

Table 4. Summary table for the overall, permanent, and late spinal cord ischemia incidence according to the implemented approach.

Incidence	Technique	Range	Reference Studies
Overall	Open	1.4–33.5% (prevalent value around 10%)	Rocha, 2019 [4]; Lella, 2022 [9]; Muston, 2023 [3]
	Endovascular	0–35% (prevalent value around 3.5%)	Wong, 2012 [14]; Rocha, 2019 [4]; Pini, 2022 [20]; Zhang, 2022 [19]; Lella, 2022 [9]; Cheng-Hao, 2023 [21]; Frankort, 2023 [7]; Muston, 2023 [3]
	Not defined	3.8–33%	Cina, 2004 [8]; Lella, 2022 [9]; Muston, 2023 [3]
Permanent	Open	3.3–11%	Rocha, 2019 [4]; Alzghari, 2024 [2]
	Endovascular	2.9–6.7%	Rocha, 2019 [4]; Lella, 2022 [9]; Alzghari, 2024 [2]
	Not defined	2–7–5.8%	Thet, 2024 [25]
Late	Open	NR	NR
	Endovascular	1.9% (95% CI: 1.2–25%)	Cheng-Hao, 2023 [21]
	Not defined	1.3–12%	Sef, 2023 [23]

Malloy et al.'s systematic review highlighted the variability in the indications and use of CSFD and the absence of a standard protocol [17]. Some studies indicated CSFD as a prophylactic measure for all patients, others in patients undergoing TEVAR, and the remaining primarily used it only in high-risk, selected patients [17]. Their review stated that the ideal timing, duration, and drainage parameters to maximize the benefits of CSFD remain unestablished, necessitating further studies in order to define an optimal CSFD protocol [17].

Zheng et al. were also among those who aimed to determine whether prophylactic use of CSFD contributes to a lower rate of SCI (SCI) after thoracic endovascular aortic repair (TEVAR) for Type B aortic dissection (TBAD) [6]. Based on a total of 34 studies involving 2749 patients, once again, the authors reported no reduction in the occurrence of permanent SCI with poutine or selective CSFD, and no difference in overall mortality between the two groups [6]. It is worth noting that the definition of "selective" CSFD was used inconsistently throughout the review, as it has been interchangeably used to refer to prophylactic drainage only in high-risk patients and drains placed after SCI [6].

According to Lella et al. CSFD, either routinely employed or in selected high-risk patients, was the most common measure to mitigate SCI after aortic repair [9]. High-risk patients included patients with longer aortic coverage, prior aortic surgery, and coverage of the subclavian and hypogastric vessels [9]. CSFD was set to a set pressure of 10 mmHg and 0 mmHg in asymptomatic and symptomatic patients [9]. Once again, the importance of TASP and MISAGE was shown, but the supporting evidence was scarce [9]. Regarding the perioperative care measures, the authors noticed an increased interest in optimizing hemodynamic flow parameters, including mean arterial blood pressure, as well as hemoglobin concentration and oxygen delivery [9]. The arterial pressure was maintained above 90 mmHg by either withholding antihypertensive medications or rarely using vasopressors, and the hemoglobin was kept above 10 g/dL [9]. Systemic or intrathecal steroids and intravenous naloxone were reported in a couple of studies without robust data on their safety and effectiveness [9].

3.7. Complications Associated with CSFD (Q5)

Seven studies reported complications associated with CSFD. Eight studies reported complications associated with CSFD. Khan et al. reported complications of CSFD during

TAAA repair, including two patients requiring external ventricular drains, four experiencing intracranial hypotension, two instances of catheter occlusion or dislodgement, and one case of persistent cerebrospinal fluid leak requiring an epidural blood patch [5]. However, the exact complication rates could not be determined [5].

According to Zhang et al., the complications of CSFD included 1 case of subarachnoid hemorrhage, 1 case of epidural hematoma, 4 cases of intracranial hypotension, and 12 cases of headache, out of a total of 435 patients [19]. However, their review notes that the incidence of other complications, such as CSF leakage, infection, and entrapped drain, was not reported, so their specific rates remain unknown [19].

According to Chen et al., several additional complications were reported after prophylactic CSFD, including spinal headache (4.3%), meningitis (0.6%), CSF leak requiring re-intervention (0.7%), insertion site bleeding (0.7%), retained catheter tip (0.7%), epidural or spinal hematoma (0.9%), intracranial or subdural hemorrhage (0.8%), and significant paraparesis or paraplegia not attributable to ischemia (0.8%) [21]. This review also highlights two drain-related deaths following large intracranial bleeds, emphasizing the potential severity of CSFD complications [21]. The authors suggest that a larger total volume drained could be a risk factor for intracranial hemorrhage [21].

Frankort et al. attempted to quantify the incidence of complications associated with CSFD [7]. Their review estimated an overall complication rate of 13.6%, with a random-effects model estimate of 10% and a 3.4% rate in low-risk bias studies [7]. However, the review did not provide details on specific complication types due to limited reporting in the source studies [7].

Alzghari et al. categorized the complications of CSFD into three groups: severe (1.95%, including subdural hematoma and intracranial hemorrhage), moderate (0.38%, including spinal headache), and minor (1.81%, including puncture site bleeding) [2]. The authors noted that the rates were pooled estimates that may have varied across studies [2].

A review by Zheng et al. focuses on the impact of prophylactic CSFD on outcomes like SCI and mortality rather than comprehensively analyzing CSFD-related complications [6]. While the review does not quantify complication rates, it acknowledges the potential for adverse events [6]. The discussion mentions complications like intracranial hypotension and meningitis, but the included studies did not consistently report these, limiting detailed analysis [6].

According to the review by Malloy et al., the pertinent literature commonly reported low-severity complications associated with CSFD, such as spinal headache and puncture site pain, with a reported incidence rate as high as 23% [17]. While fewer studies detailed complications requiring intervention, the available evidence suggests that more serious issues, including spinal hematomas, an entrapped drain, and cerebrospinal fluid leaks, did occur in some cases [17]. Importantly, no studies reported persistent morbidity or mortality directly attributed to CSFD procedures [17].

Leone et al. identified seven CSFD-related deaths among 365 patients in three publications [24]. The authors estimated the crude mortality rate and the random effects model mortality to be as high as 1.9% and 1.4%, respectively, both of which are non-negligible figures [24]. Notably, all deaths occurred after massive intracranial hemorrhage during hospitalization or within 30 days after surgery [24].

3.8. Treatment (Q6)

None of the studies reviewed directly focused on summarizing the evidence on managing postoperative SCI. Similarly, no review addressed the management of delayed SCI. However, two studies did discuss relevant aspects of SCI treatment as a secondary aim.

Postoperative SCI management, according to Lella et al., focuses on prompt diagnosis and treatment [9]. Strategies for managing postoperative SCI include hemodynamic optimization, which involves maintaining adequate mean arterial pressure, often above 80 mmHg or higher, depending on patient-specific factors [9]. Permissive hypertension may be employed, in the sense of withholding antihypertensive medication [9]. Continuing or initiating CSF drainage to reduce pressure on the spinal cord is a common practice, with target pressures generally below 10–15 mmHg [9]. Surgical intervention, such as decompression or revascularization, may be considered in cases of persistent or worsening neurological deficits [9]. Supportive care, which includes maintaining adequate oxygenation, managing fluid and electrolyte balance, and providing appropriate pain control, is also crucial. Regular neurological assessments are essential to monitor for changes in neurological status and guide treatment decisions [9]. The review emphasizes the importance of a multidisciplinary approach involving vascular surgeons, neurologists, and critical care specialists. It also highlights the need for further research to optimize postoperative SCI management strategies [9].

Pini et al. focused on the occurrence of SCI after endovascular repair of TAAA and mentioned certain measures, such as pharmacologic blood pressure support, direct usage of CSFD, and intensive physiotherapy, as being clinically useful [20]. Significant clinical amelioration was observed in selected patients after stenting a stenotic hypogastric artery [20].

3.9. Prognosis (Q7)

Most of the systematic reviews mentioned the overall mortality rates in the context of open surgical or endovascular repair but did not primarily address mortality specifically associated with SCI. Tanaka et al. reported that the total mortality rate across the included studies was 6.9% (54/782 patients) [15]. Likewise, Algzhari et al. (2023) distinguish between operative mortality, which is death during the initial hospital stay or within 30 days of the operation if the stay was shorter, in up to 6.2% of cases, and late mortality, defined as death occurring after the initial hospital stay or after 30 days post-operation, without a single pooled late mortality rate but presenting data for different follow-up periods [2]. Muston et al. added that the 36-month survival rates were as follows: the hybrid group had the highest survival at 88.7%, the open group had a survival of 61.7%, while the endovascular group had insufficient data for meaningful interpretation [3].

Wong et al. were among those to comment on the negative impact of SCI on medium-term survival [14]. The review references a single study which found that perioperative SCI after thoracic aortic interventions is associated with impaired medium-term survival [14]. Once again, the review does not provide precise mortality rates attributable to SCI [14]. Likewise, Lella et al. noted that patients with permanent paraplegia due to SCI were characterized by a poorer prognosis and had a mortality rate as high as 75% for DTA, and 44% for TAAA within the first year after surgery [9].

On the other hand, Moulakakis et al. focused on 25 cases with SCI from 18 studies regarding neurological improvement [1]. Their review included patients with variable presentation, ranging from mild sensory deficits to complete paraplegia, and mentions that common symptoms include motor weakness (paraparesis or paraplegia), sensory disturbances, and bowel or bladder dysfunction [1]. The specific neurological deficits depended on the level and extent of spinal cord involvement and are indicative of the definition of SCI variability [1]. In half of these cases, patients exhibited only modest improvement at follow-up. In a quarter of the cases, no improvement was observed, while a quarter of cases demonstrated near-complete recovery [1].

3.10. Results of Quality Appraisal

Of the studies, twenty-three were rated as being "critically low" and two as "low" quality according to AMSTAR-2. It is worth noting that no study reported the list of the excluded records except one [7], and no study considered the role of funding or the risk of bias while discussing their results (Figure 2). Furthermore, the clinical heterogeneity of the available data precluded performing an umbrella meta-analysis that could help us estimate the risk of publication bias.

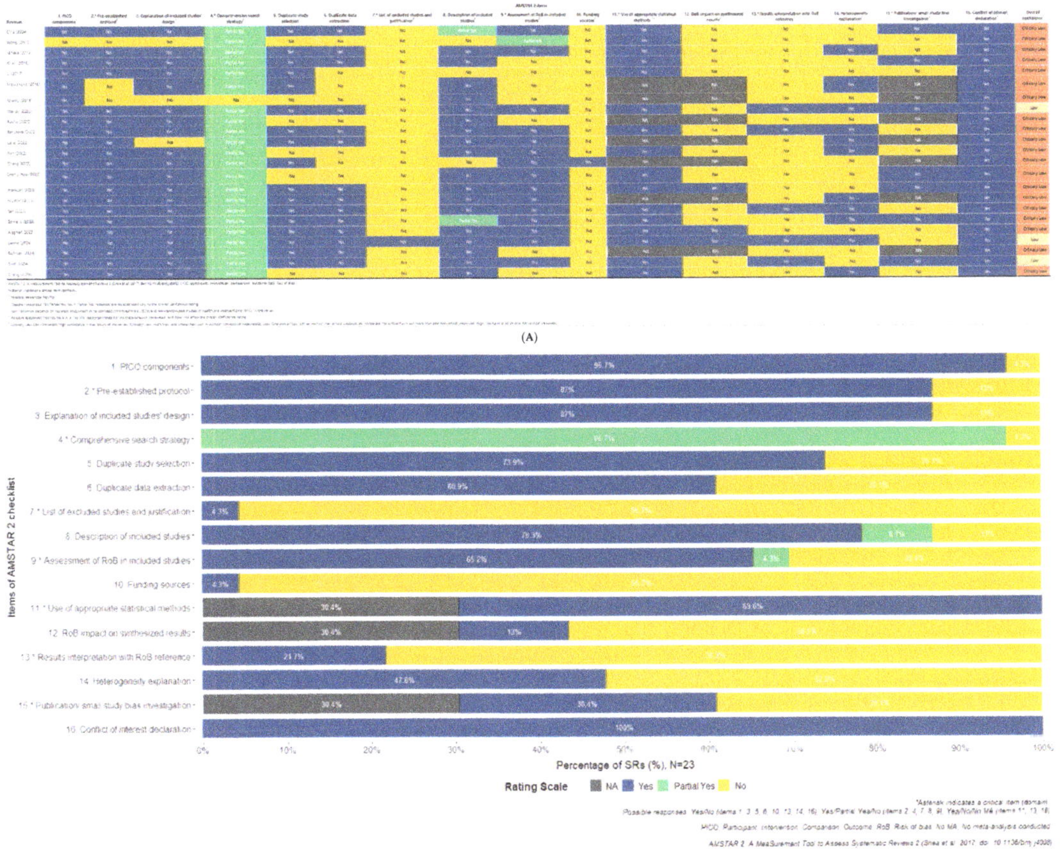

Figure 2. AMSTAR-2 grading for each review study individually (**A**) and for the whole dataset (**B**) [1–9,11,14–26].

The eligible reviews and meta-analyses of our study were largely characterized by a high risk of bias, frequent inconsistencies or conflicting findings, and a lack of direct evidence on numerous topics (Table 5). It is also notable that only a few studies controlled for potential moderators. Thus, according to the GRADE recommendations, the overall quality of evidence was moderate for Q1, Q4, and Q5, low for Q3, and very low for Q2, Q6, and Q7, suggesting that further research is still needed to better characterize the underlying pathogenesis, methods for early SCI detection, and treatment strategies for perioperative SCI (Table 6).

Table 5. Quality of evidence according to GRADE.

Q	Question	Study Design	Risk of Bias	Inconsistency	Indirectness	Publication Bias	Magnitude of Effect	Dose Response	Testing Modera-tors	Overall Quality	Grade
Q1	Incidence and risk factors	4	−1	−1	0	0	0	0	1	3	Moderate
Q2	Pathogenesis	2	−1	0	−1	0	0	0	0	0	Very low
Q3	Early detection	4	−1	−1	0	0	0	0	0	2	Low
Q4	Prevention	4	−1	−1	0	0	0	0	1	3	Moderate
Q5	Complications associated with CSFD	4	−1	0	0	0	0	0	0	3	Moderate
Q6	Treatment	2	−1	−1	0	0	0	0	0	0	Very low
Q7	Prognosis	2	−1	−1	0	0	0	0	0	0	Very low

GRADE, Grading of Recommendations Assessment, Development and Evaluation.

Table 6. Summary of the evidence.

Q	Question	Findings	Grade	Areas of Future Research
Q1	Incidence and risk factors	Open: 10%; endovascular up to 3.5%; permanent: 3.5%	Moderate	High-quality studies are needed
Q2	Pathogenesis	Disruption of the spinal cord's blood supply at some point, leading to hypoxia, metabolic arrest, and ischemia	Very low	Pathogenetic mechanisms at the cellular and molecular level
Q3	Early detection	Neuromonitoring could be an option	Low	Optimization of neuromonitoring intraoperative, and maybe early postoperatively
Q4	Prevention	CSFD seems to work in open aortic repair, LSA F/B EVAR	Moderate	High-quality studies are needed
Q5	Complications associated with CSFD	Morbidity between 10 and 23%, non-negligible mortality	Moderate	Identify high-risk patients
Q6	Treatment	Selective CSFD, optimize perfusion and hemodynamic parameters	Very low	Study the role of several drugs, including steroids, calcium channel blockers, fasudil, and milrinone
Q7	Prognosis	Mortality of up to 75% in the first year	Very low	Studies focusing on the morbidity and mortality associated with SCI after aortic repair

4. Discussion

4.1. Overview of Our Findings

This paper includes systematic reviews and studies that provide a comprehensive overview of the current evidence on diagnosing, preventing, and managing SCI in the context of thoracic and thoraco-abdominal aortic interventions. SCI has been found to occur with a reported incidence ranging from 1.4% to 10% for open repair and 3% to 10% for endovascular procedures. Permanent paraplegia remains in less than 5% of the cases. Among the risk factors of SCI, extensive aortic coverage, poor collateral blood perfusion, reoperation, and hemodynamic instability have been identified (Q1). The reviewed studies also highlight the effectiveness of various interventions, such as CSFD, pharmacologic blood pressure support, and selective revascularization, in preventing postoperative issues (Q4). Finally, CSFD seems to have non-negligible morbidity and mortality, and its use should weigh the benefits against the potential risks (Q7).

4.2. Prevention and Treatment of SCI in the Guidelines

Several clinical guidelines were published in 2024, including the "2024 ESC Guidelines for the management of peripheral arterial and aortic diseases", the "European Society for Vascular Surgery (ESVS) 2024 Clinical Practice Guidelines on the Management of Abdominal Aorto-Iliac Artery Aneurysms", and the "AO Spine & Praxis Spinal Cord Institute Guidelines for the Management of Acute Spinal Cord Injury". These guidelines provide comprehensive recommendations to prevent and manage spinal cord injury [27,28].

The ESVS recommendations support the assertion that SCI is more common after the open or endovascular repair of TAAAs, types I, II, and III [29]. The endovascular repair of complex AAAs may triple the SCI risk compared to open surgery, although recent studies show varying incidences [29]. Preventive strategies include staging the procedure, maintaining high blood pressure and oxygenation, preserving collateral circulation, CSFD, and neuromonitoring [29]. Prophylactic CSFD is proven for open TAAA repair but lacks evidence for complex AAA EVAR [29]. Due to potential complications, routine prophylactic CSFD is not recommended for complex AAA repair, but may be considered in high-risk patients [29]. Rapid post-operative extubation for neurological assessment is desirable, and a rescue drainage policy is often preferred over prophylactic drainage [29].

According to the ESC guidelines, SCI is reported in 11% to 15% of cases, and is often linked to the severity of aortic pathology [30]. However, thoracic endovascular aortic repair has been associated with an increased risk of SCI, underscoring the need for a prudent approach to revascularization strategies [30]. This may involve the prior surgical or concurrent endovascular revascularization of the left subclavian artery in elective settings [30]. The guidelines do not comment on neuromonitoring or the use of CSFD and provide no treatment strategy in the event of SCI [30].

AO Spine defines intraoperative spinal cord injury as a new or worsening neurological deficit due to spinal cord dysfunction diagnosed during surgery, using neuromonitoring, wake-up tests, or immediate post-operative clinical assessment [31]. The reported frequency of intraoperative SCI varies widely from 0% to 61%, with risk factors including older age, male sex, cardiovascular disease, severe myelopathy, blood loss, osteotomy, and spinal deformities [31]. Conversely, better preoperative neurological status and intraoperative neuromonitoring are associated with decreased ISCI risk [31]. Multimodal monitoring can achieve high sensitivity (83.5%) and specificity (93.8%) [32]. The authors recommend a comprehensive checklist of surgical, technical, and anesthetic measures to prevent and manage ISCI, emphasizing communication between surgeons and anesthesiologists [32]. In the event of persistent neurophysiologic changes, options include steroids, consulting colleagues, wake-up tests, and potentially aborting the procedure [32]. Post-operative management involves close monitoring, steroids, blood pressure control, and further imaging [32]. AO Spine also recommended maintaining the mean arterial blood pressure between 75 and 80 mmHg, but not exceeding 90–95 mmHg, in order to optimize spinal cord perfusion in patients with acute traumatic SCI [28]. This recommendation is for a time period of at least three to seven days [28]. However, the attending physician should use their discretion in selecting the appropriate vasopressor or inotrope to achieve the target mean arterial pressure goals in these patients [28]. The guidelines do not provide any commentary on the use of CSFD, and they also lack a clear definition of the optimal steroid treatment and its recommended dosage.

4.3. Evidence Gaps and Future Perspectives

The current umbrella review identified five important gaps in the literature. Firstly, the literature does not consistently define and report SCI. Most reviews did not distinguish between permanent and temporary neurological deficits, which could have important implications for patient outcomes and management. Minor motor and sensory deficits were not registered. The absence of consistent definitions extends to the terms "temporary and "permanent" neurological deficit, a fact which adds to the complexity in understanding this disabling complication. A detailed, multifaceted definition that considers severity, timing, and other factors like neurological level should be broadly used and supported by the appropriate guideline bodies. Moreover, many of the reviewed studies did not assess long-term neurologic outcomes beyond the immediate perioperative period.

Secondly, all risk factors point towards an ischemic etiology for SCI, with the final pathway likely being, most likely, the hypoperfusion of the spinal cord during aortic surgery (Q2). The surgical manipulation, aortic cross-clamping, and coverage of the involved segmental arteries during repair can compromise spinal cord perfusion, leading to ischemia and subsequent neurological deficits. Nevertheless, the pathogenesis seems to be multifactorial and incompletely understood, implicating factors like inadequate revascularization, elevated CSF pressure, and spinal cord compression from hematomas to be less studied. Likewise, the molecular pathogenetic pathways, including spinal cord edema, neuroinflammation, excitotoxicity, spasm of the microcirculation, mitochondrial dysfunction, oxidative stress, and apoptosis, are not fully characterized. Moreover, it is not clear if the underlying mechanisms of delayed SCI are the same as in acute/peri-operative injury. Understanding the pathogenetic mechanisms is critical in the development of effective targeted preventive and therapeutic interventions.

Thirdly, no established method exists to monitor or measure spinal cord perfusion intraoperatively to guide surgical and anesthetic management (Q3). Modern techniques, like somatosensory and motor-evoked potentials, remain an established method in spine surgery. However, their accuracy in aortic repair surgery could be affected by several factors, such as hypothermia, cardiopulmonary bypass, and drug selection during anesthesia. Therefore, further comprehending the limitations and optimizing the use of neuromonitoring strategies is of utmost importance. Other methods, like CSF biochemistry and NIRS, seem to be less promising, at least in the near future.

Fourthly, a lack of consensus on the optimal treatment strategies is observed, althrough this is not to say that there are no treatment methods at all (Q6). It is clear that endovascular repair is associated with significantly less risk for SCI. Likewise, staged procedures, F/B endovascular aortic repair, and LSA revascularization have shown protective effects against SCI [33,34]. Empasis is also placed on the optimal aneurysm selection, due to inherent differences in the associated SCI risk. However, many of the implemented measures are, in fact, extensions of the preventive measures during postoperative care. Among these are the use of CSFD, blood pressure augmentation, hypothermia, pharmacologic agents, and stimulation strategies [35]. Moreover, the target CSFD remains ill-defined, with significant differences among studies. The role of steroids is also unclear. In spinal cord trauma, early high-dose methylprednisolone has been advocated for a limited period of 24 h in highly selected young patients without any underlying comorbidities, but its utility in SCI associated with aortic procedures is not proven. Likewise, specific vasodilators or other neuroprotective medications with documented benefits after cerebral aneurysmal vasospasm, like nimodipine, milrinone, or fasudil, warrant further investigation. It is of note that the "ISCOPE" trial by Papadopoulos et al. demonstrated that neurologic recovery may be more closely tied to spinal cord perfusion pressure (SCPP) than to mean arterial pressure. Future guidelines may include SCPP monitoring and management recommendations as new evidence emerges, with stratification for early and delayed SCI.

Finally, the impact of SCI on long-term functional outcomes and quality of life remains poorly characterized. While the available studies provide mortality rates, they do not systematically report on SCI-related parameters. These figures are important to guide patients and their families in the complex decision-making process surrounding the risks and benefits of thoracic or thoraco-abdominal aortic interventions. Moreover, accurate data would support future research endeavors, cost-effectiveness analyses, and healthcare policy decisions. In addition, future studies need to address several functional patient-reported data, including quality of life, overall patient functioning, psychological distress, and social parameters.

4.4. Ongoing Trials

Numerous ongoing clinical trials are poised to yield valuable insights regarding the prevention and management of SCI in the context of TAAA repair procedures. The clinical trial denoted as NCT04941157 serves as a pilot study, specifically aiming to evaluate the feasibility of conducting a larger randomized controlled trial that contrasts the prophylactic versus selective placement of CSFD for SCI prevention in patients undergoing endovascular TAAA repair. This investigation seeks to ascertain whether the implementation of prophylactic CSF drains, as part of a comprehensive SCI prevention protocol, effectively diminishes the incidence of SCI compared to a strategy of placing drains exclusively upon the manifestation of SCI.

Similarly, the SINATRA trial (NCT03074487) is focused on exploring methodologies for the early detection of SCI subsequent to open surgical interventions for TAAA. This study aims to assess the accuracy and feasibility of alternative neurophysiological assessments for the postoperative detection of SCI in sedated or partially sedated patients. Among the diagnostic modalities being evaluated are long loop reflexes (LLR) utilizing F-waves and paraspinal muscle oxygenation metrics measured through near-infrared spectroscopy (NIRS).

Conversely, the trial labeled NCT05195905 investigates the application of physician-modified endografts (PMEG) in treating pararenal and thoracoabdominal aortic aneurysms. This research intends to enroll approximately 30 participants aged 18 years and older. The primary outcomes to be measured encompass the incidence of major adverse events within 30 days post-procedure and the success of the treatment at the 12-month follow-up. Secondary outcomes include mortality rates, incidences of major adverse events, occurrences of spinal cord ischemia, treatment success, and the rate of freedom from secondary interventions.

The PAPA-ARTiS trial (NCT03434314) is designed to investigate the potential reduction in paraplegia and mortality risk associated with the minimally invasive staged aortic coiling and embolization (MISACE) procedure in patients undergoing thoracoabdominal aortic aneurysm repair. This multinational, prospective, open-label, two-arm randomized controlled trial compares two distinct treatment strategies: TAAA repair conducted with versus without MISACE pre-treatment, the latter of which involves the staged embolization of segmental arteries prior to aneurysm repair in an effort to enhance collateral blood flow to the spinal cord.

Lastly, the CASPER trial represents a multicenter initiative aimed at enrolling 100 patients diagnosed with acute traumatic cervical and thoracic SCI to explore the influence of spinal cord perfusion pressure (SCPP) management on neurological outcomes. Patients will have a lumbar intrathecal catheter placed within 24 h post injury for the purposes of intrathecal pressure (ITP) measurement and CSF sampling. The primary objective of this study is to ascertain whether the maintenance of an SCPP $\geq$ 65 mmHg yields improved neurological recovery outcomes in comparison to conventional hemodynamic management practices. Additionally, the trial will investigate the feasibility of CSF drainage to mitigate ITP while assessing the complications associated with intrathecal catheter insertion and CSF drainage in this specific patient demographic.

4.5. Key Challenges in Studying Spinal Cord Injury

The rarity of SCI and the inherent difficulties in conducting large-scale clinical trials pose significant barriers to advancing research in this field. Multidisciplinary collaboration among vascular surgeons, anesthesiologists, critical care physicians, neurosurgeons, neurologists, and rehabilitation specialists is essential to comprehensively investigate the various aspects of this complex clinical condition. Securing adequate funding and overcoming the inherent heterogeneity among SCI cases further contribute to the slow progress in this area of study. Additionally, the use of diverse definitions and outcome measures in the available literature makes it challenging to synthesize the evidence and draw firm conclusions. Despite these limitations, the past decade has witnessed a substantial increase in the volume of published research on SCI associated with aortic surgery. Establishing standardized registries with well-defined parameters would be instrumental in advancing this field of study.

4.6. The Role of CSF Drainage

The current review identifies prophylactic cerebrospinal fluid (CSF) drainage as a commonly used technique in open elective TAAA repairs to preserve spinal cord perfusion, aiming to maintain intracranial pressure below central venous pressure or 10 mmHg. Drainage rates typically fall within the range of 5 to 15 milliliters per hour (mL/h), with some centers opting for slightly higher rates, up to 20 mL/h, during the intraoperative period. Postoperatively, many protocols recommend a more conservative drainage rate, often not exceeding 10 mL/h. The total volume of CSF drained can also vary significantly, with some protocols specifying maximum volumes, such as no more than 25 mL in a four-hour period or 150 mL within a 24 h window. The overall duration of CSF drainage typically extends for 24 to 72 h following surgery in patients who do not exhibit any neurological deficits. However, in cases where SCI symptoms develop, the drainage period may be prolonged, sometimes lasting up to 5 to 7 days. This approach is often supplemented by strategies to ensure adequate blood pressure and cardiac output. However, the effectiveness of CSF drainage in thoracic endovascular aortic repair (TEVAR) is debated, with some centers recommending it for high-risk patients while others advocate for selective use only. Although intended to prevent spinal cord ischemia, the procedure carries risks, including headaches and infections, necessitating careful patient selection and monitoring. To optimize the use of prophylactic CSF drainage, further investigation into specific drainage parameters from medical associations and the detailed exploration of patient selection criteria is crucial, along with recommendations for future randomized controlled trials to provide more definitive evidence.

4.7. The Role of Neuromonitoring

The adjustment for confounding variables such as operation duration and aortic coverage, disturbances in oxygenation and core body temperature is paramount for the accurate interpretation of intraoperative recordings in abdominal aortic repair surgery. Within this context, multimodal neuromonitoring—specifically the integration of MEPs and SSEPs—emerges as a significant tool for the intraoperative evaluation of spinal cord functionality during surgery. This combinatorial approach is characterized by enhanced sensitivity and specificity, which may facilitate the improved identification of risks associated with SCI. Nevertheless, the literature surrounding the definitive impact of neuromonitoring on the reduction in paraplegia rates presents conflicting evidence, likely attributable to variability in monitoring protocols and the influence of multiple external factors. Therefore, it is essential to embed neuromonitoring within a comprehensive strategy for SCI prevention, which should include the implementation of CSFD, distal aortic perfusion, and the selective re-implantation of intercostal arteries. To elucidate the role of neuromonitoring and refine its application in enhancing neurological outcomes for patients undergoing abdominal aortic repair, further empirical research, particularly well-structured randomized controlled trials that adequately account for possible confounders, is warranted. In addition, intraoperative neuromonitoring might help identify patients at risk of developing delayed SCI. Given the dynamic nature of both open and endovascular surgical techniques, a continuous reassessment of optimal neuromonitoring strategies is necessary, alongside the recognition that the presence of proficient multidisciplinary teams is critical for the successful adoption and interpretation of these advanced monitoring techniques.

4.8. Limitations

The current umbrella review is limited by the shortcomings of primary and secondary studies. Firstly, it is based on small-sized, single-center, retrospective studies, which carry a risk of bias. Secondly, the reporting clarity of the secondary reviews and meta-analyses is often suboptimal, limiting the ability to assess methodological quality. Thirdly, there is substantial clinical heterogeneity among the included studies in terms of definitions of SCI, patient population, surgical procedures, and reported outcomes. Fourthly, the limited available evidence precludes the stratification of the findings according to the implemented technique, patients' age and gender, aneurysm extent, and studies from low- or middle-income countries. Finally, as in every umbrella review, there is an obvious bias against newer techniques and devices.

5. Conclusions

SCI remains a devastating complication after aortic repair surgery with a variable rate depending on several factors, including the type of repair and the adopted prophylactic measures. To effectively address the existing gaps in our understanding of SCI related to thoracic and thoraco-abdominal aortic procedures, future research should prioritize standardizing definitions of SCI and associated neurological deficits to ensure consistency across studies, thereby enhancing communication and collaboration within the research community. Furthermore, a deeper examination of the pathogenic mechanisms of SCI at the cellular and molecular levels is necessary to identify potential therapeutic targets. Optimizing neuromonitoring techniques through multimodal approaches could significantly improve the intraoperative and early postoperative detection of SCI. Conducting high-quality studies, particularly randomized controlled trials, is vital for assessing the effectiveness of preventive strategies such as CSFD, staged procedures, and meticulous hemodynamic management, alongside establishing evidence-based treatment protocols that explore pharmacological interventions and surgical decompression strategies. Identifying high-risk patients who may be susceptible to CSFD-related complications and developing strategies to mitigate these risks is crucial, as is a thorough assessment of the long-term morbidity and mortality linked to SCI after aortic repair, which will provide valuable insights for patient management and prognostication. By addressing these research priorities, we can significantly enhance our ability to prevent, diagnose, and manage SCI, leading to improved outcomes for patients undergoing aortic surgery.

Author Contributions: Conceptualization, M.M. and A.G.B.; methodology, A.G.B. and A.K.; validation, K.N.F., E.A. and M.M.; formal analysis, A.G.B. and A.K.; data curation, K.N.F., M.M., A.G.B. and E.A.; writing—original draft preparation, A.G.B., K.S. and A.K.; writing—review and editing, K.N.F., M.M., E.A., K.S., M.B., A.G.B. and A.K.; supervision, K.N.F. and M.M.; project administration, A.G.B. All authors have read and agreed to the published version of the manuscript.

Funding: This research received no external funding.

Institutional Review Board Statement: All patient-related data were anonymized. Finally, no experimental or other novel interventions took place. No ethical committee approval was required.

Data Availability Statement: No new data were created or analyzed in this study.

Conflicts of Interest: The authors declare no conflicts of interest.

Abbreviations

The following abbreviations are used in this manuscript:

BMT	Best medical treatment
CSF	Cerebrospinal fluid
CSFD	Cerebrospinal fluid drain
CT	Computerized tomography
CNIHE	Canadian National Institute of Health Economics
DTA	Descending thoracic aortic
F/B-EVAR	Fenestrated or branched endovascular repair
GRADE	Grading of Recommendations Assessment
LSA	Left subclavian artery
MA	Meta-analysis
MEPs	Motor evoked potentials
MICACE	Minimally invasive segmental spinal artery coil embolization
MRI	Magnetic resonance imaging
NIRS	Near-infrared spectroscopy
NOS	Newcastle Ottawa scale
OS	Open surgery
SCI	Spinal cord ischemia
SR	Systematic review
SSEPs	Somatosensory evoked potentials
QUADAS-2	Quality Assessment of Diagnostic Accuracy Studies—2
TAAAs	Thoracoabdominal aortic aneurysms
TASP	Temporary aneurysm sac perfusion
TBAD	Type B aortic dissection
TCD	Transcranial Doppler
TEVAR	Thoracic endovascular aneurysm repair
US	Ultrasound
W/O	Without

References

1. Moulakakis, K.G.; Alexiou, V.G.; Karaolanis, G.; Sfyroeras, G.S.; Theocharopoulos, G.N.; Lazaris, A.M.; Kakisis, J.D.; Geroulakos, G. Spinal Cord Ischemia Following Elective Endovascular Repair of Infrarenal Aortic Aneurysms: A Systematic Review. *Ann. Vasc. Surg.* **2018**, *52*, 280–291. [CrossRef]
2. Alzghari, T.; An, K.R.; Harik, L.; Rahouma, M.; Dimagli, A.; Perezgorvas-Olaria, R.; Demetres, M.; Cancelli, G.; Soletti, G., Jr.; Lau, C.; et al. Spinal Cord Injury After Open and Endovascular Repair of Descending Thoracic Aneurysm and Thoracoabdominal Aortic Aneurysm: An Updated Systematic Review and Meta-Analysis. *Ann. Cardiothorac. Surg.* **2023**, *12*, 409–417. [CrossRef] [PubMed]
3. Muston, B.T.; Bilbrough, J.; Bushati, Y.; Wilson-Smith, A.R.; Misfeld, M.; Yan, T. Open, Closed or a Bit of Both: A Systematic Review and Meta-Analysis of Staged Thoraco-Abdominal Aortic Aneurysm Repair. *Ann. Cardiothorac. Surg.* **2023**, *12*, 418–428. [CrossRef]
4. Rocha, R.V.; Lindsay, T.F.; Friedrich, J.O.; Shan, S.; Sinha, S.; Yanagawa, B.; Al-Omran, M.; Forbes, T.L.; Ouzounian, M. Systematic Review of Contemporary Outcomes of Endovascular and Open Thoracoabdominal Aortic Aneurysm Repair. *J. Vasc. Surg.* **2020**, *71*, 1396–1412.e12. [CrossRef] [PubMed]
5. Khan, N.R.; Smalley, Z.; Nesvick, C.L.; Lee, S.L.; Michael, L.M. The Use of Lumbar Drains in Preventing Spinal Cord Injury Following Thoracoabdominal Aortic Aneurysm Repair: An Updated Systematic Review and Meta-Analysis. *J. Neurosurg. Spine* **2016**, *25*, 383–393. [CrossRef]
6. Zheng, H.; Lin, D.; Cheng, Y.; Yan, C.; Yu, S.; Li, J.; Cheng, W. Systematic Review of the Effect of Cerebrospinal Fluid Drainage on Outcomes After Endovascular Type B Aortic Dissection Repair. *J. Cardiothorac. Surg.* **2024**, *19*, 116. [CrossRef] [PubMed]
7. Frankort, J.; Mees, B.; Doukas, P.; Keszei, A.; Kontopodis, N.; Antoniou, G.A.; Jacobs, M.J.; Gombert, A. Systematic Review of the Effect of Cerebrospinal Fluid Drainage on Outcomes After Endovascular Descending Thoracic/Thoraco-Abdominal Aortic Aneurysm Repair. *Eur. J. Vasc. Endovasc. Surg.* **2023**, *66*, 501–512. [CrossRef]
8. Cinà, C.S.; Abouzahr, L.; Arena, G.O.; Laganà, A.; Devereaux, P.J.; Farrokhyar, F. Cerebrospinal Fluid Drainage to Prevent Paraplegia during Thoracic and Thoracoabdominal Aortic Aneurysm Surgery: A Systematic Review and Meta-Analysis. *J. Vasc. Surg.* **2004**, *40*, 36–44. [CrossRef]
9. Lella, S.K.; Waller, H.D.; Pendleton, A.; Latz, C.A.; Boitano, L.T.; Dua, A. A Systematic Review of Spinal Cord Ischemia Prevention and Management After Open and Endovascular Aortic Repair. *J. Vasc. Surg.* **2022**, *75*, 1091–1106. [CrossRef]
10. Ouzzani, M.; Hammady, H.; Fedorowicz, Z.; Elmagarmid, A. Rayyan—A Web and Mobile App for Systematic Reviews. *Syst. Rev.* **2016**, *5*, 210. [CrossRef]
11. Li, L.; Asemota, I.; Liu, B.; Gomez-Valencia, J.; Lin, L.; Arif, A.W.; Siddiqi, T.J.; Usman, M.S. AMSTAR 2 Appraisal of Systematic Reviews and Meta-Analyses in the Field of Heart Failure from High-Impact Journals. *Syst. Rev.* **2022**, *11*, 147. [CrossRef] [PubMed]
12. Shea, B.J.; Reeves, B.C.; Wells, G.; Thuku, M.; Hamel, C.; Moran, J.; Moher, D.; Tugwell, P.; Welch, V.; Kristjansson, E.; et al. AMSTAR 2: A Critical Appraisal Tool for Systematic Reviews That Include Randomised or Non-Randomised Studies of Healthcare Interventions, or Both. *BMJ* **2017**, *358*, j4008. [CrossRef]
13. Prasad, M. Introduction to the GRADE Tool for Rating Certainty in Evidence and Recommendations. *Clin. Epidemiol. Glob. Health* **2024**, *25*, 101484. [CrossRef]
14. Wong, C.S.; Healy, D.; Canning, C.; Coffey, J.C.; Boyle, J.R.; Walsh, S.R. A Systematic Review of Spinal Cord Injury and Cerebrospinal Fluid Drainage After Thoracic Aortic Endografting. *J. Vasc. Surg.* **2012**, *56*, 1438–1447. [CrossRef]
15. Tanaka, Y.; Kawaguchi, M.; Noguchi, Y.; Yoshitani, K.; Kawamata, M.; Masui, K.; Nakayama, T.; Yamada, Y. Systematic Review of Motor Evoked Potentials Monitoring during Thoracic and Thoracoabdominal Aortic Aneurysm Open Repair Surgery: A Diagnostic Meta-Analysis. *J. Anesth.* **2016**, *30*, 1037–1050. [CrossRef] [PubMed]
16. Harky, A.; Fok, M.; Fraser, H.; Howard, C.; Rimmer, L.; Bashir, M. Could Cerebrospinal Fluid Biomarkers Offer Better Predictive Value for Spinal Cord Ischaemia Than Current Neuromonitoring Techniques During Thoracoabdominal Aortic Aneurysm Repair—A Systematic Review. *Braz. J. Cardiovasc. Surg.* **2019**, *34*, 464–471. [CrossRef]
17. Malloy, P.C.; Raghavan, A.; Elder, T.; Wright, J.; Wright, C.H.; Burant, C.; Sajatovic, M.; Hoffer, A. Cerebrospinal Fluid Drainage During Endovascular Aortic Aneurysm Repair: A Systematic Review of the Literature and Treatment Recommendations. *Vasc. Endovasc. Surg.* **2020**, *54*, 205–213. [CrossRef] [PubMed]
18. Batubara, E.A.D.; Nugraha, R.A.; Amshar, M.; Siddiq, T.; Indriani, S.; Adiarto, S. Ischemic Complications Following Thoracic Endovascular Aortic Repair with and Without Revascularization of Left Subclavian Artery: A Systematic Review and Meta-Analysis. *Ann. Vasc. Surg.* **2022**, *86*, 417–427. [CrossRef] [PubMed]
19. Zhang, Z.; Zhou, Y.; Lin, S.; Xiao, J.; Ai, W.; Zhang, W.W. Systematic Review and Meta-Analysis of Association of Prophylactic Cerebrospinal Fluid Drainage in Preventing Spinal Cord Ischemia After Thoracic Endovascular Aortic Repair. *J. Vasc. Surg.* **2022**, *75*, 1478–1489.e5. [CrossRef]

20. Pini, R.; Faggioli, G.; Paraskevas, K.I.; Alaidroos, M.; Palermo, S.; Gallitto, E.; Gargiulo, M. A Systematic Review and Meta-Analysis of the Occurrence of Spinal Cord Ischemia After Endovascular Repair of Thoracoabdominal Aortic Aneurysms. *J. Vasc. Surg.* **2022**, *75*, 1466–1477.e8. [CrossRef]
21. Chen, C.-H.J.; Jiang, H.; Nguyen, V.D.D. Prophylactic Cerebrospinal Fluid Drainage and Spinal Cord Ischemia in Thoracic and Thoracoabdominal Endovascular Procedures: A Systematic Review and Meta-Analysis. *Ann. Cardiothorac. Surg.* **2023**, *12*, 392–408. [CrossRef] [PubMed]
22. Spinella, P.C.; Wade, C.E.; Blackbourne, L.H.; Borgman, M.A.; Zarzabal, L.A.; Du, F.; Perkins, J.G.; Maegele, M.; Schreiber, M.; Hess, J.R.; et al. The Association of Blood Component Use Ratios with the Survival of Massively Transfused Trauma Patients with and Without Severe Brain Injury. *J. Trauma-Inj. Infect. Crit. Care* **2011**, *71*, S343–S352. [CrossRef] [PubMed]
23. Sef, D.; Thet, M.S.; Miskolczi, S.; Velissaris, T.; De Silva, R.; Luthra, S.; Turina, M.I. Perioperative Neuromonitoring during Thoracoabdominal Aortic Aneurysm Open Repair: A Systematic Review. *Eur. J. Cardiothorac. Surg.* **2023**, *63*, ezad221. [CrossRef] [PubMed]
24. Leone, N.; D'Oria, M.; Mani, K.; Oderich, G.; Maleti, G.; Bartolotti, L.A.M.; Silingardi, R.; Lepidi, S.; Gennai, S. Systematic Review and Meta-Analysis of Cerebrospinal Fluid Drain-Related Mortality and Morbidity After Fenestrated-Branched Endovascular Aortic Repair. *J. Vasc. Surg.* **2024**, *80*, 586–594.e5. [CrossRef]
25. Thet, M.S.; D'Oria, M.; Sef, D.; Klokocovnik, T.; Oo, A.Y.; Lepidi, S. Neuromonitoring during Endovascular Thoracoabdominal Aortic Aneurysm Repair: A Systematic Review. *Ann. Vasc. Surg.* **2024**, *109*, 206–215. [CrossRef]
26. Soliman, M.A.; Ramadan, A.; Shah, A.S.; Corr, S.J.; Abdelazeem, B.; Rahimi, M. Postoperative Spinal Cord Ischemia Monitoring: A Review of Techniques Available After Endovascular Aortic Repair. *Ann. Vasc. Surg.* **2024**, *106*, 438–466. [CrossRef]
27. Spratt, J.R.; Walker, K.L.; Neal, D.; Arnaoutakis, G.J.; Martin, T.D.; Back, M.R.; Zasimovich, Y.; Franklin, M.; Shahid, Z.; Upchurch, G.R.; et al. Rescue Therapy for Symptomatic Spinal Cord Ischemia After Thoracic Endovascular Aortic Repair. *J. Thorac. Cardiovasc. Surg.* **2024**, *168*, 15–25.e11. [CrossRef]
28. Kwon, B.K.; Tetreault, L.A.; Martin, A.R.; Arnold, P.M.; Marco, R.A.W.; Newcombe, V.F.J.; Zipser, C.M.; McKenna, S.L.; Korupolu, R.; Neal, C.J.; et al. A Clinical Practice Guideline for the Management of Patients with Acute Spinal Cord Injury: Recommendations on Hemodynamic Management. *Glob. Spine J.* **2024**, *14*, 187S–211S. [CrossRef]
29. Wanhainen, A.; Van Herzeele, I.; Bastos Goncalves, F.; Bellmunt Montoya, S.; Berard, X.; Boyle, J.R.; D'Oria, M.; Prendes, C.F.; Karkos, C.D.; Kazimierczak, A.; et al. Editor's Choice—European Society for Vascular Surgery (ESVS) 2024 Clinical Practice Guidelines on the Management of Abdominal Aorto-Iliac Artery Aneurysms. *Eur. J. Vasc. Endovasc. Surg.* **2024**, *67*, 192–331. [CrossRef]
30. Mazzolai, L.; Teixido-Tura, G.; Lanzi, S.; Boc, V.; Bossone, E.; Brodmann, M.; Bura-Rivière, A.; De Backer, J.; Deglise, S.; Della Corte, A.; et al. 2024 ESC Guidelines for the Management of Peripheral Arterial and Aortic Diseases. *Eur. Heart J.* **2024**, *45*, 3538–3700. [CrossRef]
31. Fehlings, M.G.; Quddusi, A.; Skelly, A.C.; Brodt, E.D.; Moghaddamjou, A.; Malvea, A.; Hejrati, N.; Srikandarajah, N.; Alvi, M.A.; Stabler-Morris, S.; et al. Definition, Frequency and Risk Factors for Intra-Operative Spinal Cord Injury: A Knowledge Synthesis. *Glob. Spine J.* **2024**, *14*, 80S–104S. [CrossRef] [PubMed]
32. Srikandarajah, N.; Hejrati, N.; Alvi, M.A.; Quddusi, A.; Tetreault, L.A.; Evaniew, N.; Skelly, A.C.; Douglas, S.; Rahimi-Movaghar, V.; Arnold, P.M.; et al. Prevention, Diagnosis, and Management of Intraoperative Spinal Cord Injury in the Setting of Spine Surgery: A Proposed Care Pathway. *Glob. Spine J.* **2024**, *14*, 166S–173S. [CrossRef] [PubMed]
33. Heidemann, F.; Tsilimparis, N.; Rohlffs, F.; Debus, E.S.; Larena-Avellaneda, A.; Wipper, S.; Kölbel, T. Staged Procedures for Prevention of Spinal Cord Ischemia in Endovascular Aortic Surgery. *Gefasschirurgie* **2018**, *23*, 39–45. [CrossRef] [PubMed]
34. Sickels, A.D.; Novak, Z.; Schanzer, A.; Farber, M.A.; Sweet, M.P.; Oderich, G.S.; Schneider, D.B.; Eagleton, M.J.; Timaran, C.; Gasper, W.J.; et al. Evolving Practices of Spinal Drain Use for Branch/Fenestrated Endovascular Aortic Repair Patients in the United States Aortic Research Consortium. *J. Vasc. Surg.* 2025; *ahead of print*. [CrossRef]
35. Rosvall, L.; Karelis, A.; Sonesson, B.; Dias, N.V. A Dedicated Preventive Protocol Sustainably Avoids Spinal Cord Ischemia After Endovascular Aortic Repair. *Front. Cardiovasc. Med.* **2024**, *11*, 1440674. [CrossRef]

brain sciences

Case Report

Delayed Intracerebral Hemorrhage 15 Years After Indirect Revascularization in Moyamoya Disease: A Case Report and Review of the Literature

Merih C. Yilmaz * and Kerametttin Aydin

Department of Neurosurgery, VM Medical Park Hospital, Samsun 55200, Turkey
* Correspondence: merihcanyilmaz@gmail.com

Abstract

Background and Clinical Significance: Moyamoya disease (MMD) is a progressive intracranial vasculopathy characterized by stenosis or occlusion of the terminal internal carotid arteries and the development of fragile collateral networks. It predisposes patients to ischemic and hemorrhagic strokes. Although both direct and indirect revascularization procedures are recommended to restore cerebral blood flow, recurrent cerebrovascular events may still occur, and delayed hemorrhage following revascularization is particularly uncommon. **Case Description**: We report the case of a 42-year-old woman who presented with seizure, syncope, and aphasia. Cranial computed tomography (CT) revealed a large left temporal–insular intraparenchymal hematoma with a midline shift. Computed tomography angiography (CTA) demonstrated bilateral internal carotid artery narrowing and collateral vessel proliferation, without aneurysm. Her history indicated a hemorrhagic stroke 15 years earlier, at which time MMD was diagnosed by magnetic resonance angiography (MRA) and managed with multiple burr hole surgeries. She remained free of cerebrovascular events until the current presentation. The patient underwent emergent hematoma evacuation, followed by intensive care management. Postoperatively, she demonstrated neurological improvement, though with residual motor aphasia and right-sided weakness, and was discharged for rehabilitation. **Conclusions**: This case underscores the rare occurrence of delayed intracerebral hemorrhage 15 years after indirect revascularization in MMD. Although revascularization surgery remains the standard therapeutic approach, this report highlights the importance of sustained long-term surveillance, strict risk factor management, and careful postoperative follow-up. The key point is that late hemorrhagic complications, though uncommon, must be considered in the long-term care of MMD patients following revascularization.

Keywords: moyamoya disease; indirect revascularization; delayed intracerebral hemorrhage; multiple burr hole technique

1. Introduction

Moyamoya disease (MMD) represents a cerebrovascular disorder that increases susceptibility to stroke due to progressive narrowing of the intracranial internal carotid arteries and their major proximal branches. Individuals who exhibit the distinctive moyamoya angiopathy in conjunction with additional underlying conditions are classified as having moyamoya syndrome [1]. MMD results in diminished cerebral perfusion, the development of collateral circulation, and a heightened susceptibility to transient ischemic attacks, ischemic strokes, and intracranial hemorrhage [1,2].

 https://doi.org/10.3390/brainsci15101077

Epidemiological data indicate a higher incidence in people of Asian ancestry; however, cases are likewise observed in Western populations, including the Americas and Europe [3]. It was observed that the incidence peaked in the age group of 5 and 40 years [4,5]. MMD shows a female predominance, with an incidence about twice that in males. In the Japanese population, it is most frequently identified during childhood, and overall, the rate in Japan is estimated to be ten times greater than in European countries [4–6].

The etiology of MMD remains incompletely understood, but genetic factors, such as mutations in the ring finger protein 213 (RNF213) gene, have been implicated in disease susceptibility, particularly among East Asian patients [7].

Imaging modalities such as cranial computed tomography angiography (CTA), magnetic resonance angiography (MRA), and digital subtraction angiography (DSA) are employed for evaluation. The distinctive angiographic pattern of the collateral vessels, reminiscent of a "puff of smoke" in Japanese, led to the designation moyamoya.

Antiplatelet and anticoagulant agents are used in cases where surgery is not possible, but the primary treatment for MMD is revascularization surgery. Given its progressive nature and significant risk of ischemic and hemorrhagic complications, early recognition and appropriate management of MMD are critical to improving long-term neurological outcomes.

MMD, both ischemic and hemorrhagic strokes may occur following revascularization surgery. These complications are typically associated with certain etiological factors, such as hyperperfusion syndrome, hemodynamic alterations at the anastomosis site, or underlying vasculopathies. However, late-onset hemorrhagic stroke cases are reported to be quite rare in the literature. In this report, we present a rare case of delayed hemorrhagic stroke occurring long after revascularization and discuss it in the context of the existing literature.

2. Case Description

A 42-year-old female patient was admitted to the emergency department with complaints of seizure and syncope, initially presenting with aphasia. Upon admission, the patient's blood pressure was recorded at 170/110 mmHg, with no prior history of hypertension. Laboratory investigations, including coagulation parameters, revealed no abnormalities.

Neurological examination showed impaired consciousness, with no anisocoria. She localized painful stimuli with the left extremities, whereas no movement was detected on the right side. There was no eye opening in response to verbal or painful stimuli (GKS 7).

An emergent brain CT demonstrated a 48 mm × 75 mm intraparenchymal hematoma in the left temporal and insular lobes, with a 16 mm midline shift to the right, as well as multiple burr hole defects (Figure 1).

CT angiography revealed reduced calibers of the bilateral internal carotid arteries, along with prominent revascularization at the hematoma base and contralateral hemisphere. No aneurysms were identified (Figure 2).

According to the history obtained from her husband, the patient had experienced a hemorrhagic stroke 15 years earlier, at which time MR angiography had confirmed the diagnosis of MMD, and she underwent multiple burr hole surgery (Figures 3 and 4).

She had remained free of ischemic or hemorrhagic stroke for 15 years and had no comorbidities, including hypertension, except for Sjögren's syndrome. Two years after the revascularization surgery performed 15 years ago, the patient was diagnosed with Sjögren's syndrome following rheumatologic assessment for complaints of dry eyes and mouth. She was managed with symptomatic therapy, and her medical history indicated no evidence of disease progression.

The patient's husband was informed, and written consent was obtained. The patient underwent a fronto-temporo-parietal skin incision, followed by the creation of an 8 cm × 6 cm craniotomy flap. Adhesions between the galea and dura from the previous revascularization were carefully dissected. Evacuation of the intraparenchymal hematoma exposed an area of atypical vascularization at its base, from which tissue samples were obtained for pathological analysis. The patient was subsequently transferred to the postoperative intensive care unit. In the postoperative period, the patient showed a favorable response to antihypertensive therapy with an angiotensin II blocker, diuretic, and calcium channel blocker, regaining consciousness and cooperative ability 34 h after surgery. Following a three-day stay in the intensive care unit, she was moved to the neurosurgery ward.

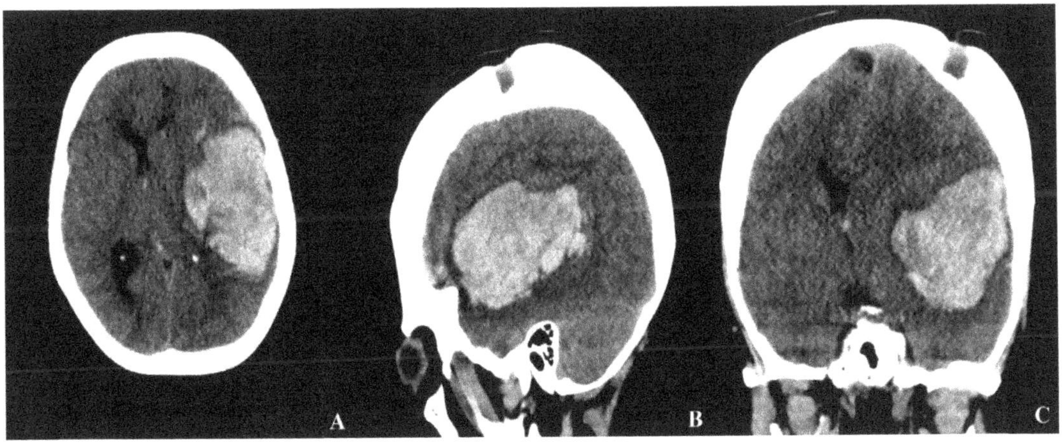

Figure 1. Initial brain CT obtained at the patient's presentation to the emergency department ((**A**) axial, (**B**) sagittal, (**C**) coronal view). The scan demonstrates a large intraparenchymal hematoma in the left temporal and insular lobes, accompanied by a significant midline shift to the right and mass effect with compression of the adjacent ventricular structures. Multiple burr hole defects from the previous revascularization procedure are also visible.

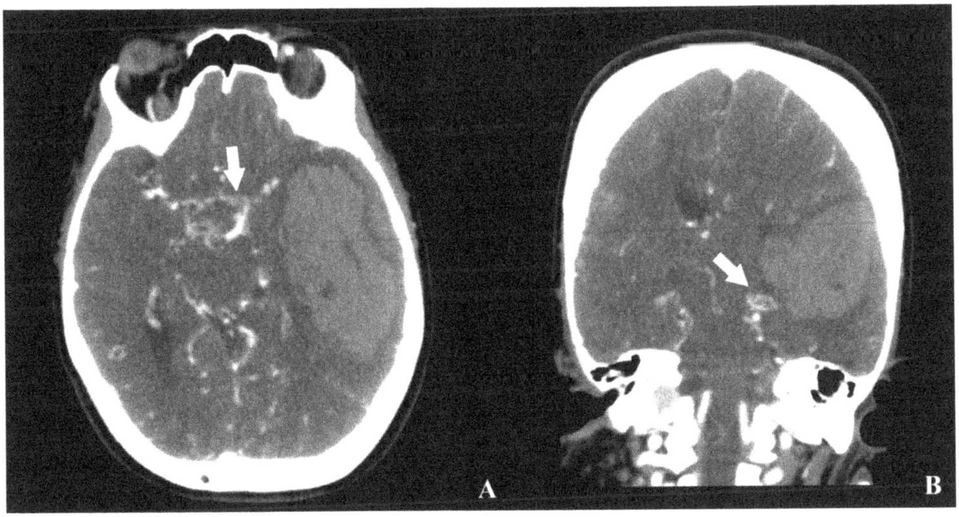

Figure 2. Preoperative brain CTA of the patient ((**A**) axial, (**B**) coronal, white arrow: revascularized region adjacent to the hemorrhage).

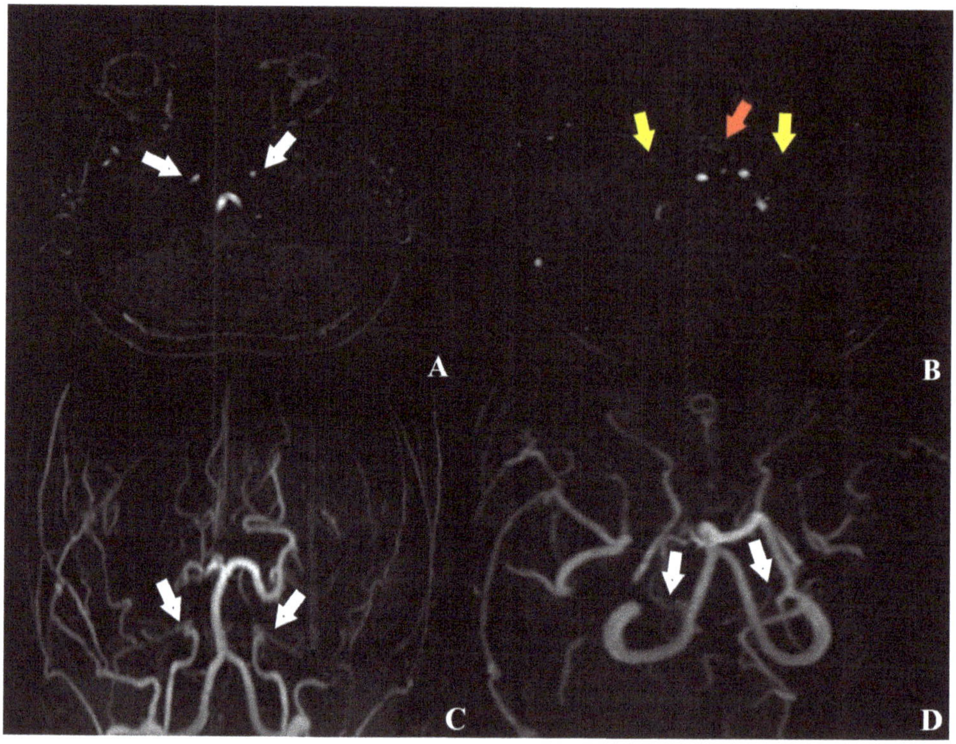

Figure 3. Pre-revascularization MR angiography obtained 15 years earlier ((**A**,**B**) axial planes; (**C**,**D**) 3D reconstructions). White arrow: decreased caliber of the internal carotid artery (ICA); yellow arrow: attenuated caliber of the middle cerebral artery (MCA); red arrow: reduced diameter of the anterior cerebral artery (ACA).

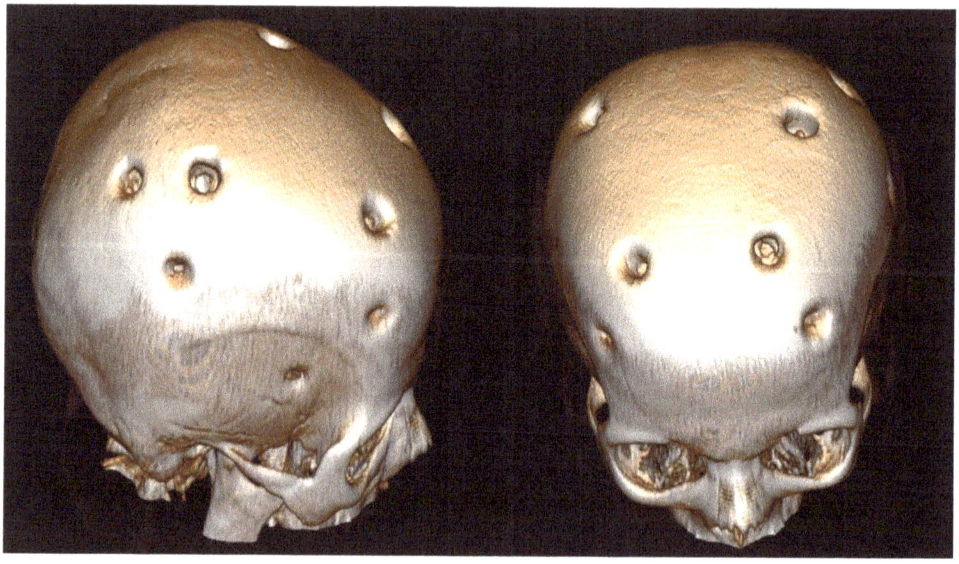

Figure 4. Three-dimensional brain CT reconstruction obtained 15 years after indirect revascularization, demonstrating the patient's appearance following the multiple burr hole (MBH) procedure.

During her ward stay, the patient developed diabetes insipidus, which was well-controlled with desmopressin therapy. Control CT and MRI obtained on postoperative day 7 demonstrated resolution of the midline shift and a decrease in cerebral edema compared with the preoperative findings (Figure 5). Histopathological evaluation revealed no evidence of vascular malformations.

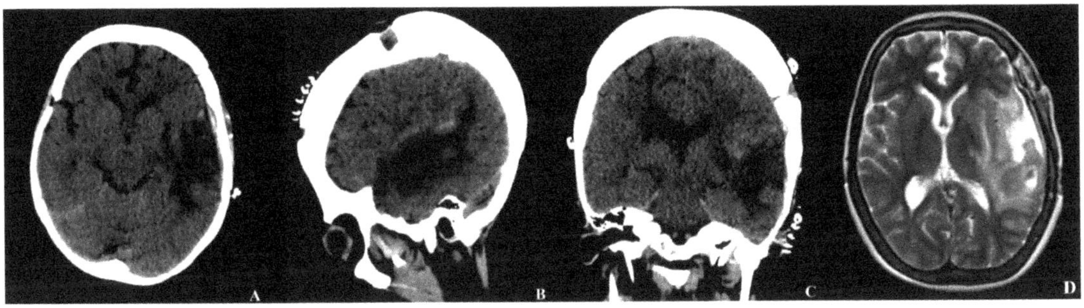

Figure 5. Brain CT and MRI obtained on the seventh postoperative day ((**A**) axial, (**B**) sagittal, (**C**) coronal view, (**D**) axial T2-weighted image). The postoperative CT demonstrates resolution of the previously observed midline shift and a marked decrease in perilesional cerebral edema. No new hemorrhage or ischemic changes are evident. The corresponding MRI sequences confirm a reduction in the mass effect, an improvement in ventricular compression, and postoperative changes consistent with hematoma evacuation.

At the time of discharge, the patient was maintained on antihypertensive therapy, including an angiotensin II receptor blocker, a diuretic, and a calcium channel blocker, with stable blood pressure. He was alert but exhibited motor aphasia, with right upper limb strength graded 2/5 and right lower limb strength 3/5 (mRS 3). He was discharged to continue physical therapy and rehabilitation.

3. Discussion

MMD impacts both children and adults, with clinical presentation ranging from cerebral ischemia and infarction to hemorrhagic lesions. Common manifestations include impaired cognition, migraine-type headaches, epileptic episodes, and motor disturbances such as abnormal contractions, muscular rigidity, and cramps [1,8–10]. In clinical series of MMD, the prevalence of ischemic stroke ranges from 50–75%, transient ischemic attacks from 50–75%, and intracranial hemorrhage from 10–40% [1]. In adult patients with MMD, enlargement and atypical branching of the anterior choroidal artery and/or posterior communicating artery serve as significant predictors of hemorrhagic episodes [11].

The etiology and mechanisms underlying MMD remain poorly understood. In the absence of an identifiable cause, it is considered an idiopathic disorder. Nevertheless, recent research has focused on clarifying potential genetic and immunological contributors.

MMD, previously regarded as a predominant genetic disorder, has also been linked to autoimmune mechanisms. A competitive endogenous RNA network centered on the long non-coding RNA MALAT1 was identified, involving 15 key mRNA targets. Immune profiling showed increased microvascular endothelial cells and reduced CD4+ memory and regulatory T cells, with MALAT1-associated gene expression correlating positively with endothelial changes and inversely with T-cell subsets. These findings indicate MALAT1 as a potential biomarker and therapeutic target in MMD [12].

MMD is most strongly linked to genetic alterations in RNF213, a founder mutation predominantly observed in East Asian populations. Emerging evidence demonstrates that RNF213 variants are also overrepresented in non-moyamoya intracranial vasculopathies, including large-artery atherosclerotic stroke and intracranial arterial stenosis or occlusion, particularly among East Asian individuals with early-onset or cryptogenic stroke [13]. Investigations of the RNF213 Arg4810Lys mutation have revealed that it disrupts angiogenic signaling, endothelial function, vascular remodeling, and immune regulation, effects worsened by stressors such as hypoxia and inflammation, and is implicated in MMD, intracranial stenosis, ischemic stroke, and atherosclerosis [7].

A ceRNA regulatory network was established to explore potential therapeutic targets in MMD, leading to the identification of AKT1, CLDN3, ISG20, and TGFB2 as critical hypoxia-immune–related genes implicated in disease mechanisms. These genes are believed to contribute to MMD pathogenesis through their involvement in processes such as epithelial–mesenchymal transition, angiogenic signaling, and cellular adhesion. Elucidating the function of hypoxia-immune genes in MMD not only provides insight into possible pathogenic mechanisms but also paves the way for novel diagnostic strategies and targeted therapeutic interventions [14].

Although the exact cause of MMD remains unclear, evidence indicates that immune dysregulation, alongside genetic predisposition, plays a key role. T and B lymphocytes, macrophages, and dendritic cells contribute to inflammation and vascular remodeling, promoting arterial stenosis and ischemic risk. Genetic and environmental factors influence immune activation, linking immune responses to disease progression. Targeting these pathways may offer therapeutic potential, but further research is needed to clarify mechanisms and optimize treatments [15].

Complement C3 levels are typically reduced in patients with MMD and show a further decline in the advanced stages as defined by Suzuki grading. Factors such as age, diastolic blood pressure, and circulating complement C3 levels have been associated with the progression of vasculopathy, supporting the hypothesis that the complement system may contribute to the pathogenesis of MMD [16].

Reports of MMD occurring in association with multiple sclerosis (MS) are rare, largely due to overlapping clinical features between the two conditions [17]. Although the characteristic angiographic findings enable the diagnosis of MMD, they do not exclude the possibility of concomitant central nervous system disorders. Without careful assessment of the clinical and neuroradiological profile, this coexistence may easily be overlooked. Therefore, in MMD patients presenting with atypical MRI lesions, cerebrospinal fluid analysis and spinal cord imaging are recommended to evaluate for potential accompanying pathologies [18].

In the differential diagnosis of MMD, it is important to consider conditions such as autoimmune disorders (e.g., Sjögren's syndrome), meningitis, intracranial neoplasms, Down syndrome, Neurofibromatosis type 1, post-radiation cerebrovascular lesions, sickle cell disease, migraine, and atherosclerosis. Moreover, clinicians should remain aware that these conditions may coexist with MMD, potentially complicating the clinical and radiological assessment [19–24].

Digital subtraction angiography (DSA) remains the gold standard in diagnosing MMD. Owing to its superior spatial and temporal resolution, it is invaluable for evaluating stenosis or occlusion of the terminal internal cerebral artery (ICA) and the patency of collateral pathways. Additionally, DSA provides the most reliable means of visualizing collateral vessel development, which is essential for guiding therapeutic decisions and monitoring postoperative neoangiogenesis [25–27]. It is also a straightforward, efficacious, and safe approach when applied for the selective embolization of ruptured aneurysms arising within Moyamoya collateral vessels [28].

Computed tomography angiography (CTA) enables clear visualization of the circle of Willis as well as the anterior, middle, and posterior cerebral arteries and their main branches, offering a valuable diagnostic tool for detecting occlusive vascular pathology. Owing to its rapid acquisition and fast image reconstruction, CTA is often the preferred modality in emergency settings [29]. Computed tomography perfusion (CTP) is commonly utilized as the primary modality for evaluating postoperative cerebral hemodynamic alterations, owing to its rapid acquisition and superior spatial resolution [30].

Magnetic resonance angiography (MRA) provides a noninvasive and radiation-free alternative to DSA and CTA for evaluating bypass patency and allows assessment of arterial diameter to predict the formation of surgical collaterals [31]. Among available methods, 3D time-of-flight (TOF) MRA is the most frequently employed for cerebral vascular imaging, owing to its high spatial resolution, favorable signal-to-noise ratio, and capability of generating very thin slices. Nonetheless, TOF-MRA has demonstrated limitations compared with CTA, including reduced accuracy in visualizing trephination bypass segments and the tendency to overestimate focal pseudo-occlusive changes in this region [32]. Intracranial vessel wall imaging (IVWI) serves as a complementary technique to conventional MRA and holds significant promise for the morphological evaluation of revascularization in MMD. High-resolution MRI–based IVWI is valuable in distinguishing MMD from intracranial atherosclerotic stenosis [33,34]. In addition, preoperative assessments suggest that IVWI may act as a predictive marker for postoperative stroke within the affected vascular territory following revascularization [35]. The "Ivy sign," characterized by leptomeningeal hyperintensity on fluid-attenuated inversion recovery MRI (FLAIR-MRI), is considered a distinctive radiological marker of MMD, reflecting sluggish flow within dilated pial vessels supplying leptomeningeal collaterals and regions of compromised perfusion [36]. Clinical studies have demonstrated that regression of the "ivy sign" on postoperative FLAIR-MRI correlates with improved cerebral hemodynamics and symptomatic relief, whereas the emergence of a new "ivy sign" may serve as an early indicator of postoperative cerebral hyperperfusion syndrome [37].

Blood oxygen level–dependent functional MRI (BOLD-fMRI) is a neuroimaging modality that exploits deoxyhemoglobin within cerebral vessels as an intrinsic contrast mechanism to generate functional activation maps. It is extensively applied to evaluate cerebrovascular reserve, alterations in neurovascular coupling, and to determine the effectiveness of surgical revascularization [38–40]. BOLD-fMRI also shows promise as a standardized tool for both pre- and postoperative assessment of MMD patients, particularly in the pediatric population. Nonetheless, enhancing the reliability and reproducibility of BOLD imaging remains a significant challenge in clinical practice [29].

Single-photon emission computed tomography (SPECT) is regarded as the gold standard for evaluating cerebral perfusion [41]. Reduced cerebrovascular reserve, detected either at baseline or following acetazolamide stimulation in postoperative MMD patients, is associated with an unfavorable prognosis, including ongoing neurological deficits and recurrent ischemic events [42]. Furthermore, alterations in cerebral blood flow measured by SPECT have been linked to cognitive recovery in both adult and pediatric populations with MMD [43].

Positron emission tomography (PET) is regarded as the reference functional imaging modality for evaluating metabolic processes associated with vascular function in MMD patients following bypass surgery [29]. Literature evidence suggests that PET provides more precise assessments for carefully selected patients who are most likely to derive benefit from surgical intervention [44–46]. Nonetheless, its widespread clinical application is constrained by limited availability, high cost, and prolonged acquisition times [29].

A novel scoring system, the MRI-Based Assessment of Risk for Stroke in Moyamoya Angiopathy (MARS-MMA), was created to evaluate hemodynamic status in patients with Moyamoya prior to revascularization and was compared with DSA and PET imaging. The

MARS-MMA score demonstrated a strong correlation with cerebral perfusion reserve. This fully MRI-based scoring system represents a potentially valuable tool for predicting stroke risk in MMD patients [47].

Suzuki and Takaku proposed a grading system for MMD based on angiographic findings, outlining the progressive stages of vascular changes. In Grade I, there is initial narrowing at the internal carotid artery (ICA) apex. Grade II is characterized by the emergence of moyamoya collateral networks, while Grade III reflects further stenosis of the ICA accompanied by intensification of these abnormal collateral vessels. In Grade IV, collateral circulation begins to develop from the external carotid artery (ECA). Grade V demonstrates prominent ECA collateral formation alongside regression of moyamoya-related vessels. Finally, Grade VI represents complete occlusion of the ICA with the disappearance of moyamoya collaterals. This staging system provides a structured framework for evaluating disease progression and guiding clinical management [48].

In the surgical management of MMD, the ECA commonly serves as the donor source for augmenting blood supply to the ischemic cerebral hemisphere. Revascularization can be achieved through either direct or indirect approaches. In direct bypass, a branch of the ECA is surgically anastomosed to a cortical artery, thereby providing immediate blood flow augmentation. In contrast, indirect techniques involve placing vascularized tissue supplied by the ECA in contact with the brain surface, stimulating angiogenesis and the subsequent penetration of new vessels into the underlying cerebral cortex [1].

Another investigation reported that the combined revascularization strategy offers the advantage of direct anastomosis, ensuring an immediate increase in cerebral blood flow, while simultaneously promoting the gradual development of indirect collateral circulation. Nonetheless, it has been proposed that patients presenting with stenosis of the ICA or middle cerebral artery (MCA), but without complete occlusion, may be more suitable candidates for indirect bypass, as an immediate augmentation of blood supply is not essential in this subgroup [49].

A review of the literature highlights multiple studies comparing the outcomes of direct and indirect revascularization techniques. A systematic analysis demonstrated that postoperative stroke incidence following direct or combined bypass is comparable to that observed after indirect procedures [50].

In a cohort study involving 559 patients with MMD who underwent direct, indirect, or combined revascularization, a prior history of intracranial hemorrhage was identified as a predictor of postoperative hemorrhagic stroke. Moreover, comorbid conditions such as hypertension and diabetes were recognized as risk factors for postoperative ischemic stroke [51–53].

The periventricular anastomosis theory has been proposed to explain the hemorrhagic mechanism in MMD. Although direct bypass reduces the risk of intracranial bleeding, a modified approach termed "personalized targeting bypass" aims specifically at hemorrhage prevention by using multimodal imaging to select the target vessel at the site of medullary artery extension from the periventricular anastomosis. In a series of eight patients, marked postoperative stenosis of the targeted anastomosis was achieved, and no recurrent hemorrhage was observed during follow-up [54]. Moreover, five days of postoperative bed rest following direct bypass markedly lowered the risk of intracerebral hemorrhage and neurological decline [55].

Revascularization surgery has been shown to decrease the formation of moyamoya collateral vessels, thereby more effectively reducing the risk of hemorrhage compared with conservative management. In adult patients with MMD, direct bypass is particularly crucial for preventing rebleeding, as indirect techniques demonstrate lower efficacy than in pediatric cases [56]. Nevertheless, certain reports have suggested the presence of hemorrhagic complications following direct or indirect revascularization procedures in both the early and late postoperative periods. In addition, although these techniques have demonstrated efficacy in decreasing ischemic events related to MMD, they do not appear to increase the incidence of postoperative hemorrhage, and additional research is warranted to clarify the potential risk factors [57].

In a study evaluating the impact of hypertension on recurrent hemorrhage and long-term survival in patients with hemorrhagic MMD treated with indirect revascularization, strict blood pressure management was shown to markedly reduce hematoma recurrence but did not affect overall survival. These findings suggest that blood pressure optimization alone is insufficient in the management of hypertensive patients with hemorrhagic MMD [58,59].

The multiple burr holes (MBH) approach provides several benefits compared to craniotomy, such as reduced operative duration, lower intraoperative blood loss, fewer post-operative adverse events, and similar perfusion as well as functional results. In addition, MBH represents a safe and effective option for anterior cerebral artery revascularization in pediatric MMD patients [60]. Another investigation demonstrated that the MBH method could lower the likelihood of recurrent cerebrovascular events and decrease the incidence of pseudomeningocele [61]. The adjunctive use of erythropoietin (EPO) with the MBH procedure has been reported to decrease the incidence of long-term cerebrovascular events in MMS patients following either hemorrhagic or ischemic stroke [62].

Although reports of delayed intracerebral hemorrhage following direct or indirect revascularization are uncommon [63–65], our case involved hemorrhage occurring 15 years after indirect revascularization. This rare occurrence is examined in the context of existing literature.

In limitation, this study is constrained by its single-case design, which precludes generalization to broader patient populations. Genetic analysis, particularly regarding RNF213 or other susceptibility loci, was not performed, limiting insights into potential hereditary contributions. Advanced hemodynamic and functional imaging modalities, such as SPECT, PET, or BOLD-fMRI, were not obtained because the patient required urgent intervention, and only emergent CT angiography was performed. Detailed longitudinal neurocognitive and functional assessments were also unavailable, restricting evaluation of recovery beyond motor outcomes. Finally, given the rarity of delayed hemorrhage after indirect revascularization, further accumulation of similar cases and multicenter analyses are necessary to better understand risk factors and optimize long-term management strategies in MMD.

4. Conclusions

MMD is an intracerebral vasculopathy that may present with either hemorrhagic or ischemic stroke. Although genetic and immunological factors have been implicated in its etiology, the precise underlying cause remains unknown. Therapeutic options with conservative management are limited, and both direct and indirect revascularization procedures are generally recommended. Nevertheless, recurrent ischemic or hemorrhagic events may occur following revascularization surgery. In this report, we present a rare case of hemorrhagic stroke occurring 15 years after indirect revascularization and discuss the diagnosis, etiology, and postoperative complications of MMD in light of the current literature. Importantly, long-term follow-up should include monitoring of collateral vessel remodeling, the hemodynamic reserve, episodic hypertension, and the presence of coexisting autoimmune conditions such as Sjögren's syndrome, as these factors may influence the risk of delayed hemorrhage and guide optimal patient management.

Author Contributions: Conceptualization M.C.Y. and K.A.; methodology, M.C.Y.; software, M.C.Y.; validation, M.C.Y.; formal analysis, M.C.Y. and K.A.; investigation, M.C.Y. and K.A.; resources, M.C.Y.; data curation, M.C.Y.; writing—original draft preparation, M.C.Y. and K.A.; writing—review and editing, M.C.Y. and K.A.; visualization, M.C.Y.; supervision, M.C.Y.; project administration, M.C.Y. All authors have read and agreed to the published version of the manuscript.

Funding: This research received no external funding.

Institutional Review Board Statement: This study is a retrospective case report and does not involve any clinical trial or experimental procedure, we confirm that ethical approval from an institutional review board is not required.

Informed Consent Statement: All data used in the study were obtained with written informed consent from the patient and their family, in full compliance with ethical standards and privacy regulations.

Data Availability Statement: The data presented in this study are available on request from the corresponding author due to the inclusion of personal radiological information in the case report.

Conflicts of Interest: The authors declare no conflicts of interest.

Abbreviations

The following abbreviations are used in this manuscript:

MMD	Moyamoya disease
CTA	Computed tomography angiography
MRA	Magnetic resonance angiography
DSA	Digital subtraction angiography
GKS	Glasgow coma scale
mRS	Modified Rankin scale
TOF	Time of flight
FLAİR	Fluid-attenuated inversion recovery
IVWI	Intracranial vessel wall imaging
CTP	Computed tomography perfusion
BOLD-fMRI	Blood oxygen level–dependent functional MRI
SPECT	Single-photon emission computed tomography
PET	Positron emission tomography
MARS-MMA	MRI-Based Assessment of Risk for Stroke in Moyamoya Angiopathy
MBHs	Multiple burr holes

References

1. Scott, R.M.; Smith, E.R. Moyamoya disease and moyamoya syndrome. *N. Engl. J. Med.* **2009**, *360*, 1226–1237. [CrossRef]
2. Kuroda, S.; Houkin, K. Moyamoya disease: Current concepts and future perspectives. *Lancet Neurol.* **2008**, *7*, 1056–1066. [CrossRef]
3. Suzuki, J.; Kodama, N. Moyamoya disease–A review. *Stroke* **1983**, *14*, 104–109. [CrossRef]
4. Baba, T.; Houkin, K.; Kuroda, S. Novel epidemiological features of moyamoya disease. *J. Neurol. Neurosurg. Psychiatry* **2008**, *79*, 900–904. [CrossRef]
5. Wakai, K.; Tamakoshi, A.; Ikezaki, K.; Fukui, M.; Kawamura, T.; Aoki, R.; Kojima, M.; Lin, Y.; Ohno, Y. Epidemiological features of moyamoya disease in Japan: Findings from a nationwide survey. *Clin. Neurol. Neurosurg.* **1997**, *99*, S1–S5. [CrossRef] [PubMed]
6. Yonekawa, Y.; Ogata, N.; Kaku, Y.; Taub, E.; Imhof, H.-G. Moyamoya disease in Europe, past and present status. *Clin. Neurol. Neurosurg.* **1997**, *99*, S58–S60. [CrossRef] [PubMed]
7. Bagyinszky, E.; Yang, Y.; An, S.S.A. Multisystemic Impact of RNF213 Arg4810Lys: A Comprehensive Review of Moyamoya Disease and Associated Vasculopathies. *Int. J. Mol. Sci.* **2025**, *26*, 7864. [CrossRef] [PubMed]
8. Chen, S.T.; Liu, Y.H.; Hsu, C.Y.; Hogan, E.L.; Ryu, S.J. Moyamoya disease in Taiwan. *Stroke* **1988**, *19*, 53–59. [CrossRef]
9. Kraemer, M.; Trakolis, L.; Platzen, J.; Schwitalla, J.C.; Bersano, A.; Albrecht, P.; Schlamann, M.; Berlit, P. Movement symptoms in European Moyamoya angiopathy—First systematic questionnaire study. *Clin. Neurol. Neurosurg.* **2017**, *152*, 52–56. [CrossRef]

10. Viteva, E.; Vasilev, P.; Vasilev, G.; Chompalov, K. Clinical Case of a 23-Year-Old Patient with Moyamoya Disease and Epilepsy in Bulgaria. *Neurol. Int.* **2024**, *16*, 869–879. [CrossRef]
11. Morioka, M.; Hamada, J.-I.; Kawano, T.; Todaka, T.; Yano, S.; Kai, Y.; Ushio, Y. Angiographic dilatation and branch extension of the anterior choroidal and posterior communicating arteries are predictors of hemorrhage in adult moyamoya patients. *Stroke* **2003**, *34*, 90–95. [CrossRef]
12. Liu, W.; Fu, H.; Fang, S.; Ni, J.; Peng, B. Construction and Analysis of Immune Infiltration and Competing Endogenous RNA Network in Moyamoya Disease. *Int. J. Mol. Sci.* **2025**, *26*, 7957. [CrossRef]
13. Yoshimoto, T.; Okune, S.; Tanaka, S.; Yamagami, H.; Matsumaru, Y. RNF213-Related Vasculopathy: An Entity with Diverse Phenotypic Expressions. *Genes* **2025**, *16*, 939. [CrossRef]
14. Tan, C.; Wang, X.; Zhou, Z.; Liu, Y.; He, S.; Zhao, Y. A Machine Learning-Based Diagnostic Nomogram for Moyamoya Disease: The Validation of Hypoxia-Immune Gene Signatures. *Bioengineering* **2025**, *12*, 577. [CrossRef] [PubMed]
15. Wang, S.; Jiang, Q.; Liu, Y.; Zhang, X.; Huang, Y.; Zhang, H. The Role of Immune Cells in Moyamoya Disease. *Brain Sci.* **2025**, *15*, 137. [CrossRef] [PubMed]
16. Wang, M.-J.; Wang, J.; Zhang, H.; Hao, F.-B.; Gao, G.; Liu, S.-M.; Wang, X.-P.; Li, J.-J.; Zou, Z.-X.; Guo, Q.-B. High level of serum complement C3 expression is associated with postoperative vasculopathy progression in moyamoya disease. *J. Inflamm. Res.* **2024**, *2024*, 1721–1733. [CrossRef]
17. Si, X.; Li, L.; Fang, Y.; Yan, Y.; Pu, J. A patient with multiple sclerosis and coexisting Moyamoya disease: Why and how. *Front. Neurol.* **2020**, *11*, 516587. [CrossRef]
18. Canavero, I.; Rifino, N.; Antozzi, C.; Caldiera, V.; Colombo, E.; Carrozzini, T.; Ganci, G.; Ferroli, P.; Acerbi, F.; Storti, B. Blurred by a "Puff of Smoke"—A Case-Based Review on the Challenging Recognition of Coexisting CNS Demyelinating Disease and Moyamoya Angiopathy. *Int. J. Mol. Sci.* **2025**, *26*, 5030. [CrossRef]
19. Tominaga, T.; Suzuki, N.; Miyamoto, S.; Koizumi, A. Recommendations for the management of moyamoya disease: A statement from research committee on spontaneous occlusion of the circle of Willis (moyamoya disease). *Surg. Cereb. Stroke* **2018**, *46*, 1–24. [CrossRef]
20. Karsonovich, T.; Lui, F. Moyamoya Disease. In *StatPearls*; StatPearls Publishing LLC.: Treasure Island, FL, USA, 2025.
21. Zedde, M.; Quaresima, M.; Capodanno, I.; Grisendi, I.; Assenza, F.; Napoli, M.; Moratti, C.; Pavone, C.; Bonacini, L.; Di Cecco, G. Neurovascular manifestations of sickle cell disease. *Hemato* **2024**, *5*, 277–320. [CrossRef]
22. Lehman, L.L.; Ullrich, N.J. Cerebral vasculopathy in children with neurofibromatosis type 1. *Cancers* **2023**, *15*, 5111. [CrossRef]
23. Matsuki, Y.; Kawakami, M.; Ishizuka, T.; Kawaguchi, Y.; Hidaka, T.; Suzuki, K.; Nakamura, H. SLE and Sjögren's syndrome associated with unilateral moyamoya vessels in cerebral arteries. *Scand. J. Rheumatol.* **1997**, *26*, 392–394. [CrossRef]
24. Asai, Y.; Nakayasu, H.; Fusayasu, E.; Nakashima, K. Moyamoya disease presenting as thalamic hemorrhage in a patient with neuromyelitis optica and Sjögren's syndrome. *J. Stroke Cerebrovasc. Dis.* **2012**, *21*, 619.e7–619.e9. [CrossRef]
25. Ge, P.; Zhang, Q.; Ye, X.; Liu, X.; Deng, X.; Wang, J.; Wang, R.; Zhang, Y.; Zhang, D.; Zhao, J.Z. Digital subtraction angiographic characteristics of progression of moyamoya disease 6 months prior to surgical revascularisation. *Stroke Vasc. Neurol.* **2020**, *5*, 97–102. [CrossRef]
26. Ge, P.; Zhang, Q.; Ye, X.; Liu, X.; Deng, X.; Wang, J.; Wang, R.; Zhang, Y.; Zhang, D.; Zhao, J. Postoperative collateral formation after indirect bypass for hemorrhagic moyamoya disease. *BMC Neurol.* **2020**, *20*, 28. [CrossRef] [PubMed]
27. Fukui, M. Guidelines for the diagnosis and treatment of spontaneous occlusion of the circle of Willis ('moyamoya' disease). Research Committee on Spontaneous Occlusion of the Circle of Willis (Moyamoya Disease) of the Ministry of Health and Welfare, Japan. *Clin. Neurol. Neurosurg.* **1997**, *99*, S238–S240. [CrossRef]
28. Ryška, P.; Lojík, M.; Habalová, J.; Kajzrová, C.; Česák, T.; Vítková, E.; Bartoš, M.; Bělobrádek, Z.; Krajina, A. Endovascular Therapy of Ruptured Aneurysms on Moyamoya Collateral Vessels: Two Cases. *Medicina* **2024**, *60*, 1499. [CrossRef] [PubMed]
29. Du, L.; Jiang, H.; Li, J.; Duan, T.; Zhou, C.; Yan, F. Imaging methods for surgical revascularization in patients with moyamoya disease: An updated review. *Neurosurg. Rev.* **2022**, *45*, 343–356. [CrossRef]
30. Chen, Y.; Xu, W.; Guo, X.; Shi, Z.; Sun, Z.; Gao, L.; Jin, F.; Wang, J.; Chen, W.; Yang, Y. CT perfusion assessment of Moyamoya syndrome before and after direct revascularization (superficial temporal artery to middle cerebral artery bypass). *Eur. Radiol.* **2016**, *26*, 254–261. [CrossRef]
31. Uchino, H.; Yamamoto, S.; Kashiwazaki, D.; Akioka, N.; Kuwayama, N.; Noguchi, K.; Kuroda, S. Using postoperative remodeling of donor arteries on MR angiography to predict the development of surgical collaterals in moyamoya disease. *J. Neurosurg.* **2019**, *134*, 1–9. [CrossRef] [PubMed]
32. Chen, Q.; Qi, R.; Cheng, X.; Zhou, C.; Luo, S.; Ni, L.; Huang, W. Assessment of extracranial-intracranial bypass in Moyamoya disease using 3T time-of-flight MR angiography: Comparison with CT angiography. *Vasa* **2014**, *43*, 278–283. [CrossRef]
33. Ryoo, S.; Cha, J.; Kim, S.J.; Choi, J.W.; Ki, C.-S.; Kim, K.H.; Jeon, P.; Kim, J.-S.; Hong, S.-C.; Bang, O.Y. High-resolution magnetic resonance wall imaging findings of Moyamoya disease. *Stroke* **2014**, *45*, 2457–2460. [CrossRef]

34. Ya, J.; Zhou, D.; Ding, J.; Ding, Y.; Ji, X.; Yang, Q.; Meng, R. High-resolution combined arterial spin labeling MR for identifying cerebral arterial stenosis induced by moyamoya disease or atherosclerosis. *Ann. Transl. Med.* **2020**, *8*, 87. [CrossRef]
35. Haas, P.; Hauser, T.-K.; Wiggenhauser, L.M.; Zerweck, L.; Tatagiba, M.; Khan, N.; Roder, C. Coincidence of Concentric Vessel-Wall Contrast Enhancement in Moyamoya Disease and Acute Postoperative Ischemic Stroke During Revascularization Procedures. *Brain Sci.* **2024**, *14*, 1190. [CrossRef]
36. Kaku, Y.; Iihara, K.; Nakajima, N.; Kataoka, H.; Fukushima, K.; Iida, H.; Hashimoto, N. The leptomeningeal ivy sign on fluid-attenuated inversion recovery images in moyamoya disease: Positron emission tomography study. *Cerebrovasc. Dis.* **2013**, *36*, 19–25. [CrossRef]
37. Horie, N.; Morikawa, M.; Morofuji, Y.; Hiu, T.; Izumo, T.; Hayashi, K.; Nagata, I. De novo ivy sign indicates postoperative hyperperfusion in moyamoya disease. *Stroke* **2014**, *45*, 1488–1491. [CrossRef]
38. Sam, K.; Poublanc, J.; Sobczyk, O.; Han, J.S.; Battisti-Charbonney, A.; Mandell, D.M.; Tymianski, M.; Crawley, A.P.; Fisher, J.A.; Mikulis, D.J. Assessing the effect of unilateral cerebral revascularisation on the vascular reactivity of the non-intervened hemisphere: A retrospective observational study. *BMJ Open* **2015**, *5*, e006014. [CrossRef]
39. Garbani Nerini, L.; Bellomo, J.; Höbner, L.M.; Stumpo, V.; Colombo, E.; van Niftrik, C.H.B.; Schubert, T.; Kulcsár, Z.; Wegener, S.; Luft, A. BOLD cerebrovascular reactivity and NOVA quantitative MR angiography in adult patients with moyamoya vasculopathy undergoing cerebral bypass surgery. *Brain Sci.* **2024**, *14*, 762. [CrossRef] [PubMed]
40. Sebök, M. BOLD Cerebrovascular Reactivity as a Novel Marker for Hemodynamic Impairment in Symptomatic Cerebrovascular Steno-Occlusive Disease. Ph.D. Thesis, University of Zurich, Zurich, Switzerland, 2022.
41. Setta, K.; Kojima, D.; Shimada, Y.; Yoshida, J.; Oshida, S.; Fujimoto, K.; Tsutsui, S.; Chiba, T.; Fujiwara, S.; Terasaki, K. Accuracy of brain perfusion single-photon emission computed tomography for detecting misery perfusion in adult patients with symptomatic ischemic moyamoya disease. *Ann. Nucl. Med.* **2018**, *32*, 611–619. [CrossRef] [PubMed]
42. So, Y.; Lee, H.-Y.; Kim, S.-K.; Lee, J.S.; Wang, K.-C.; Cho, B.-K.; Kang, E.; Lee, D.S. Prediction of the clinical outcome of pediatric moyamoya disease with postoperative basal/acetazolamide stress brain perfusion SPECT after revascularization surgery. *Stroke* **2005**, *36*, 1485–1489. [CrossRef] [PubMed]
43. Kazumata, K.; Tokairin, K.; Sugiyama, T.; Ito, M.; Uchino, H.; Osanai, T.; Kawabori, M.; Nakayama, N.; Houkin, K. Association of cognitive function with cerebral blood flow in children with moyamoya disease. *J. Neurosurg. Pediatr.* **2019**, *25*, 62–68. [CrossRef]
44. Ikezaki, K.; Matsushima, T.; Kuwabara, Y.; Suzuki, S.O.; Nomura, T.; Fukui, M. Cerebral circulation and oxygen metabolism in childhood moyamoya disease: A perioperative positron emission tomography study. *J. Neurosurg.* **1994**, *81*, 843–850. [CrossRef] [PubMed]
45. Hara, S.; Kudo, T.; Hayashi, S.; Inaji, M.; Tanaka, Y.; Maehara, T.; Ishii, K.; Nariai, T. Improvement in cognitive decline after indirect bypass surgery in adult moyamoya disease: Implication of 15 O-gas positron emission tomography. *Ann. Nucl. Med.* **2020**, *34*, 467–475. [CrossRef]
46. Roder, C.; Haas, P.; Fudali, M.; Milian, M.; Ernemann, U.; Meyer, P.T.; Tatagiba, M.; Khan, N. Neuropsychological impairment in adults with moyamoya angiopathy: Preoperative assessment and correlation to MRI and H215O PET. *Neurosurg. Rev.* **2020**, *43*, 1615–1622. [CrossRef]
47. Zerweck, L.; Roder, C.; Blazhenets, G.; Martus, P.; Thurow, J.; Haas, P.; Estler, A.; Gohla, G.; Ruff, C.; Selo, N. MRI-Based Assessment of Risk for Stroke in Moyamoya Angiopathy (MARS-MMA): An MRI-Based Scoring System for the Severity of Moyamoya Angiopathy. *Diagnostics* **2024**, *14*, 1437. [CrossRef] [PubMed]
48. Suzuki, J.; Takaku, A. Cerebrovascular moyamoya disease: Disease showing abnormal net-like vessels in base of brain. *Arch. Neurol.* **1969**, *20*, 288–299. [CrossRef]
49. Liu, J.J.; Steinberg, G.K. Direct versus indirect bypass for moyamoya disease. *Neurosurg. Clin.* **2017**, *28*, 361–374. [CrossRef]
50. Kazumata, K.; Ito, M.; Tokairin, K.; Ito, Y.; Houkin, K.; Nakayama, N.; Kuroda, S.; Ishikawa, T.; Kamiyama, H. The frequency of postoperative stroke in moyamoya disease following combined revascularization: A single-university series and systematic review. *J. Neurosurg.* **2014**, *121*, 432–440. [CrossRef]
51. Liu, W.; Huang, K.; Zhang, J.; Zhou, D.; Chen, J. Clinical features and risk factors of postoperative stroke in adult moyamoya disease. *Brain Sci.* **2023**, *13*, 1696. [CrossRef]
52. Chen, Y.; Ma, L.; Lu, J.; Chen, X.; Ye, X.; Zhang, D.; Zhang, Y.; Wang, R.; Zhao, Y. Postoperative hemorrhage during the acute phase after direct or combined revascularization for moyamoya disease: Risk factors, prognosis, and literature review. *J. Neurosurg.* **2019**, *133*, 1450–1459. [CrossRef] [PubMed]
53. Tokairin, K.; Kazumata, K.; Uchino, H.; Ito, M.; Ono, K.; Tatezawa, R.; Shindo, T.; Kawabori, M.; Nakayama, N.; Houkin, K. Postoperative intracerebral hemorrhage after combined revascularization surgery in moyamoya disease: Profiles and clinical associations. *World Neurosurg.* **2018**, *120*, e593–e600. [CrossRef]
54. Funaki, T.; Kataoka, H.; Yoshida, K.; Kikuchi, T.; Mineharu, Y.; Okawa, M.; Yamao, Y.; Miyamoto, S. The targeted bypass strategy for preventing hemorrhage in moyamoya disease. *Neurol. Med.-Chir.* **2019**, *59*, 517–522. [CrossRef] [PubMed]

55. Nomura, S.; Kawashima, A.; Ishiguro, T.; Hashimoto, K.; Hodotsuka, K.; Nakamura, A.; Kuwano, A.; Tanaka, Y.; Murakami, M.; Shiono, T. Five-day bed rest reduces postoperative intracerebral hemorrhage after direct bypass for moyamoya disease. *World Neurosurg.* **2022**, *159*, e267–e272. [CrossRef]
56. Houkin, K.; Kamiyama, H.; Abe, H.; Takahashi, A.; Kuroda, S. Surgical therapy for adult moyamoya disease: Can surgical revascularization prevent the recurrence of intracerebral hemorrhage? *Stroke* **1996**, *27*, 1342–1346. [CrossRef]
57. Ryan, R.W.; Chowdhary, A.; Britz, G.W. Hemorrhage and risk of further hemorrhagic strokes following cerebral revascularization in Moyamoya disease: A review of the literature. *Surg. Neurol. Int.* **2012**, *3*, 72. [CrossRef]
58. Guo, Q.; Xie, M.; Ji, H.; Wang, Q.N.; Bao, X.; Duan, L. Long-Term Outcomes in Patients with Hemorrhagic Moyamoya Disease Combined with Hypertension After Encephaloduroarteriosynangiosis. *J. Am. Heart Assoc.* **2025**, *14*, e039054. [CrossRef]
59. Lucia, K.; Acker, G.; Rubarth, K.; Beyaztas, D.; Vajkoczy, P. The development and effect of systemic hypertension on clinical and radiological outcome in adult Moyamoya angiopathy following revascularization surgery: Experience of a single European institution. *J. Clin. Med.* **2023**, *12*, 4219. [CrossRef]
60. Kim, J.W.; Phi, J.H.; Lee, J.Y.; Koh, E.J.; Kim, K.H.; Kim, H.-S.; Kim, S.-K. Comparison of bifrontal craniotomy and multiple burr hole encephalogaleoperiosteal-synangiosis for pediatric moyamoya disease: An experience of 346 patients. *Neurosurgery* **2023**, *93*, 824–834. [CrossRef] [PubMed]
61. Soler-Rico, M.; Di Santo, M.; Vaz, G.; Joris, V.; Fomekong, E.; Guillaume, S.; Van Boven, M.; Raftopoulos, C. How to reduce the complication rate of multiple burr holes surgery in moyamoya angiopathy. *Acta Neurochir.* **2023**, *165*, 3613–3622. [CrossRef] [PubMed]
62. Lee, Y.; Lee, J.S.; Lee, S.-J.; Hong, J.M.; Lim, Y.C. Multiple burr hole and erythropoietin combination therapy: Optimal early surgical intervention for patients with acute stroke episode of moyamoya disease or moyamoya syndrome. *Front. Neurol.* **2024**, *15*, 1479379. [CrossRef]
63. Aoki, N. Cerebrovascular bypass surgery for the treatment of Moyamoya disease: Unsatisfactory outcome in the patients presenting with intracranial hemorrhage. *Surg. Neurol.* **1993**, *40*, 372–377. [CrossRef] [PubMed]
64. Otawara, Y.; Ogasawara, K.; Seki, K.; Kibe, M.; Kubo, Y.; Ogawa, A. Intracerebral hemorrhage after prophylactic revascularization in a patient with adult moyamoya disease. *Surg. Neurol.* **2007**, *68*, 335–337. [CrossRef] [PubMed]
65. Nishimoto, T.; Yuki, K.; Sasaki, T.; Murakami, T.; Kodama, Y.; Kurisu, K. A ruptured middle cerebral artery aneurysm originating from the site of anastomosis 20 years after extracranial-intracranial bypass for moyamoya disease: Case report. *Surg. Neurol.* **2005**, *64*, 261–265. [CrossRef] [PubMed]

brain sciences

MDPI

Brief Report

The Impact of Revascularization Surgery on Headaches in Association with Cerebrovascular Reactivity in Patients with Moyamoya Angiopathy

Francy D. Gallego Moyano [1], Helena C. Janssen [1], Lashmi Venkatraghavan [2], David J. Mikulis [3], Hugo Andrade Barazarte [4], Ivan Radovanovic [4], Eef J. Hendriks [3] and Joanna D. Schaafsma [1,*]

1 Department of Medicine, Division of Neurology, University Health Network (UHN), 399 Bathurst St., Toronto, ON M5T 2S8, Canada; d.gallegomoyano@hotmail.com (F.D.G.M.); helena.janssen@uhn.ca (H.C.J.)
2 Department of Anesthesiology, University Health Network (UHN), Toronto, ON M5T 2S8, Canada; lashmi.venkatraghavan@uhn.ca
3 Division of Neuroradiology, Joint Department of Medical Imaging, University Health Network (UHN), Toronto, ON M5T 2S8, Canada; david.mikulis@uhn.ca (D.J.M.); eef.hendriks@uhn.ca (E.J.H.)
4 Department of Surgery, Division of Neurosurgery, University Health Network (UHN), Toronto, ON M5T 2S8, Canada; hugo.andradebarazarte@uhn.ca (H.A.B.); ivan.radovanovic@uhn.ca (I.R.)
* Correspondence: joanna.schaafsma@uhn.ca

Abstract: Background/Objectives: Headaches in Moyamoya angiopathy are common but poorly understood. We aimed to investigate if headaches in Moyamoya angiopathy improve after revascularization surgery and whether this is associated with improvement in cerebrovascular reactivity on MRI (CVR-MRI). Methods: We included consecutive adult patients with Moyamoya angiopathy who had chart data on headaches, CVR-MRI, and underwent extracranial–intracranial bypass surgery between January 2010 and September 2022 at a tertiary neurovascular referral center. Clinical and CVR-MR imaging data of all patients were collected through systematic chart review, complemented by standard-of-care headache questionnaires from patients who were operated between 2018 and 2022. We evaluated headache features and explored the association between headaches and CVR before and after revascularization surgery. Results: Fifty-nine patients were included (mean age 47 ± 14 years, 43 females (73%)); among them, 41/59 (69%) reported headaches pre-surgery. Headache improved in 28/41 (68%) patients after revascularization surgery with a reduction in pain severity (median VAS-score from 5/10 to 2.5/10; $p = 0.002$), analgesic use (from 84% to 40%; $p = 0.007$), and sick leave (from 60% to 16%; $p < 0.001$). Improvement in headaches was associated with improvement in CVR (OR 5.3; 95% CI: 1.2–23.5) and sick leave reduction (OR 1.4; 95% CI: 1.6–121.4). Conclusions: Headaches in Moyamoya angiopathy are common and disabling. They may improve in most patients after revascularization surgery and seem to be associated with improvement in CVR, supporting the hypothesis of a potential vascular origin of the headaches.

Keywords: moyamoya angiopathy; headaches; hemodynamic; cerebrovascular insufficiency; extracranial intracranial arterial bypass

1. Introduction

Moyamoya angiopathy is characterized by a progressive stenosis of the terminal portion of the internal carotid artery and its main branches with development of compensatory collaterals, so-called Moyamoya vessels [1,2]. Moyamoya angiopathy comprises both Moyamoya disease and Moyamoya syndrome, where the first is idiopathic and the latter occurs in association with another medical condition [2]. Moyamoya angiopathy can cause hemodynamic insufficiency resulting in ischemic stroke and intracranial hemorrhage caused by rupture of frail collaterals, both associated with a high rate of disability and even death [2,3]. Treatment in adults consists of medical management and in selected cases, revascularization surgery through a direct extracranial–intracranial arterial (EC–IC) bypass, with or without an indirect bypass, to prevent ischemic or hemorrhagic stroke [4,5]. To decide on revascularization surgery, an assessment of the hemodynamic status is part of the standard work-up [4,5]. An advanced technique to assess the hemodynamic reserve capacity is blood-oxygenation-level-dependent (BOLD)-MRI in response to carbon dioxide (CO_2), a vasodilatory stimulus. This cerebrovascular reactivity MRI (CVR-MRI) is increasingly being offered to patients with chronic steno-occlusive disease [6,7].

In patients with Moyamoya angiopathy, the clinical focus is on stroke-like symptoms [4,5]. Headaches in Moyamoya patients are common, but limited data are available on their pathophysiology, characteristics, impact on quality of life, and response to revascularization surgery [8].

We aimed to investigate the presence and features of headaches in patients with Moyamoya angiopathy, their association with hemodynamic reserve capacity on CVR-MRI, and response to revascularization surgery to enhance recognition and improve understanding of this potentially disabling symptom.

2. Materials and Methods

From a prospective database of adult patients with cerebrovascular disease, who had at least one CVR-MRI study at our neurovascular tertiary referral center, we included consecutive patients with unilateral or bilateral Moyamoya angiopathy who underwent direct EC–IC bypass with or without indirect bypass surgery between January 2010 and September 2022 and had data on the presence or absence of headaches documented on their chart (Figure 1). We collected data on demographics, headache characteristics, CVR-MR imaging results, and type of flow augmentation surgery through systematic chart review.

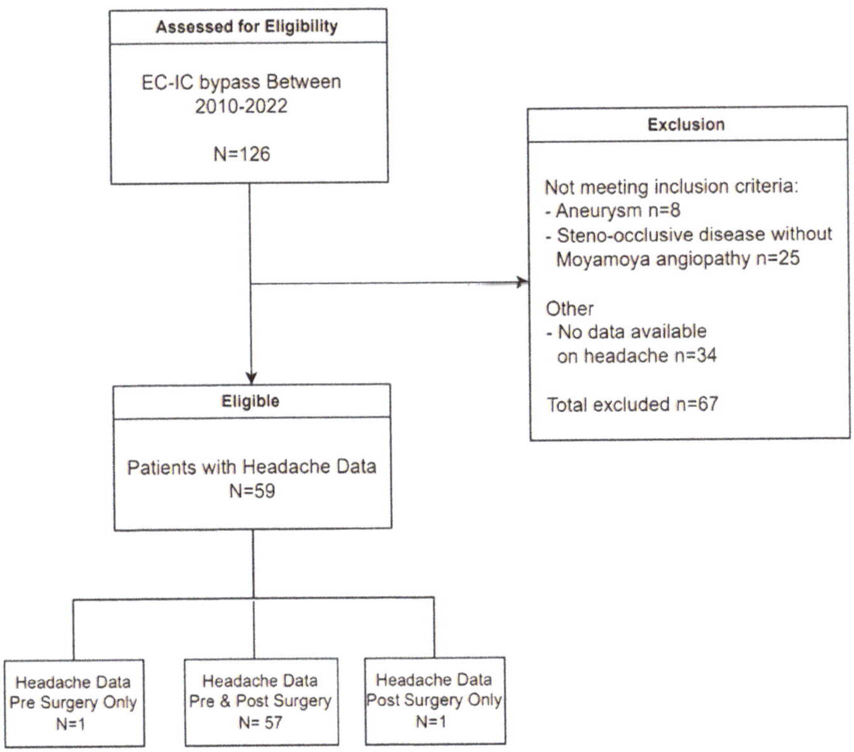

Figure 1. Patient selection. EC–IC bypass = extracranial–intracranial arterial bypass surgery.

CVR-MR imaging involved controlled end-tidal partial pressure of CO_2 ($P_{ET}CO_2$) as a vasoactive stimulus delivered through a sealed mask (RespirAct, Thornhill Medical, Toronto, ON, Canada), and BOLD MRI at a 3.0-Tesla system. Full brain BOLD MR images were acquired using a T2*-weighted two-dimensional gradient-echo sequence with standard echo-planar readout. Three-dimensional T1-weighted anatomical MR images were acquired for co-registration with BOLD MR images using an inversion-recovery fast spoiled gradient-echo sequence. The calculated CVR was based on the BOLD-MR signal intensity related to the $P_{ET}CO_2$. This technique has been described previously in further detail [6,7]. A clinic visit followed CVR-MR imaging.

Patients who had surgery between 2018 and 2022 also completed a structured headache questionnaire as part of standard clinical practice. This questionnaire comprises the presence, localization, and types of headaches, headache triggers, accompanying symptoms, as well as analgesic use and the impact of headaches on mood and sick leave before and after surgery. It includes a Visual Analog Scale (VAS) score on a scale from 0 (no pain) to 10 (maximal pain).

The Institutional Research Ethics Board approved the study before data collection. The need for informed consent was waived.

Statistical Analysis

In addition to descriptive analyses, we used the McNemar–Bowker test to compare proportions and the Wilcoxon signed rank test to compare VAS scores before and after surgery. A p-value < 0.05 was considered statistically significant. We explored the association between headache improvement and improvement of cerebrovascular reactivity after surgery using odds ratios with corresponding 95% confidence intervals (95% CI). Subsequently, a logistic regression analysis was employed to identify potential confounders for this association and examine other factors related to headache improvement after surgery. The data were statistically analyzed using SPSS version 28 software.

3. Results

Fifty-nine patients met the inclusion criteria (mean age 47 ± 14 years, 73% females) (Figure 1). Most patients (70%) were diagnosed with Moyamoya disease and 30% with Moyamoya syndrome. Thirty-eight patients (64%) were diagnosed with bilateral Moyamoya angiopathy, and 19 (50%) of them underwent bilateral flow augmentation surgery (Table 1). o

Table 1. Baseline characteristics.

	n = 59
Age (yr)	47 ± 14
Female sex	43/59 (73%)
Moyamoya disease	41/59 (70%)
Unilateral	11/41 (27%)
Bilateral	30/41 (73%)
Moyamoya syndrome	18/59 (31%)
Unilateral	10/18 (56%)
Bilateral	8/18 (44%)
History of stroke	
Only ischemic	35/59 (59%)
Only hemorrhagic	6/59 (10%)
Ischemic and hemorrhagic	9/59 (15%)
No history of stroke	9/59 (15%)

Table 1. *Cont.*

	n = 59
Bypass surgery n (%)	
EC–IC bypass left	22/59 (37%)
EC–IC bypass right	18/59 (31%)
EC–IC bypass bilateral	19/59 (32%)
EC–IC bypass + EDAS	4/59 (7%)
Interval CVR-MRI & bypass surgery (median (IQR), months)	5 (3–8)
Interval bypass surgery & CVR-MRI (median (IQR), months)	6 (3–12)

EC–IC bypass: extracranial–intracranial arterial bypass surgery (direct); EDAS: encephaloduroarteriosynangiosis (indirect). IQR: interquartile range.

3.1. Headaches before and after Flow Augmentation Surgery

Data on headaches both before and after surgery were available for 57/59 (97%) patients (Figure 1). Most patients (72%) reported headaches before bypass surgery, which improved in more than two-thirds (68%) of patients after surgery. Two patients developed new headaches after surgery (Table 2). The lateralization of the headache was not correlated with the side of Moyamoya arteriopathy ($p = 0.317$) nor with the side of surgery ($p = 0.754$).

Table 2. Headaches before and after flow augmentation surgery.

	n (%)
Headaches before surgery	41/57 (72%)
Headaches improved after surgery	28/41 (68%)
Headaches were unchanged after surgery	11/41 (27%)
Headaches worsened after surgery	2/41 (5%)
New onset headaches after surgery	2/57 (4%)

Thirty-one patients who underwent flow augmentation surgery between 2018 and 2022 completed the headache questionnaire. Twenty-five (25/31; 81%) reported mostly throbbing or pressure-type headaches before surgery with a median headache severity of 5/10 on the VAS. Among these patients, 17/25 (68%) reported one or more headache triggers, and 15/25 (60%) described one or more accompanying symptoms, predominantly nausea/vomiting and a preceding aura. Most patients (84%) used one or more classes of analgesics. Almost half of the patients felt depressed due to their headaches, and nearly two-thirds of patients missed work or quit their jobs because of headaches (Table 3).

Table 3. Headache characteristics before and after flow augmentation surgery.

	Before Surgery n (%)	After Surgery n (%)
Completed questionnaires	31/59 (53%)	31/59 (53%)
Presence of headaches	25/31 (81%)	19/31 (61%)
Types of Headaches		
Throbbing headache	9/25 (36%)	6/19 (32%)
Pressure-type headache	7/25 (28%)	6/19 (32%)
Dull headache	6/25 (24%)	6/19 (32%)
Sharp headache	4/25 (16%)	2/19 (11%)

Table 3. *Cont.*

	Before Surgery n (%)	After Surgery n (%)
Localization of Headaches		
Bilateral	19/25 (76%)	14/19 (74%)
Unilateral	6/25 (24%)	5/19 (26%)
Headache Triggers		
Lack of sleep	6/25 (24%)	5/19 (26%)
Menses	4/25 (16%)	4/19 (21%)
Exercise	3/25 (12%)	1/19 (5%)
Mental stress	3/25 (12%)	2/19 (11%)
Weather changes	1/25 (4%)	1/19 (5%)
Accompanying Symptoms		
Preceding aura	6/25 (24%)	6/19 (32%)
Nausea/vomiting	9/25 (36%)	9/19 (47%)
Photo-/phonophobia	4/25 (16%)	3/19 (16%)
Dizziness	4/25 (16%)	2/19 (11%)
Transient focal weakness/sensory symptoms	2/25 (8%)	0/19 (0%)
Analgesic Use	21/25 (84%)	10/25 (40%) *
Acetaminophen	16/25 (64%)	5/25 (20%)
Non-steroidal anti-inflammatory drugs	5/25 (20%)	2/25 (8%)
Triptans	3/25 (12%)	1/25 (4%)
Anticonvulsants	5/25 (20%)	2/25 (8%)
Opioids (codeine, caffeine, morphine)	3/25 (12%)	3/25 (12%)
Multiple drug classes	7/25 (28%)	3/25 (12%)
Headache impact		
Pain severity: VAS-score (median (IQR))	5 (0–9)	2.5 (0–5) *
Feelings of depression	11/25 (44%)	8/25 (32%)
Sick leave/quit job	15/25 (60%)	4/25 (16%) *

VAS: Visual Analog Scale (0–10). IQR: interquartile range. * Statistically significant difference.

After surgery, sick leave decreased significantly, from 60% (15/25) to 16% (4/25) ($p < 0.001$), which was associated with headache improvement (OR 1.4; 95% CI: 1.6–121.4). Headache severity improved with a reduction in VAS score from 5/10 to 2.5/10 after surgery ($p = 0.002$), resulting in a reduction in analgesic use from 84% to 40% ($p = 0.007$) after surgery (Table 3).

3.2. Cerebrovascular Reserve before and after Flow Augmentation Surgery

Pre-operative CVR-MRI results were available for 57/59 patients (97%). Most patients (39/57 (68%)) had bilateral decreased CVR. Post-operative CVR-MRI results were available for 53/59 patients (90%). CVR improved in 36/53 patients (68%) and worsened in 6/53 patients (11%) after surgery. Improvement of CVR was associated with an improvement in headaches (OR 5.3; 95%CI: 1.2–23.5).

4. Discussion

In this cohort of patients with Moyamoya angiopathy, headaches were common, disabling, and associated with a high rate of sick leave. Following flow augmentation surgery, most patients experienced a reduction in headaches, along with observed improvement in cerebrovascular reserve on MRI. This led to a decreased use of analgesics and a reduction in sick leave.

Headaches in Moyamoya angiopathy are common but often remain unaddressed in clinical practice due to insufficient awareness of their impact on quality of life and a limited understanding of the underlying pathophysiology [8,9].

In a prior study including 55 patients with Moyamoya angiopathy, of whom 34 had flow augmentation surgery, a similar headache frequency before surgery was described [8]. Headaches improved after surgery in around two-thirds of the patients, consistent with our findings. Additionally, our analysis showed an association between headache reduction and improved cerebrovascular reserve on MRI after surgery, potentially offering insights into its underlying pathophysiological mechanism. When the cerebrovascular reserve capacity is compromised due to Moyamoya angiopathy, leptomeningeal collateral arteries typically dilate to compensate for reduced flow, which may cause headaches by stimulation of dural nociceptors [8,10,11]. The vasoactive hypothesis in migraine supports this theory and would explain the migraine-like headaches in Moyamoya angiopathy patients [12,13]. Another explanation for headaches in this patient population could be hypoxia and microvascular ischemia induced by chronic cerebral hypoperfusion and impaired hemodynamics from progressive intracranial steno-occlusive disease. Microvascular ischemia could generate cortical spreading depression, as is also seen in migraine with aura [8,10,14]. To support this hypothesis, future studies could focus on headaches and chronic ischemic changes on MRI in patients with Moyamoya angiopathy.

Another potential explanation for headaches in this patient population could be concomitant depression. Psychological well-being, including depression, can improve after revascularization surgery in Moyamoya disease patients [15]. Feelings of depression improved after revascularization surgery in our cohort, though not significantly, and they were not associated with headache improvement, potentially because of lack of power.

Not only in adults, but also in pediatric patients with Moyamoya disease, headaches are common and respond to indirect revascularization surgery [9,16,17].

Interestingly, contrasting findings were reported by a Chinese observational study, which showed no differences in long-term outcomes of headaches between Moyamoya angiopathy patients who underwent revascularization surgery and those with conservative treatment [13]. It could be argued that patients receiving conservative management had less advanced disease compared to patients who required revascularization surgery and therefore had fewer headaches, potentially masking a positive effect of surgery on headaches.

As demonstrated in this study, the impact of headaches on the daily routine of patients with Moyamoya angiopathy is significant, which warrants increased awareness in clinical practice. In children with headaches caused by Moyamoya disease, a decrease in school attendance was seen [16]. The effect of revascularization surgery on headache severity and reduction in sick leave is significant and, therefore, patients and their families should be informed about these benefits when discussing surgery.

A strength of this study is the relatively large cohort size of Moyamoya angiopathy patients and the available standard-of-care headache questionnaire, both providing robust data on their clinical and radiographic status before and after revascularization surgery.

A limitation of this study is its retrospective nature and the potential introduction of reporting bias concerning the presence of headaches and recall bias regarding headache characteristics and changes. This limits the ability to establish causality and warrants careful drawing of conclusions.

These study results need to be validated prospectively in a larger cohort of patients with Moyamoya angiopathy to mitigate recall and reporting bias. Once the pathophysiology of these disabling headaches is better understood, specific medical treatment targets may be identified to tailor headache management in this patient population.

5. Conclusions

Headaches in Moyamoya angiopathy were common and disabling, although they often improved after revascularization surgery, resulting in a better quality of life. Their association with improved cerebrovascular reactivity post-surgery supports the postulation that headaches in patients with Moyamoya angiopathy may have a vascular origin.

Author Contributions: Conceptualization, H.C.J., I.R., D.J.M. and J.D.S.; methodology, F.D.G.M., H.C.J., L.V., D.J.M., I.R., H.A.B., E.J.H. and J.D.S.; software, F.D.G.M. and J.D.S.; validation, H.C.J. and J.D.S.; formal analysis, F.D.G.M. and J.D.S.; investigation, F.D.G.M., H.C.J. and J.D.S.; resources, L.V. and J.D.S.; data curation, F.D.G.M., H.C.J., L.V. and J.D.S.; writing—original draft preparation, F.D.G.M.; writing-review and editing, H.C.J., L.V., D.J.M., H.A.B., I.R., E.J.H. and J.D.S.; visualization, F.D.G.M. and J.D.S.; supervision, H.C.J. and J.D.S.; project administration, F.D.G.M., H.C.J. and J.D.S. All authors have read and agreed to the published version of the manuscript.

Funding: This research received no external funding.

Institutional Review Board Statement: The study was conducted in accordance with the Declaration of Helsinki and was approved by the Institutional Review Board of the University Health Network (protocol code 22-5779, approved on 5 October 2022).

Informed Consent Statement: Patient consent was waived due to the retrospective nature of this study.

Data Availability Statement: The data that support the findings of this study are available from the corresponding author, J.D.S., upon reasonable request. The data are not publicly available due to privacy and ethical restrictions.

Conflicts of Interest: The authors declare no conflicts of interest.

References

1. Shang, S.; Zhou, D.; Ya, J.; Li, S.; Yang, Q.; Ding, Y.; Ji, X.; Meng, R. Progress in Moyamoya disease. *Neurosurg. Rev.* **2020**, *43*, 371–382. [CrossRef] [PubMed]
2. Scott, R.M.; Smith, E.R. Moyamoya disease and Moyamoya syndrome. *N. Engl. J. Med.* **2009**, *360*, 1226–1237. [CrossRef] [PubMed]
3. Guzman, R.; Lee, M.; Achrol, A.; Bell-Stephens, T.; Kelly, M.; Do, H.M.; Marks, M.P.; Steinberg, G.K. Clinical outcome after 450 revascularization procedures for Moyamoya disease. *J. Neurosurg.* **2009**, *111*, 927–935. [CrossRef] [PubMed]
4. Bersano, A.; Khan, N.; Fuentes, B.; Acerbi, F.; Canavero, I.; Tournier-Lasserve, E.; Vajcoczy, P.; Zedde, M.L.; Hussain, S.; Lémeret, S.; et al. European Stroke Organisation (ESO) Guidelines on Moyamoya angiopathy endorsed by Vascular European Reference Network (VASCERN). *Eur. Stroke J.* **2023**, *8*, 55–84. [CrossRef] [PubMed]
5. Gonzalez, N.R.; Amin-Hanjani, S.; Bang, O.Y.; Coffey, C.; Du, R.; Fierstra, J.; Fraser, J.F.; Kuroda, S.; Tietjen, G.E.; Yaghi, S.; et al. Adult Moyamoya disease and Syndrome: Current Perspectives and Future Directions: A Scientific Statement from the American Heart Association/American Stroke Association. *Stroke* **2023**, *54*, e465–e479. [CrossRef] [PubMed]
6. Van Niftrik, C.H.B.; Sebok, M.; Germans, M.R.; Halter, M.; Pokorny, T.; Stumpo, V.; Bellomo, J.; Piccirelli, M.; Pangalu, A.; Katan, M.; et al. Increased risk of recurrent stroke in symptomatic large vessel disease with impaired BOLD cerebrovascular reactivity. *Stroke* **2024**, *55*, 613–621. [CrossRef] [PubMed]
7. Raghavan, V.; Sobczyk, O.; Sayin, E.S.; Poublanc, J.; Skanda, A.; Duffin, J.; Venkatraghavan, L.; Fisher, J.A.; Mikulis, D.J. Assessment of cerebrovascular reactivity using CO_2-BOLD MRI: A 15-year, single center experience. *J. Magn. Reson. Imaging* **2024**, *60*, 954–961. [CrossRef] [PubMed]
8. Kraemer, M.; Lee, S.I.; Ayzenberg, I.; Schwitalla, J.C.; Diehl, R.R.; Berlit, P.; Bosche, B.; Katsarava, Z.; Obermann, M. Headache in Caucasian patients with Moyamoya angiopathy—A systematic cohort study. *Cephalalgia* **2017**, *37*, 496–500. [CrossRef] [PubMed]
9. Kim, S.K.; Cho, B.K.; Phi, J.H.; Lee, J.Y.; Chae, J.H.; Kim, K.J.; Hwang, Y.S.; Kim, I.O.; Lee, D.S.; Lee, J.; et al. Pediatric Moyamoya disease: An analysis of 410 consecutive cases. *Ann. Neurol.* **2010**, *68*, 92–101. [CrossRef] [PubMed]
10. Zach, V.; Bezov, D.; Lipton, R.B.; Ashina, S. Headache associated with Moyamoya disease: A case story and literature review. *J. Headache Pain.* **2010**, *11*, 79–82. [CrossRef] [PubMed]
11. Fujimura, M.; Tominaga, T. Diagnosis of Moyamoya disease: International standard and regional differences. *Neurol. Med. Chir.* **2015**, *55*, 189–193. [CrossRef] [PubMed]
12. Amin, F.M.; Ashgar, M.S.; Hougaard, A.; Hansen, A.E.; Larsen, V.A.; de Koning, P.J.; Larsson, H.B.; Olesen, J.; Ashina, M. Magnetic resonance angiography of intracranial and extracranial arteries in patients with spontaneous migraine without aura: A cross-sectional study. *Lancet Neurol.* **2013**, *12*, 454–461. [CrossRef] [PubMed]
13. Gao, B.; Kang, K.; Zhang, J.; Zhang, D.; Zhao, X. Clinical Characteristics and long-term outcome of headaches associated with Moyamoya disease in the Chinese population—A cohort study. *Front. Neurol.* **2020**, *11*, 605636. [CrossRef] [PubMed]
14. Chiang, C.C.; Shahid, A.H.; Harriott, A.M.; Tietjen, G.E.; Savastano, L.E.; Klaas, J.P.; Lanzino, G. Evaluation and treatment of headache associated with Moyamoya disease—A narrative review. *Cephalalgia* **2022**, *42*, 542–552. [CrossRef] [PubMed]
15. Haas, P.; Kittelberger, B.B.; Hurth, H.; Wang, S.; Tellermann, J.; Tatagiba, M.; Khan, N.; Roder, C. Health-related quality of life and neuropsychological outcome after EC-IC bypass revascularization in adult patients with Moyamoya disease. *Neurosurgery* **2024**, *94*, 1107–1115. [CrossRef] [PubMed]

16. Kawabori, M.; Kuroda, S.; Nakayama, N.; Hirata, K.; Shiga, T.; Houkin, K.; Tamaki, N. Effective surgical revascularization improves cerebral hemodynamics and resolves headache in pediatric Moyamoya disease. *World Neurosurg.* **2013**, *80*, 612–619. [CrossRef] [PubMed]
17. Bohara, M.; Sugata, S.; Nishimuta, Y.; Karki, P.; Nagayama, T.; Sakamoto, S.; Tokimura, H.; Arita, K. Effect of revascularization on headache associated with Moyamoya disease in pediatric patients. *Hiroshima J. Med. Sci.* **2015**, *64*, 39–44. [PubMed]

brain sciences

MDPI

Article

Comparative Analysis of AI Models in Predicting Treatment Strategies for Unruptured Intracranial Aneurysms

Manou Overstijns [1], Sameer Nazeeruddin [1], Pierre Scheffler [1], Roland Roelz [1], Jürgen Beck [1,*] and Amir El Rahal [1,2]

1 Department of Neurosurgery, Faculty of Medicine, Medical Centre, University of Freiburg, Breisacher-Str. 64, 79106 Freiburg, Germany; manou.overstijns@uniklinik-freiburg.de (M.O.); sameer.nazeeruddin@uniklinik-freiburg.de (S.N.); pierre.scheffler@uniklinik-freiburg.de (P.S.); roland.roelz@uniklinik-freiburg.de (R.R.); amir.elrahal@uniklinik-freiburg.de (A.E.R.)

2 Faculty of Medicine of Geneva, University of Geneva, 1201 Geneva, Switzerland

* Correspondence: j.beck@uniklinik-freiburg.de; Tel.: +49-761-270-50010; Fax: +49-761-270-50240

Abstract

Objectives: The increasing incidence of unruptured intracranial aneurysms (UIAs) has led to significant demands on neurovascular boards. Large language models (LLMs), such as ChatGPT-4, ChatGPT-3.5, Claude, and Atlas GPT, have emerged as tools to support clinical decision-making. This study compares treatment recommendations from these AI models with those of an interdisciplinary neurovascular board to evaluate their accuracy and alignment. **Methods:** We retrospectively included all 57 patients with UIAs discussed by the neurovascular board in 2023. The board's consensus decision served as the reference standard. Key clinical and radiographic data, including PHASES, ELAPSS, and UIATS scores, were provided to the AI models. Each model was tasked with recommending either conservative or operative management and specifying the treatment modality (clipping, coiling, flow diverter, or WEB device/flow diverter) where appropriate. AI model recommendations were compared with the board's decisions for management and the specific treatment modality of the UIA. **Results:** ChatGPT-4 achieved the highest accuracy in correctly predicting conservative or operative management (89%) and specific treatment types (73%), followed by Atlas GPT (74% accuracy in conservative/operative decisions and 55% accuracy in specific treatment types), Claude (70% accuracy in conservative/operative decisions and 50% accuracy in specific treatment types), and ChatGPT-3.5 (82% accuracy in conservative/operative decisions and 27% accuracy in specific treatment types). ChatGPT-3.5 displayed a strong preference for clipping (94.3%). ELAPSS scores significantly influenced AI recommendations and decision-making, particularly for ChatGPT-4 and ChatGPT-3.5. Follow-up recommendations for conservative management were shorter among AI models, with Claude suggesting the shortest interval (7.72 months) compared to the neurovascular board's 13.36 months. **Conclusions:** AI models, particularly ChatGPT-4, align closely with expert neurovascular board decisions and offer promising support for initial clinical decision-making, particularly in resource-limited settings. However, interdisciplinary neurovascular boards remain unreplaceable for UIA management, and AI should be viewed as a complementary tool. The observed improvement from ChatGPT-3.5 to ChatGPT-4 underscores the rapid evolution of AI technology, and further advancements are expected to enhance both performance and accuracy in the future.

Keywords: artificial intelligence; unruptured intracranial aneurysm; treatment prediction; AI model comparison; predictive accuracy

1. Introduction

Unruptured intracranial aneurysms (UIAs) affect approximately 3% of the general population, often remaining asymptomatic and undetected until discovered incidentally through neuroimaging performed for unrelated reasons [1,2]. The increasing accessibility of advanced imaging techniques has led to a higher incidence of incidental UIA detection, posing significant challenges in clinical decision-making regarding their management [3]. The primary dilemma revolves around whether to intervene or manage the aneurysm conservatively, a decision that necessitates a careful balance between the risk of aneurysm rupture and the potential complications associated with treatment [4–6].

Management strategies for UIAs are inherently complex and require close interdisciplinary collaboration between neurosurgeons, neuroradiologists, and neurologists. A range of patient-specific factors, including age, comorbidities, family history, and aneurysm characteristics such as size, location, morphology, and documented growth patterns, guide decisions [4,7]. Treatment options encompass conservative treatment, surgical clipping, endovascular coiling, flow diversion, and the use of WEB (Woven EndoBridge) devices, each with its risk–benefit profile [8–10].

To aid in the decision-making process, predictive scoring systems have been developed. The PHASES score estimates the 5-year risk of aneurysm rupture based on population, hypertension, age, aneurysm size, a history of earlier subarachnoid hemorrhage from another aneurysm, and aneurysm site [11]. The ELAPSS score predicts the risk of aneurysm growth based on factors such as patient age, aneurysm size, and location [12]. The Unruptured Intracranial Aneurysm Treatment Score (UIATS) integrates both patient- and aneurysm-related factors to provide a comprehensive assessment for recommending either intervention or observation [13].

Even with established decision-making aids, the rising number of incidental UIA detections can place a considerable burden on neurovascular teams, sometimes leading to resource constraints and delayed specialist consultations [14]. In many clinical settings, immediate access to an interdisciplinary neurovascular board may not be readily available, highlighting the need for supplementary forms of preliminary decision support. In this context, artificial intelligence (AI), particularly Large Language Models (LLMs), has emerged as a promising adjunct. Models such as ChatGPT-4 (OpenAI), ChatGPT-3.5. Claude (Anthropic) and Atlas GPT (Atlas Meditech) utilize deep learning algorithms and extensive medical literature to generate human-like language outputs that can aid in guiding initial clinical decisions [15].

Recent studies have explored the application of AI and LLMs in neurosurgical decision-making, particularly in neuro-oncology. For instance, investigations into ChatGPT's ability to provide diagnoses and treatment plans for brain tumors have demonstrated its potential to assist in clinical evaluation [16]. However, the use of LLMs in determining management strategies for UIAs has not been extensively studied. This study aims to compare the decisions made by an interdisciplinary neurovascular board with those generated by four different LLMs—ChatGPT-4, ChatGPT-3.5, Claude, and Atlas GPT—regarding the optimal management of unruptured intracranial aneurysms.

2. Methods

2.1. Study Design

Ethical approval was obtained from the local ethics committee (protocol code EK-Freiburg: 24-1429-S1, approval date 12 November 2024). The requirement for individual informed consent was waived because the study involved a retrospective analysis of pseudonymized patient data, which did not allow direct identification of individuals. We adhered to the STROBE (Strengthening the Reporting of Observational Studies in

Epidemiology) checklist guidelines to ensure comprehensive and transparent reporting [17]. All data is available on reasonable request to the authors.

Patients were included if (i) UIA was confirmed using neuroimaging (either digital subtraction angiography, computed tomography angiography, or magnetic resonance angiography), (ii) they were discussed in our interdisciplinary neurovascular board between 1 January 2023, and 31 December 2023, and (iii) were aged 18 years or above. Patients were excluded if (i) other vascular pathologies were present (e.g., arteriovenous malformation), (ii) patients had ruptured aneurysms, and iii) patients without definitive management decisions from the board (3 patients in total). Excluding these cases ensured that all included patients had clear expert decisions, which was essential for accurate comparison with the Large Language Models (LLMs).

2.2. Expert Decision

All cases were reviewed in our institutional interdisciplinary neurovascular board, which is convened on a weekly basis. For each case, at least one senior specialist from each core discipline was present: a neuroradiologist, a neurointerventionalist, a neurologist, and a neurosurgeon. The estimated 5-year aneurysm rupture risk, primarily assessed using the PHASES score, was weighed against the estimated treatment risk, taking into account patient age, comorbidities (with special consideration of severe comorbidities defined as ASA $\geq$ 3), aneurysm morphology (saccular or fusiform), size, location, irregularity, and documented growth [11]. In cases where rupture risk exceeded expected procedural risk, interventional treatment was favored. Additional factors included the ELAPSS score to estimate growth risk, anatomical considerations for surgical versus endovascular feasibility, and any history of previous subarachnoid hemorrhage. The final decision reflected consensus among all present board members, integrating quantitative risk scores with qualitative expert judgment in accordance with current international guidelines [4,18].

2.3. Data Collection

We collected key patient characteristics essential for determining the management of unruptured intracranial aneurysms (Figure 1). These data were subsequently entered into four Large Language Models (LLMs) to obtain management recommendations: ChatGPT-4 (OpenAI, GPT-4.0), ChatGPT-3.5 (OpenAI, GPT-3.5-turbo), Claude (Anthropic, Claude 2.1), and Atlas GPT (Atlas Meditech, Atlas GPT v1.3). All models were accessed and queried in October 2024, ensuring that each was evaluated in the same time frame. Specifying the exact model versions and access date is essential for reproducibility, as LLM performance and outputs can change substantially with updates. The collected data included patient age, presence of severe comorbidities, aneurysm morphology (saccular or fusiform), and aneurysm irregularity. We also recorded whether the aneurysm was intradural or extradural, its maximum size in millimeters, anatomical location, presence of multiple aneurysms, size ratio, aspect ratio, and whether an aneurysmal growth was identified. Additionally, we calculated key risk assessment scores for each patient, including PHASES, ELAPSS, UIATS, and American Society of Anesthesiology (ASA) score, to create a comprehensive profile that guides management decision [11–13].

To ensure consistency, we prompted each Large Language Model (LLM), ChatGPT-4, ChatGPT-3.5, Claude, and Atlas GPT, with a standardized request (Supplementary data S1). We instructed the models to analyze each patient's clinical and radiographic data and to recommend either conservative management or treatment for unruptured intracranial aneurysms. When recommending treatment, the models were asked to specify the modality (surgical or endovascular) and, if endovascular, to further detail the specific technique (coiling with or without stenting, flow diverter, or web device). For conservative management recommendations, we asked the models to indicate a suggested follow-up time.

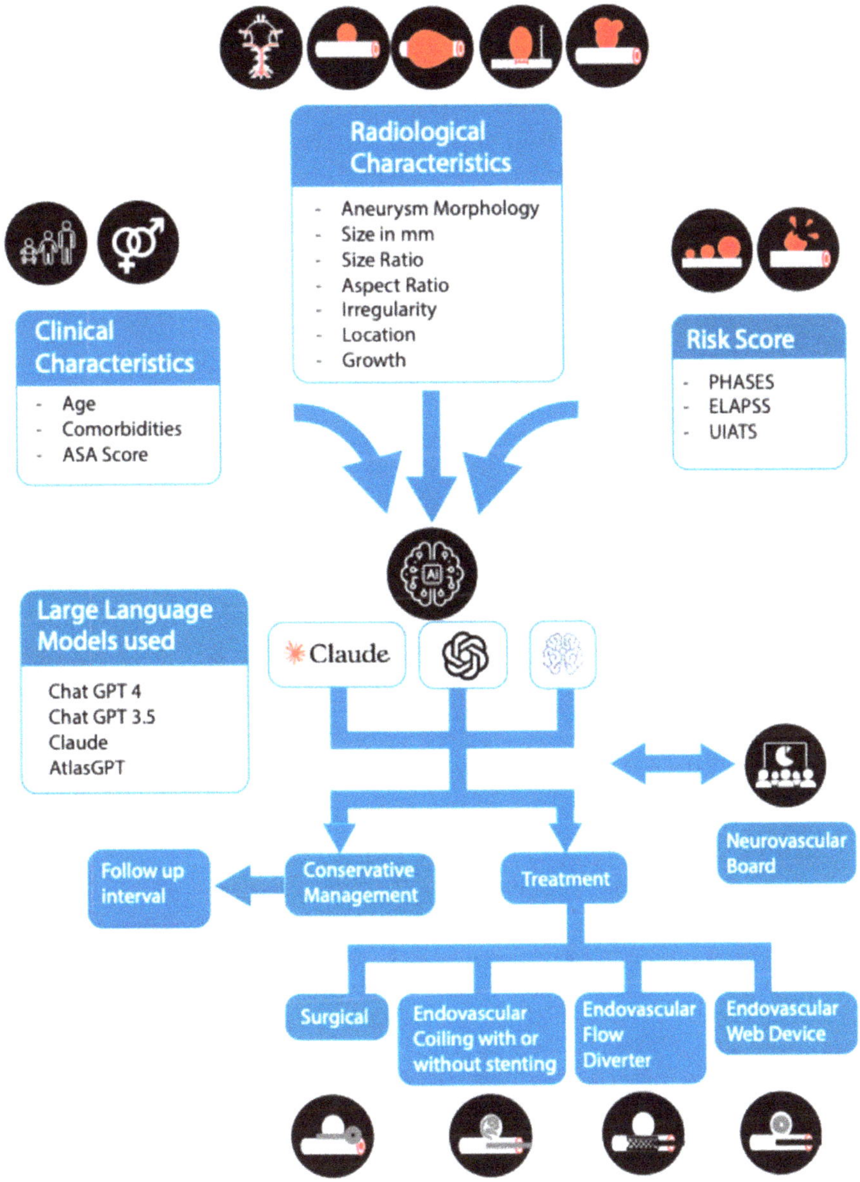

Figure 1. Flowchart depicting clinical, radiological, and risk-score data fed into Large Language Models (GPT-4, GPT-3.5, Claude, Atlas GPT) to generate recommendations for UIA management. The models propose either conservative follow-up or interventional treatment (surgical or endovascular), which is then compared against the expert neurovascular board's decisions.

2.4. Data Input and Prompt Design

To ensure consistency and minimize variability in the AI-generated recommendations, we developed a standardized input format that was uniformly presented to each Large

Language Model (LLM). This standardized format included key patient and aneurysm characteristics, as well as relevant risk scores (e.g., PHASES, ELAPSS), mirroring the clinical data used in neurovascular board discussions. By providing an identical dataset and prompt wording to each model, we aimed to obtain responses that could be directly compared with one another and with the decisions of our neurovascular board.

Because LLMs like ChatGPT-4 and ChatGPT-3.5, as well as other models, are heavily influenced by the nature and detail of the input provided, adopting a methodical and structured input design was critical for generating reproducible outputs. Each case was presented in tabular form, describing patient demographics, aneurysm morphology and metrics, as well as the scoring systems for rupture risk and growth risk. Each model was queried with a standardized prompt that explicitly asked for a single preferred management decision. Outputs were subsequently mapped into five predefined categories: conservative management, surgical clipping, endovascular coiling, flow diverter, or WEB device. If a model proposed several options but expressed a preference (for example, "clipping would be preferred, though coiling could also be considered"), the preferred option was coded. In cases where hedging language was used, a follow-up clarification was requested, and the final stated preference was recorded. Free-text terminology was standardized to the closest category (for example, "microsurgical occlusion" was classified as clipping, and "endovascular embolization with coils" was classified as coiling). With this structured approach, each model ultimately provided a clear recommendation that could be assigned consistently to one of the predefined treatment categories.

2.5. Statistical Analysis

Statistical analysis was performed using SPSS, version 24 (IBM Corp, Armonk, NY, USA). To assess the accuracy of each LLM, we used a binary outcome (1 = correct, 0 = incorrect) to indicate alignment with the neurovascular board's decision. We then used Cochran's Q test to evaluate the significance of differences in accuracy across the four models. Subsequently, pairwise comparisons between the LLMs were performed using the McNemar test. Given the multiple comparisons, we applied a Bonferroni correction to control for Type I error.

3. Results

3.1. Demographics and Aneurysm Characteristics

A total of 57 patients with unruptured intracranial aneurysms (UIAs) were included in the study after applying the inclusion and exclusion criteria (Table 1). The mean age of the patients was 66.2 years. In total, 53 (93.0%) aneurysms were saccular in morphology, with 3 (5.3%) cases classified as fusiform. Forty-eight aneurysms (84.2%) were located intradurally, while nine cases (15.8%) were extradural [19].

The median maximum aneurysm size was 6.0 mm, ranging from 2.0 to 25.0 mm. In terms of location, aneurysms were found in the middle cerebral artery (MCA) in 16 cases (28.1%), anterior communicating artery (ACOM) in 13 cases (22.8%), internal carotid artery (ICA), including posterior communicating artery, in 15 cases (26.3%), vertebral artery and posterior cerebral artery in 3 cases (5.3%), basilar artery in 7 cases (12.3%), and other locations in 3 cases (5.3%). Thirteen patients (22.8%) had multiple aneurysms, and 4 patients (7.0%) showed documented growth of the aneurysm over time.

The calculated risk scores for each patient provided additional context for management decisions. The mean PHASES score was 6.9, ranging from 0 to 16, while the mean ELAPSS score was 12.1, with a range from 2 to 29. The Unruptured Intracranial Aneurysm Treatment Score (UIATS) favored intervention in 30 patients (52.6%) and conservative management in 27 patients (47.4%).

Table 1. Descriptive Statistics of Patient Demographics, Aneurysm Characteristics, and Risk Scores.

Demographics	Range	Median (IQR)/Mean ± SD/n (%)
Age (years)	31–95	65.40 ± 12.51
Severe Comorbidities		15 (26.3%)
Aneurysm saccular Morphology		53 (93.0%)
Irregular Aneurysm		2 (4%)
Aneurysm location - Middle cerebral artery - Anterior cerebral artery - Internal carotid artery - Vertebral/posterior cerebral artery		 14 (24.6%) 17 (29.8%) 24 (42.1%) 2 (3.5%)
Intradural aneurysm location		48 (84.2%)
Growth under conservative treatment		4 (7.0%)
Aneurysm Size (mm)	2.0–25.0	6 (2.2–9.8)
Size Ratio	1.00–6.60	2.0 (0.5–3.5)
Aspect Ratio	0.66–8.50	3.0 (1.29–4.71)
PHASES Score	0–23	6.0 (1.0–11.0)
ELAPSS Score	2–29	14.63 ± 7.11
UIATS Favors Repair	2–15	8.0 (4.0–12.0)
Conservative treatment		26 (45.6%)
Treatment method - Operative clipping - Endovascular coiling - Endovascular flow diverter -Endovascular WEB device/coiling		 14 (24.6%) 13 (22.8%) 2 (3.5%) 2 (3.5%)

Expert interdisciplinary consensus recommended conservative treatment for 26 (45.6%) patients, and 31 (54.3%) patients were recommended for treatment of the aneurysm. Among those advised to undergo treatment, 14 patients (24.6%) were recommended for operative clipping, and 13 patients (22.8%) were advised to undergo endovascular coiling. Additionally, 2 patients (3.5%) received recommendations for treatment with a flow diverter, and another 2 patients (3.5%) were advised to use the WEB device/flow diverter.

ChatGPT-3.5 advocated treatment of the aneurysm the most (61.4%), followed by ChatGPT-4 (57.9%), Claude (52.6%), and Atlas GPT (49.1%). Regarding treatment types, ChatGPT-3.5 showed a strong preference for clipping (57.9%), whereas ChatGPT-4 demonstrated a more balanced distribution between clipping (22.8%) and coiling (29.9%). Claude and Atlas GPT leaned toward coiling (33.3% and 29.9%, respectively) and conservative management (42.1% and 50.9%, respectively).

For follow-up recommendations in conservative management, the neurovascular board suggested a mean interval of 13.36 months (SD = 5.84). ChatGPT-3.5 consistently recommended a 12-month follow-up (SD = 0), while GPT-4 and Atlas GPT proposed shorter intervals of 10.00 months (SD = 2.89) and 10.76 months (SD = 2.47), respectively. Claude advised the shortest follow-up period, with a mean of 7.72 months (SD = 3.60) (Table 2).

Table 2. Comparison of treatment decisions and follow-up recommendations between the neurovascular board and AI models. ChatGPT-3.5 favored clipping, whereas ChatGPT-4 demonstrated a more balanced approach. Claude and Atlas GPT leaned toward coiling and other endovascular treatments. AI models generally recommended shorter follow-up intervals for conservative management. All percentages are calculated using the entire study cohort (n = 57) as the denominator. Both absolute numbers (N) and percentages (%) are reported.

Model	Conservative (%)	WEB Device/ Coiling (%)	Clipping (%)	Coiling (%)	Flow Diverter (%)	Mean Follow-Up in Months
Neurovascular Board	26 (45.6)	2 (3.5)	14 (24.6)	13 (41.9)	2 (3.5)	13.36
ChatGPT-4	24 (42.1)	3 (5.3)	13 (22.8)	17 (29.9)	0 (0.0)	10.00
ChatGPT-3.5	22 (38.6)	0 (0.0)	33 (57.9)	2 (3.5)	0 (0.0)	12.00
Claude	27 (42.1)	10 (17.5)	1 (1.8)	19 (33.3)	0 (0.0)	7.72
Atlas GPT	29 (50.9)	9 (15.78)	2 (3.5)	17 (29.9)	0 (0.0)	10.76

3.2. Accuracy of AI Models in Predicting Conservative Treatment

In predicting the possibility for conservative treatment, ChatGPT-4 had the highest accuracy, correctly aligning with the neurovascular board's recommendation 89% of the time, followed by ChatGPT-3.5 at 82%, Atlas at 74%, and Claude at 70% (Table 3A and Figure 2A). Cochran's Q test demonstrated a statistically significant difference among the models ($p = 0.003$). Pairwise comparisons with the Bonferroni adjustment indicated that ChatGPT-4 was significantly more accurate than both Claude ($p < 0.001$) and Atlas ($p = 0.002$). At the same time, the differences between GPT-4 and GPT-3.5, as well as between GPT-3.5 and Claude, were not statistically significant.

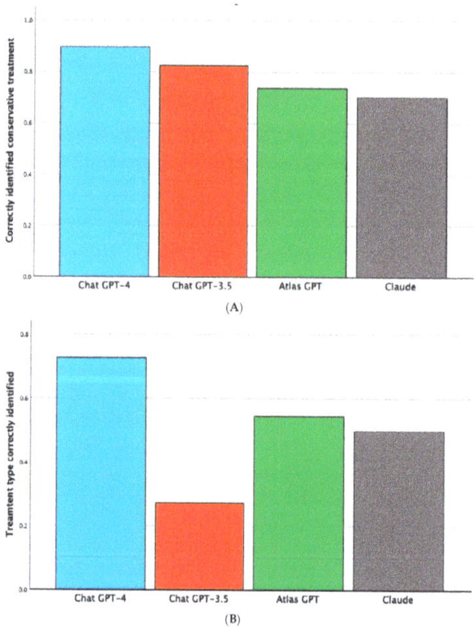

Figure 2. (**A**) Accuracy of each AI model in correctly identifying conservative treatment recommendations for unruptured intracranial aneurysms. ChatGPT-4 achieved the highest accuracy, followed by ChatGPT-3.5, Atlas GPT, and Claude. (**B**) Accuracy of each AI model in correctly identifying the specific treatment type for unruptured intracranial aneurysms.

Table 3. (**A**) Left column: Accuracy of each AI model in correctly predicting conservative management for unruptured intracranial aneurysms. ChatGPT-4 achieved the highest accuracy at 89%, followed by ChatGPT-3.5, Atlas, and Claude. Right column: Pairwise comparisons of accuracy between AI models, with Bonferroni-adjusted *p*-values. ChatGPT -4 demonstrated significantly higher accuracy than Claude and Atlas, while the other comparisons were not statistically significant. (**B**) Left columns: Accuracy of each AI model in correctly predicting treatment type for unruptured intracranial aneurysms with ChatGPT-4 achieving the highest accuracy at 73%, followed by Atlas, Claude, and ChatGPT-3.5. Right columns: Pairwise comparisons of accuracy between AI models with Bonferroni-adjusted *p*-values. ChatGPT-4 demonstrated significantly higher accuracy than ChatGPT-3.5, while other comparisons were not statistically significant.

(A)

AI Model	Mean Accuracy Conservative Prediction	Std. Deviation	Pair Comparison	*p*-Value	Significant with Bonferroni Adjustment?
ChatGPT-4	0.89	0.310	ChatGPT-4 vs. ChatGPT-3.5	0.160	No
ChatGPT-3.5	0.82	0.384	ChatGPT-4 vs. Claude GPT	< 0.001	Yes
Atlas GPT	0.74	0.444	Chatgpt-4 vs. Atlas GPT	0.002	Yes
Claude	0.70	0.462	GPT-3.5 vs. Claude	0.070	No
Cochran's Q *p*-value	0.003		ChatGPT-3.5 vs. Atlas GPT	0.230	No
			Claude vs. Atlas GPT	0.310	No

(B)

AI Model	Mean Accuracy (Treatment Type)	Std. Deviation	Pair Comparison	*p*-Value	Significant with Bonferroni Adjustment?
ChatGPT-4	0.73	0.456	ChatGPT-4 vs. ChatGPT-3.5	0.002	Yes
ChatGPT-3.5	0.27	0.456	ChatGPT-4 vs. Claude	0.157	No
Claude	0.50	0.512	ChatGPT-4 vs. Atlas GPT	0.317	No
Atlas GPT	0.55	0.510	ChatGPT-3.5 vs. Claude	0.071	No
Cochran's Q *p*-value	0.008		ChatGPT-3.5 vs. Atlas GPT	0.023	No
			Claude vs. Atlas GPT	0.564	No

The recommendations for follow-up intervals among patients advised to undergo conservative management varied across the neurovascular board and each AI model. The neurovascular board recommended a mean follow-up interval of 13.36 months (SD = 5.84). ChatGPT-4 suggested a slightly shorter follow-up period, with a mean of 10 months (SD = 2.89), while ChatGPT-3.5 consistently recommended a 12-month interval for all cases (resulting in a standard deviation of 0). Claude advised a shorter follow-up interval than the others, with a mean of 7.72 months (SD = 3.60). Atlas GPT's recommendations were closer to ChatGPT-4, with a mean follow-up interval of 10.76 months (SD = 2.47). Compared with the neurovascular board, this represents significant mean reductions of approximately 3.4 months for ChatGPT-4, 1.4 months for ChatGPT-3.5, 5.6 months for Claude, and 2.6 months for Atlas GPT (all $p < 0.001$).

There was no significant difference in the percentage of conservative treatment recommendations between the neurovascular board and the AI models (ChatGPT-4, ChatGPT-3.5, Claude, and Atlas GPT). Cochran's Q test showed a result of 5.214 (df = 4, $p = 0.266$). The mean rates of conservative recommendations were 45.6% for the neurovascular board, 42.1% for ChatGPT-4, 38.6% for ChatGPT-3.5, 42.1% for Claude, and 50.9% for Atlas GPT. These results suggest that the AI models were neither more conservative nor more aggressive compared to the neurovascular board.

3.3. Accuracy of AI Models in Predicting Specific Treatment Type

The accuracy of each AI model in correctly matching the neurovascular board's recommendation for the specific treatment modality (Operative clipping, endovascular coiling, flow diverter, or WEB device) is shown in Table 3B and Figure 2B. ChatGPT-4 again achieved the highest accuracy at 73%, followed by Atlas GPT (55%) and Claude (50%). ChatGPT-3.5 had the lowest accuracy at 27%. Cochran's Q test revealed a significant difference across the models ($p = 0.008$). Pairwise comparisons with Bonferroni adjustment showed that ChatGPT-4 performed significantly better than ChatGPT-3.5 ($p = 0.002$), though differences between ChatGPT-4 and Claude or Atlas GPT were not statistically significant. ChatGPT-4 again showed the highest accuracy, with Atlas GPT and Claude performing moderately well, while ChatGPT-3.5 had the lowest accuracy.

3.4. Factors Influencing AI Model Predictions for Treatment

To determine the factors influencing AI model decisions for the treatment of unruptured intracranial aneurysms, a multivariate logistic regression analysis was performed. In the multivariable analysis, the dependent variable was whether the AI model's treatment recommendation (surgical vs. conservative) matched the neurovascular board's decision for each patient. In this analysis, the ELAPSS score emerged as a significant predictor of AI model accuracy for both ChatGPT-4 (OR = 1.37, 95% CI: 1.11–1.69, $p = 0.003$) and ChatGPT-3.5 (OR = 1.40, 95% CI: 1.10–1.78, $p = 0.007$), indicating that higher ELAPSS scores, which reflect aneurysm growth risk, were strongly associated with alignment to neurovascular board decisions. For ChatGPT-3.5, the PHASES score showed a significant negative association (OR = 0.73, 95% CI: 0.55–0.97, $p = 0.029$), while severe comorbidities significantly reduced the likelihood of treatment recommendations in both models (OR = 0.047, $p = 0.014$ for ChatGPT-4 and OR = 0.002, $p < 0.001$ for ChatGPT-3.5). In contrast, no significant predictors were identified for Claude, and the analysis for Atlas GPT revealed unstable results with wide confidence intervals, suggesting lower robustness in these models.

4. Discussion

This study evaluates the performance of multiple AI models, including ChatGPT-4, ChatGPT-3.5, Claude, and Atlas GPT, in predicting treatment strategies for UIAs. Expert consensus and guideline recommendations underline the importance of multidisciplinary decision-making in the management of unruptured intracranial aneurysms. In daily practice, this is usually achieved through discussion in a dedicated neurovascular board, where neurosurgeons, neurointerventionalists, neuroradiologists, and neurologists contribute their perspectives. These boards combine established risk scores such as PHASES, ELAPSS, or UIATS with clinical judgement and patient-specific factors, allowing a balanced decision between rupture risk and treatment risk. On this basis, the neurovascular board is widely regarded as the reference standard for therapeutic recommendations in patients with UIA [7,18]. Our findings demonstrate that AI models might align with expert neurovascular board decisions, particularly in terms of overall treatment recommendations. This supports the growing evidence that AI, and specifically LLMs, can serve as valuable tools to assist in complex clinical decision-making processes and provide a first-line assessment and triage.

ChatGPT-4 achieved the highest overall accuracy, both in predicting conservative or operative therapy and in identifying the specific type of operative treatment. While ChatGPT-3.5 showed a stronger preference for clipping, and Claude and Atlas GPT leaned toward coiling, these variations reflect subtle differences in model outputs rather than significant deviations from clinical standards. Notably, the AI models demonstrated neither a conservative nor an aggressive tendency compared to the neurovascular board, reinforcing their ability to replicate expert-level decision-making.

AI models consistently recommended shorter follow-up intervals than the neurovascular board, which could have significant implications. While earlier imaging could help detect aneurysm growth or morphological change sooner and potentially lower rupture risk, it also has clear downsides. More frequent scans increase resource use and costs, place additional demands on radiology services, and, when CTA is the primary modality, add cumulative exposure to radiation and iodinated contrast [20,21]. For patients, this may translate into more outpatient clinic visits, interruptions to daily life, anxiety, and an increased chance of false positives leading to unnecessary investigations. Current guidelines emphasize individualized surveillance rather than fixed intervals, considering aneurysm and patient-specific risk [4,7]. Against this background, our findings indicate that although AI models generally agree with experts on whether to treat or observe, their tendency to suggest earlier re-imaging could shift practice toward over-surveillance if applied without modification. Integrating AI outputs with multidisciplinary board review and guideline-based protocols remains essential to balance vigilance with patient safety and efficient resource use.

The role of predictive risk scores, particularly the ELAPSS and PHASES scores, in guiding AI model outputs was also notable in our analysis. This observation reflects the importance of structured, evidence-based tools in enhancing AI performance, a finding that has been similarly reported in other AI-driven studies [15]. By integrating established clinical scoring systems, AI models can provide recommendations that are both interpretable and aligned with current standards of care.

Radiomics, the extraction of large amounts of quantitative features from medical imaging, has shown promise in characterizing aneurysm morphology, wall integrity, and other anatomical features that may correlate with rupture risk [22,23]. However, current AI-based language models are not yet capable of directly interpreting or analyzing raw imaging data. They therefore cannot independently generate radiomics-based predictions of UIA rupture risk. Our findings suggest that when provided with sufficiently detailed clinical and radiographic information, mirroring a radiomics-driven summary, AI models can offer recommendations that closely match expert decisions. This underscores the importance of integrating advanced imaging analytics with AI language models. This direction holds significant potential for improving the accuracy and reliability of rupture risk assessment in future clinical applications.

The accuracy observed in this study aligns with findings from other medical disciplines exploring AI applications. For example, recent studies have shown that GPT models can assist in neuro-oncology for diagnosing and determining treatment strategies for gliomas, with ChatGPT achieving a reasonable level of accuracy comparable to clinical experts [24]. Additionally, the use of AI in radiological interpretation and treatment planning has demonstrated its capability to support clinicians by reducing workload and enhancing efficiency [15]. Furthermore, it was shown that ChatGPT-3.5 responses on general neurosurgical topics were comparable to those of neurosurgeons with low seniority.

In contrast, the assessment of ChatGPT 4.0 was comparable to that of neurosurgeons with high seniority [25]. These studies, coupled with our results, highlight the broad applicability of AI models across various neurosurgical and medical domains.

An important aspect to consider when interpreting AI model performance is inter-user variability. While AI models like ChatGPT can generate reliable outputs, the results are often influenced by the phrasing of prompts and the level of detail provided. In this study, we sought to minimize such variability by employing a rigorous, structured input design: each of the four LLMs received the same description of the expected response, as well as the same patient data and standardized prompts. This approach allowed us to generate more detailed and uniform responses across models. Nonetheless, it is worth noting that LLMs are continually evolving and adapting as their underlying databases expand, which introduces variability over time and presents an ongoing challenge to their reliability as clinical support tools. These considerations underscore the importance of clearly defined guidelines, consistent data presentation, and standardized prompting protocols when integrating AI into clinical workflows, particularly for complex cases like UIA management.

The findings of this study suggest that AI models, particularly ChatGPT-4, have the potential to serve as a valuable first-line triage tool to support clinical decision-making in the management of unruptured intracranial aneurysms. This is especially relevant in settings where healthcare providers may not frequently encounter UIAs or lack access to experienced neurovascular teams. By rapidly synthesizing clinical and radiographic data, AI can provide a preliminary recommendation that aligns closely with expert-level decisions. Such support could be beneficial in resource-limited settings, where access to specialized care is limited, or in emergencies that require swift preliminary assessments.

Nevertheless, it is crucial to acknowledge that AI models cannot supplant the expert judgment and collaborative decision-making processes offered by an interdisciplinary neurovascular board, which remains the cornerstone of UIA management. Neurovascular boards bring together diverse clinical perspectives, patient-specific considerations, and nuanced real-time discussions, factors that current AI models do not fully replicate. While AI can streamline preliminary evaluations by rapidly synthesizing large volumes of data, its role is best viewed as complementary to human expertise. Our results suggest that AI may serve as a first-line tool to help clinicians navigate complex cases. Still, it should not replace the in-depth deliberation and collective expertise characteristic of a multidisciplinary approach.

5. Limitations

Despite the encouraging results, it is essential to recognize several limitations in this study. First, each AI model analyzed is subject to ongoing updates and refinements, meaning that both inter-model variability and intra-model evolution are inevitable as their underlying datasets expand. This can lead to evolving and sometimes inconsistent outputs over time, even if the clinical scenario remains unchanged. Second, although we used a standardized format for data input, real-world clinical decision-making encompasses dynamic, multidisciplinary interactions and patient-specific factors that are not fully captured by retrospective data alone. Third, the recommendations produced by LLMs can vary significantly based on how prompts are formulated—slight differences in phrasing or the level of detail provided can substantially alter the generated responses. Fourth, our relatively small sample size may limit the generalizability of these findings, particularly for rarer treatment modalities such as flow diverters and WEB devices, which were each used in only two cases in our cohort. The low frequency of these modalities reflects their limited application in real-world practice at our center rather than selection bias; however, this small number inevitably restricts the precision of AI performance estimates in these subgroups, and results should therefore be interpreted with caution. Finally, exploring the performance of next-generation AI models, which may feature continuous learning capabilities, along with prospectively evaluating patient outcomes, will be crucial to fully understanding the actual impact of AI on clinical decision-making. Future studies incorporating larger, multi-center cohorts, real-time data, and patient-centered outcomes will help validate and refine the clinical utility of AI-driven decision support for the management of unruptured intracranial aneurysms.

6. Conclusions

In conclusion, our findings indicate that the evaluated LLMs, particularly ChatGPT-4, demonstrated high accuracy in determining whether conservative or operative management was appropriate for unruptured intracranial aneurysms. However, there was noticeably more variability when recommending specific treatment modalities (e.g., clipping vs. coiling). These results suggest that AI-based language models can be a valuable tool for initial screening decisions, especially in settings with limited access to specialized neurosurgical expertise. Nevertheless, the multidisciplinary neurovascular board, with its comprehensive and collaborative approach, remains essential for definitive management of unruptured intracranial aneurysms.

Supplementary Materials: The following supporting information can be downloaded at: https://www.mdpi.com/article/10.3390/brainsci15101061/s1, Supplementary data S1: Search engine data entry describing clinical and radiographic parameters entered into each Large Language Model (LLM), along with the corresponding outputs and the neurovascular board's decisions.

Author Contributions: Conceptualization, M.O. and A.E.R.; methodology, M.O. and S.N.; software, S.N.; validation, M.O., P.S. and R.R.; formal analysis, M.O.; investigation, M.O. and P.S.; resources, J.B. and A.E.R.; data curation, M.O.; writing—original draft preparation, M.O.; writing—review and editing, S.N., P.S., R.R., J.B. and A.E.R.; visualization, M.O. and S.N.; supervision, R.R., J.B. and A.E.R.; project administration, A.E.R. All authors have read and agreed to the published version of the manuscript.

Funding: This research received no external funding.

Institutional Review Board Statement: The study was conducted in accordance with the Declaration of Helsinki and approved by the Ethics Committee of the Albert-Ludwigs-Universität Freiburg (protocol code EK-Freiburg: 24-1429-S1, approval date 12 November 2024).

Informed Consent Statement: The requirement for individual informed consent was waived by the Ethics Committee, as the study involved a retrospective analysis of anonymized patient data, and obtaining consent would have required a disproportionately high effort relative to the minimal risk.

Data Availability Statement: The data presented in this study are available on reasonable request from the corresponding author. The data are not publicly available due to ethical and privacy restrictions, as they contain clinical information derived from patient records.

Conflicts of Interest: The authors declare no conflicts of interest.

Abbreviations

ACA	Anterior cerebral artery
ACOM	Anterior communicating artery
AI	Artificial intelligence
ASA	American Society of Anesthesiologists physical-status score
CI	Confidence interval
DDR	Distal dural ring

ELAPSS	Aneurysm growth-risk score (Earlier SAH, Location, Age, Population, Size, Shape)
GPT	Generative Pre-Trained Transformer (e.g., GPT-4, GPT-3.5)
ICA	Internal carotid artery
LLM	Large language model
MCA	Middle cerebral artery
OR	Odds ratio
PHASES	Aneurysm rupture-risk score (Population, Hypertension, Age, Size, Earlier SAH, Site)
SAH	Subarachnoid haemorrhage
SD	Standard deviation
SPSS	Statistical Package for the Social Sciences
STROBE	Strengthening the Reporting of Observational Studies in Epidemiology
UIA	Unruptured intracranial aneurysm
UIATS	Unruptured Intracranial Aneurysm Treatment Score
WEB	Woven EndoBridge (intrasaccular flow-diversion device)

References

1. Vlak, M.H.; Algra, A.; Brandenburg, R.; Rinkel, G.J. Prevalence of unruptured intracranial aneurysms, with emphasis on sex, age, comorbidity, country, and time period: A systematic review and meta-analysis. *Lancet Neurol.* **2011**, *10*, 626–636. [CrossRef] [PubMed]
2. Vernooij, M.W.; Ikram, M.A.; Tanghe, H.L.; Vincent, A.J.; Hofman, A.; Krestin, G.P.; Niessen, W.J.; Breteler, M.M.; van der Lugt, A. Incidental findings on brain MRI in the general population. *N. Engl. J. Med.* **2007**, *357*, 1821–1828. [CrossRef]
3. Wiebers, D.O.; Whisnant, J.P.; Huston, J.; Meissner, I.; Brown, R.D.; Piepgras, D.G.; Forbes, G.S.; Thielen, K.; Nichols, D.; O'Fallon, W.M.; et al. Unruptured intracranial aneurysms: Natural history, clinical outcome, and risks of surgical and endovascular treatment. *Lancet* **2003**, *362*, 103–110. [CrossRef]
4. Thompson, B.G.; Brown, R.D.; Amin-Hanjani, S.; Broderick, J.P.; Cockroft, K.M.; Connolly, E.S.; Duckwiler, G.R.; Harris, C.C.; Howard, V.J.; Johnston, S.C.; et al. Guidelines for the Management of Patients With Unruptured Intracranial Aneurysms: A Guideline for Healthcare Professionals From the American Heart Association/American Stroke Association. *Stroke* **2015**, *46*, 2368–2400. [CrossRef]
5. Etminan, N.; Brown, R.D.; Beseoglu, K.; Juvela, S.; Raymond, J.; Morita, A.; Torner, J.C.; Derdeyn, C.P.; Raabe, A.; Mocco, J.; et al. The unruptured intracranial aneurysm treatment score. *Neurology* **2015**, *85*, 881–889. [CrossRef]
6. Hackenberg, K.A.M.; Hänggi, D.; Etminan, N. Unruptured Intracranial Aneurysms. *Stroke* **2018**, *49*, 2268–2275. [CrossRef]
7. Etminan, N.; de Sousa, D.A.; Tiseo, C.; Bourcier, R.; Desal, H.; Lindgren, A.; Koivisto, T.; Netuka, D.; Peschillo, S.; Lémeret, S.; et al. European Stroke Organisation (ESO) guidelines on management of unruptured intracranial aneurysms. *Eur. Stroke J.* **2022**, *7*, V. [CrossRef]
8. Pontes, F.G.B.; da Silva, E.M.; Baptista-Silva, J.C.; Vasconcelos, V. Treatments for unruptured intracranial aneurysms. *Cochrane Database Syst. Rev.* **2021**, *5*, CD013312. [CrossRef] [PubMed]
9. Reddy, A.; Masoud, H.E. Endovascular and Medical Management of Unruptured Intracranial Aneurysms. *Semin. Neurol.* **2023**, *43*, 480–492. [CrossRef]
10. Kashkoush, A.; El-Abtah, M.E.; Petitt, J.C.; Glauser, G.; Winkelman, R.; Achey, R.L.; Davison, M.; Abdulrazzak, M.A.; Hussain, S.M.; Toth, G.; et al. Flow diversion for the treatment of intracranial bifurcation aneurysms: A systematic review and meta-analysis. *J. Neurointerv. Surg.* **2024**, *16*, 921–927. [CrossRef] [PubMed]
11. Greving, J.P.; Wermer, M.J.; Brown, R.D.; Morita, A.; Juvela, S.; Yonekura, M.; Ishibashi, T.; Torner, J.C.; Nakayama, T.; Rinkel, G.J.; et al. Development of the PHASES score for prediction of risk of rupture of intracranial aneurysms: A pooled analysis of six prospective cohort studies. *Lancet Neurol.* **2014**, *13*, 59–66. [CrossRef]
12. Backes, D.; Rinkel, G.J.E.; Greving, J.P.; Velthuis, B.K.; Murayama, Y.; Takao, H.; Ishibashi, T.; Igase, M.; terBrugge, K.G.; Agid, R.; et al. ELAPSS score for prediction of risk of growth of unruptured intracranial aneurysms. *Neurology* **2017**, *88*, 1600–1606. [CrossRef] [PubMed]
13. Mayer, T.E. The unruptured intracranial aneurysm treatment score: A multidisciplinary consensus. *Neurology* **2016**, *86*, 792–793. [CrossRef] [PubMed]
14. Laukka, D.; Kivelev, J.; Rahi, M.; Vahlberg, T.; Paturi, J.; Rinne, J.; Hirvonen, J. Detection Rates and Trends of Asymptomatic Unruptured Intracranial Aneurysms From 2005 to 2019. *Neurosurgery* **2024**, *94*, 297–306. [CrossRef]
15. Esteva, A.; Robicquet, A.; Ramsundar, B.; Kuleshov, V.; DePristo, M.; Chou, K.; Cui, C.; Corrado, G.; Thrun, S.; Dean, J. A guide to deep learning in healthcare. *Nat. Med.* **2019**, *25*, 24–29. [CrossRef] [PubMed]

16. Kozel, G.; Gurses, M.E.; Gecici, N.N.; Gökalp, E.; Bahadir, S.; Merenzon, M.A.; Shah, A.H.; Komotar, R.J.; Ivan, M.E. Chat-GPT on brain tumors: An examination of Artificial Intelligence/Machine Learning's ability to provide diagnoses and treatment plans for example neuro-oncology cases. *Clin. Neurol. Neurosurg.* **2024**, *239*, 108238. [CrossRef]
17. von Elm, E.; Altman, D.G.; Egger, M.; Pocock, S.J.; Gøtzsche, P.C.; Vandenbroucke, J.P.; Initiative, S. The Strengthening the Reporting of Observational Studies in Epidemiology (STROBE) statement: Guidelines for reporting observational studies. *J. Clin. Epidemiol.* **2008**, *61*, 344–349. [CrossRef]
18. Hoh, B.L.; Ko, N.U.; Amin-Hanjani, S.; Chou, S.H.-Y.; Cruz-Flores, S.; Dangayach, N.S.; Derdeyn, C.P.; Du, R.; Hänggi, D.; Hetts, S.W.; et al. 2023 Guideline for the Management of Patients With Aneurysmal Subarachnoid Hemorrhage: A Guideline From the American Heart Association/American Stroke Association. *Stroke* **2023**, *54*, e314–e370. [CrossRef]
19. Beretta, F.; Sepahi, A.N.; Zuccarello, M.; Tomsick, T.A.; Keller, J.T. Radiographic imaging of the distal dural ring for determining the intradural or extradural location of aneurysms. *Skull Base* **2005**, *15*, 253–261. [CrossRef]
20. Howard, B.M.; Hu, R.; Barrow, J.W.; Barrow, D.L. Comprehensive review of imaging of intracranial aneurysms and angiographically negative subarachnoid hemorrhage. *Neurosurg. Focus* **2019**, *47*, E20. [CrossRef]
21. Lam, D.L.; Pandharipande, P.V.; Lee, J.M.; Lehman, C.D.; Lee, C.I. Imaging-based screening: Understanding the controversies. *AJR Am. J. Roentgenol.* **2014**, *203*, 952–956. [CrossRef] [PubMed]
22. Lauric, A.; Ludwig, C.G.; Malek, A.M. Enhanced Radiomics for Prediction of Rupture Status in Cerebral Aneurysms. *World Neurosurg* **2022**, *159*, e8–e22. [CrossRef]
23. Wen, Z.; Wang, Y.; Zhong, Y.; Hu, Y.; Yang, C.; Peng, Y.; Zhan, X.; Zhou, P.; Zeng, Z. Advances in research and application of artificial intelligence and radiomic predictive models based on intracranial aneurysm images. *Front. Neurol.* **2024**, *15*, 1391382. [CrossRef]
24. Carl, N.; Schramm, F.; Haggenmüller, S.; Kather, J.N.; Hetz, M.J.; Wies, C.; Michel, M.S.; Wessels, F.; Brinker, T.J. Large language model use in clinical oncology. *npj Precis. Oncol.* **2024**, *8*, 240. [CrossRef] [PubMed]
25. Liu, J.; Zheng, J.; Cai, X.; Wu, D.; Yin, C. A descriptive study based on the comparison of ChatGPT and evidence-based neurosurgeons. *iScience* **2023**, *26*, 107590. [CrossRef] [PubMed]

brain sciences

MDPI

Article

Assessment of Interrater Reliability and Accuracy of Cerebral Aneurysm Morphometry Using 3D Virtual Reality, 2D Digital Subtraction Angiography, and 3D Reconstruction: A Randomized Comparative Study

Attill Saemann [1,*,†], Daniel de Wilde [1,†], Jonathan Rychen [1], Michel Roethlisberger [1,2], Marek Żelechowski [3], Balázs Faludi [3], Philippe Claude Cattin [3], Marios-Nikos Psychogios [2,4], Jehuda Soleman [1,2] and Raphael Guzman [1,2]

1 Department of Neurosurgery, University Hospital of Basel, 4031 Basel, Switzerland
2 Faculty of Medicine, University of Basel, 4056 Basel, Switzerland
3 Department of Biomedical Engineering, University of Basel, 4123 Allschwil, Switzerland
4 Department of Neuroradiology, University Hospital Basel, 4031 Basel, Switzerland
* Correspondence: attill.saemann@usb.ch
† These authors contributed equally to this work.

Abstract: Background/Objectives: Detailed morphometric analysis of an aneurysm and the related vascular bifurcation are critical factors when determining rupture risk and planning treatment for unruptured intracranial aneurysms (UIAs). The standard visualization of digital subtraction angiography (DSA) and its 3D reconstruction on a 2D monitor provide precise measurements but are subject to variability based on the rater. Visualization using virtual (VR) and augmented reality platforms can overcome those limitations. It is, however, unclear whether accurate measurements of the aneurysm and adjacent arterial branches can be obtained on VR models. This study aimed to assess interrater reliability and compare measurements between 3D VR, standard 2D DSA, and 3D DSA reconstructions, evaluating the reliability and accuracy of 3D VR as a measurement tool. Methods: A pool of five neurosurgeons performed three individual analyses on each of the ten UIA cases, measuring them in completely immersed 3D VR and the standard on-screen format (2D DSA and 3D reconstruction). This resulted in three independent measurements per modality for each case. Interrater reliability of measurements and morphology characterization, comparative differences, measurement duration, and VR user experience were assessed. Results: Interrater reliability for 3D VR measurements was significantly higher than for 3D DSA measurements (3D VR mean intraclass correlation coefficient [ICC]: 0.69 ± 0.22 vs. 3D DSA mean ICC: 0.36 ± 0.37, $p = 0.042$). No significant difference was observed between 3D VR and 2D DSA (3D VR mean ICC: 0.69 ± 0.22 vs. 2D DSA mean ICC: 0.43 ± 0.31, $p = 0.12$). A linear mixed-effects model showed no effect of 3D VR and 3D DSA (95% CI = −0.26–0.28, $p = 0.96$) or 3D VR and 2D DSA (95% CI = −0.02–0.53, $p = 0.066$) on absolute measurements of the aneurysm in the anteroposterior, mediolateral, and craniocaudal dimensions. Conclusions: 3D VR technology allows for reproducible, accurate, and reliable measurements comparable to measurements performed on a 2D screen. It may also potentially improve precision for measurements of non-planar aneurysm dimensions.

Keywords: augmented reality; cerebrovascular neurosurgery; intracranial aneurysm; measurement; morphometry; surgical planning; virtual reality

1. Introduction

Unruptured intracranial aneurysms (UIAs), relatively common vascular abnormalities found in 2–4% of the population [1], are increasingly detected due to the widespread use of non-invasive imaging [2]. While most UIAs remain asymptomatic, with a low risk of rupture, some may eventually rupture and lead to subarachnoid hemorrhage (SAH), which is associated with substantial morbidity and mortality [3]. The management of UIAs includes three primary approaches: conservative (with follow-up imaging), endovascular, or surgical treatment [4]. Selecting the most suitable strategy is a complex, patient-specific, and multidisciplinary decision. This decision is grounded in a comprehensive assessment comparing potential interventional and rupture risks.

Rupture risk is based on aneurysm dimensions, morphological features, and clinical patient characteristics [1,5–7]. In clinical practice, aneurysm dimensions and morphological features are necessary to calculate validated risk assessment scores such as PHASES and UIATS [7–9] and morphological parameters such as size ratio, aspect ratio, and dome-to-neck ratio, objectively quantifying rupture risk [10–12]. These scores have limits; for instance, they tend to inadequately assess small aneurysms (<7 mm), highlighting the need for a detailed evaluation of aneurysm dynamics and morphological characteristics [13–16].

Developed through different methodologies, these morphological parameters each provide a unique perspective: The aspect ratio is based on 2D digital subtraction angiography (DSA) measurements [10,17], while the size ratio and dome-to-neck ratio are derived from 3D DSA reconstruction measurements [11,12]. Ultimately, a precise assessment of the aneurysm is invaluable for planning the treatment (i.e., clip placement or fitting of an endosaccular device).

In a typical clinical routine, these measurements and characterizations are performed on 2D screens based on the primary imaging dataset, such as digital subtraction angiography (DSA), computed tomography angiography (CTA), or magnetic resonance angiography (MRA) of the UIA by neurosurgeons or neuroradiologists [18–20]. Among these methods, DSA remains the gold standard for analyzing aneurysms in clinical practice, with 3D DSA reconstruction (hereafter referred to as 3D DSA) preferred over 2D source imaging due to its ability to provide more detailed and 3D visualization of the aneurysm [10,21–23].

Virtual reality (VR) has quickly emerged as a transformative tool in the medical field, offering substantial benefits across applications, including medical education, patient education, rehabilitation, and surgical planning [24–28]. One of VR's key advantages is its ability to generate detailed 3D models of complex anatomy, which can be viewed and manipulated from multiple angles. This capability allows clinicians and students to overcome the inherent limitations of traditional 2D imaging, offering a more comprehensive understanding of anatomy and pathology. Newer VR technologies also offer intraluminal perspectives, further underscoring that VR could provide reliable measurements and characterization of UIAs compared to the 2D DSA source images and 3D reconstructions. However, despite the increasing use and availability of VR for neurosurgical planning, the validity of VR's measurement capability has yet to be confirmed, and its reliability in measurements and morphological characterization remains an area that requires further investigation.

To address this gap, we compared the interrater reliability of aneurysm measurements and morphological characterization of UIAs using 3D VR, 3D DSA, and 2D DSA. Furthermore, we aimed to investigate the comparative difference in size measurements and the duration of the measurements.

2. Materials and Methods

2.1. Study Design and Participants

Patients who underwent open surgical or endovascular treatment for UIAs at "our hospital" from 2021 to 2022 were retrospectively screened for inclusion. All of these had complete imaging and were judged to have been treated by an interdisciplinary neurovascular board consisting of neurosurgeons and interventional neuroradiologists. Ten cases were randomly selected and assigned unique identifiers. The latest 2D DSA (Siemens Healthineers, Erlangen, Germany) source images were used as baseline images for 2D DSA measurements. The vessel-injected flat-detector CTA (FD-CTA) from the same imaging session was used as a source image to reconstruct the 3D DSA and 3D VR models. Raters were randomly assigned to the UIA cases using an online randomization tool (randomlists.com, FL, USA). Each rater followed a measuring protocol (see Supplemental Digital Content S1 and S2) in the 3D VR and 2D modalities (Figure 1). The raters included five microsurgically trained neurosurgeons from the Department of Neurosurgery at the University Hospital of Basel, with various degrees of experience in vascular neurosurgery (one chief resident, three attending vascular neurosurgeons, and one chairman of vascular neurosurgery).

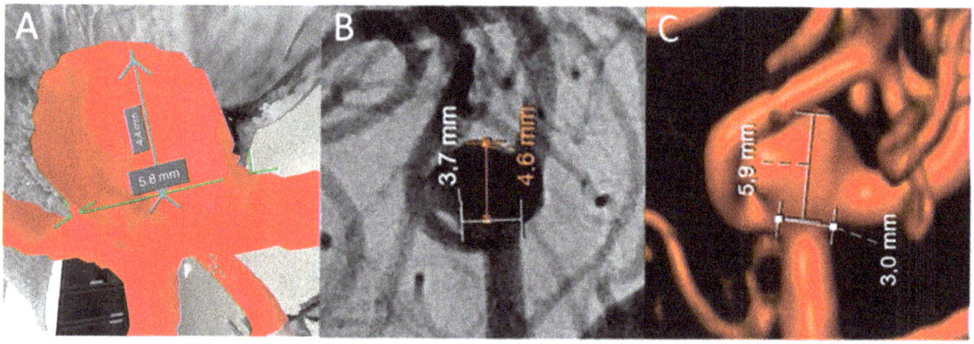

Figure 1. Comparison of 2D DSA, 3D DSA, and 3D VR measurements. (**A**) Measurement of neck diameter and maximum perpendicular aneurysm height using 3D VR. (**B**) Measurement of neck diameter and maximum perpendicular height using 2D DSA. (**C**) Measurement of neck diameter and maximum perpendicular aneurysm height using 3D DSA reconstructions.

2.2. VR Software

Each FD-CTA DICOM dataset was converted into a 3D VR model within the VR software SpectoVR (Version 5.0.0, Specto Medical AG, Basel, Switzerland). Initially, the DICOM dataset was imported into the software, followed by Hounsfield unit-based segmentation to visualize the blood vessels and the skull. Subsequently, an investigator manually removed any unnecessary noise or vessels to refine the model for accurate visualization. The geometrical and anatomical precision of SpectoVR has been established through previous validation studies [29,30]. The software was deployed on a Windows PC (Razer Blade 17 2022, Irvine, CA, USA, Intel CPU i7-12800H, 16GB DDR5 RAM, NVidia GeForce RTX 3080 Ti GPU, Santa Clara, CA, USA). Each model was subsequently saved and stored as a custom Specto file type on a password-encrypted external hard drive.

2.3. Measurements

The aneurysm dimensions measured in millimeters (mm) included the anteroposterior, mediolateral, craniocaudal, dome, neck (only if the presence of a neck was established), parent vessel diameter, maximum perpendicular height, and maximum aneurysm height. In addition to the measurements, raters were asked to assess aneurysm features, including morphological classification, the presence of a neck, spatial aneurysm orientation, and parent vessel (see Supplemental Digital Content S1). Raters first performed measurements in 3D VR, followed by measurements in 2D DSA and 3D DSA on-screen, with substantial temporal intervals between each modality.

Before the 3D VR measurements, each rater completed a questionnaire (see Supplemental Digital Content S2) containing questions about their neurosurgical experience and prior VR exposure. Raters were additionally granted the opportunity to review an overview of the aneurysm dimensions and morphological features planned to be assessed and pose any questions regarding definitions assuring standardized measurement. Subsequently, they entered a fully immersive 3D VR space using an HP Reverb G2 headset and HP motion controllers (HP Inc., Palo Alto, CA, USA). The investigator asked all raters to measure each aneurysm dimension and assess each morphological feature individually (Figure 2). Measurements in 3D VR were performed using two custom-definable points in the 3D space (Video S3, Figure 3).

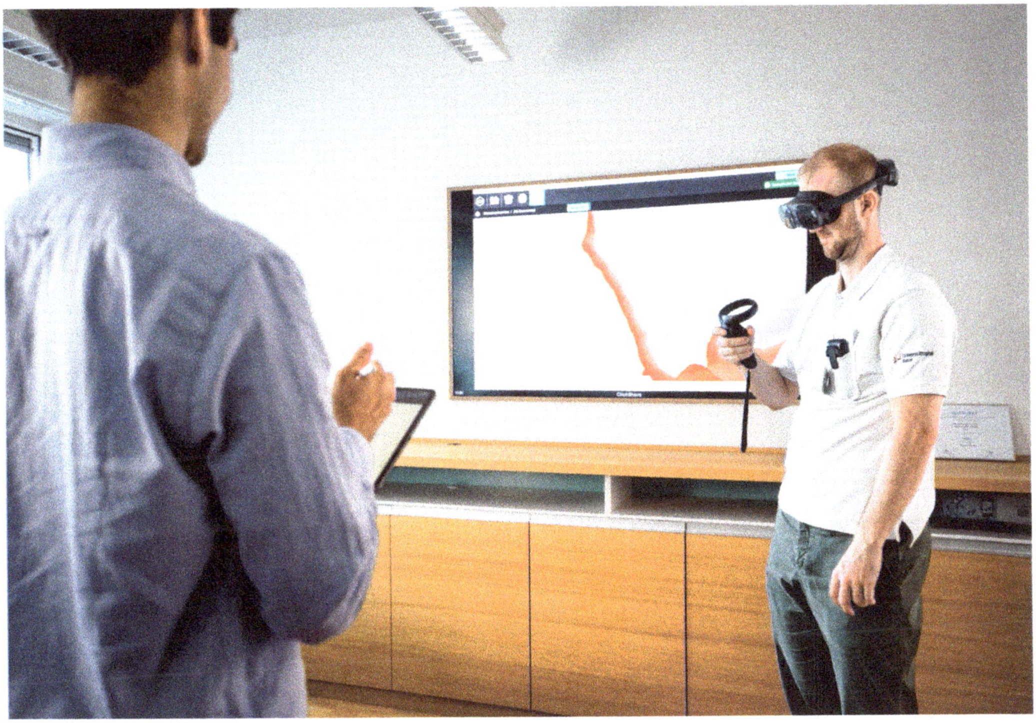

Figure 2. Investigator guiding rater through 3D VR measurements.

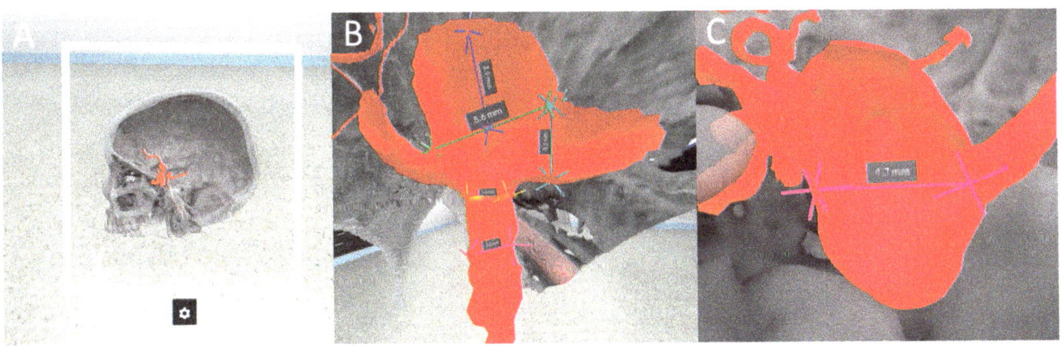

Figure 3. Various VR images from the study. (**A**) Interactive cutting plane feature for precise 3D slicing of anatomical models. (**B**) Measurement of neck diameter, maximum perpendicular height, and parent artery diameters in a 3D VR environment. (**C**) Intraluminal perspective for dome diameter measurement.

After all 3D VR measurements were completed, a questionnaire was administered to examine each rater's 3D VR measurement experience (see Supplemental Digital Content S2). Following the 3D VR measurements, all 2D and 3D DSA measurements were performed in the Sectra PACS image viewing software (Sectra AB, Linkoping, Sweden), following the same methodology outlined for the 3D VR measurements. Across all three modalities, measurements were performed with an accuracy of 0.1 mm.

2.4. Outcome Variables

The study's primary outcome was the interrater reliability in size measurement and description of aneurysm features (morphological classification, presence of neck, orientation, and parent vessel) between the three modalities (3D VR, 3D DSA, and 2D DSA).

The secondary outcomes included the comparative difference in size measurements in millimeters of the patient-specific UIA conducted in the modalities, the measurements' duration, and the VR's usability.

2.5. Statistical Analysis

All generated data were recorded in case report forms (Supplemental Digital Content S1 and S2). The data were subsequently imported as a CSV file into RStudio (Version 1.4.1106, Posit, PBC, Boston, MA, USA) for statistical analysis.

Comparative statistics were determined using the Wilcoxon signed-rank test, ANOVA, paired t-test, z-test, and linear mixed-effects model. Interrater reliability was assessed using the intraclass correlation coefficient (ICC) and Fleiss' κ. The threshold for statistical significance was set at a p value < 0.05.

3. Results

3.1. Patient Population and Rater Cohort

The study included ten patient-based cases with UIAs mostly arising from the anterior circulation, particularly the middle cerebral artery (50%, n = 5) and anterior communicating artery (30%, n = 3) (Table 1). Every case was assessed by three different raters out of a pool of five neurosurgeons. Consequently, a total of 90 measurements were acquired, 30 of which were performed using 3D VR, 30 using 3D DSA, and 30 using 2D DSA.

Table 1. Overview of unruptured intracranial aneurysm cases.

Patient ID	Parent Vessel	Side
1	MCA	Left
2	ACOM	Left
3	MCA	Right
4	MCA	Right
5	ACOM	Right
6	PCOM	Right
7	PCOM	Right
8	MCA	Right
9	ACOM	Left
10	MCA	Right

3.2. Primary Outcome

3.2.1. Interrater Reliability of Aneurysm Measurements Comparing 3D VR with 3D DSA and 2D DSA

Measurements of the anteroposterior diameter, mediolateral diameter, dome diameter, neck diameter, parent vessel diameter, and maximum perpendicular height all showed higher interrater reliability in 3D VR than in 3D DSA and 2D DSA. Craniocaudal diameter was the only dimension to demonstrate lower interrater reliability in 3D VR than both 3D DSA and 2D DSA. Maximum aneurysm height showed lower interrater reliability in 3D VR than 3D DSA alone (Table 2, Figures 4 and 5).

Overall, 3D VR exhibited higher interrater reliability than both 3D DSA and 2D DSA in aneurysm dimension measurements. The comparison between 3D VR and 3D DSA was significantly different (3D VR mean ICC: 0.69 ± 0.22 vs. 3D DSA mean ICC: 0.36 ± 0.37, p = 0.042). However, this difference did not reach significance when 3D VR was compared to 2D DSA (3D VR mean ICC: 0.69 ± 0.22 vs. 2D DSA mean ICC: 0.43 ± 0.31, p = 0.12).

Table 2. Interrater reliability of aneurysm dimensions and morphological parameters.

	3D VR (n = 30)		3D DSA (n = 30)		2D DSA (n = 30)	
Aneurysm Dimension	**ICC (95% CI)**	***p* Value**	**ICC (95% CI)**	***p* Value**	**ICC (95% CI)**	***p* Value**
Anteroposterior Diameter	0.9 (0.74–0.97)	0.000000003	0.65 (0.30–0.88)	0.00025	0.79 (0.51–0.94)	0.000007
Mediolateral Diameter	0.8 (0.55–0.94)	0.0000014	0.54 (0.16–0.84)	0.0026	0.59 (0.22–0.86)	0.00097
Cephalocaudal Diameter	0.56 (0.19–0.85)	0.0016	0.6 (0.24–0.87)	0.00075	0.73 (0.43–0.92)	0.00002
Smallest Axial Diameter	0.88 (0.71–0.97)	0.00000001	0.77 (0.49–0.93)	0.000005	0.8 (0.55–0.94)	0.0000013
Neck Diameter	0.8 (0.50–0.95)	0.000016	−0.49 (−0.50–−0.08)	0.98	0.26 (−0.26–0.91)	0.18
Parent Vessel Diameter	0.93 (0.82–0.98)	0.00000000004	0.5 (0.12–0.82)	0.0047	0.03 (−0.26–0.50)	0.41
Maximum Aneurysm Height	0.35 (−0.03–0.74)	0.037	0.57 (0.20–0.85)	0.0014	0.27 (−0.09–0.69)	0.079
Maximum Perpendicular Height	0.78 (0.50–0.93)	0.000004	0.52 (0.14–0.83)	0.0033	0.25 (−0.11–0.68)	0.099
			Morphological Parameter			
Aspect Ratio	0.33 (−0.09–0.77)	0.066	0.23 (−0.33–0.96)	0.23	0.34 (−0.21–0.92)	0.13
Dome-to-Neck Ratio	0.55 (0.13–0.87)	0.0051	0.14 (−0.36–0.95)	0.30	0.72 (0.17–0.98)	0.0067
Size Ratio	0.76 (0.47–0.93)	0.0000086	−0.04 (−0.3–0.43)	0.55	−0.04 (0.3–0.43)	0.55

VR = virtual reality, DSA = digital subtraction angiography, ICC = intraclass correlation coefficient, CI = confidence interval.

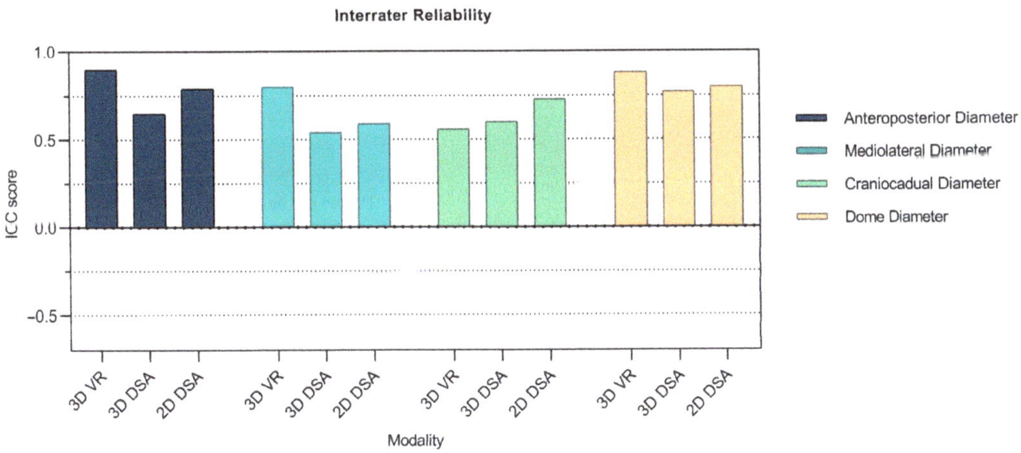

Figure 4. Bar charts showing ICC scores for 2D DSA, 3D DSA, and 3D VR measurements of various aneurysm dimensions.

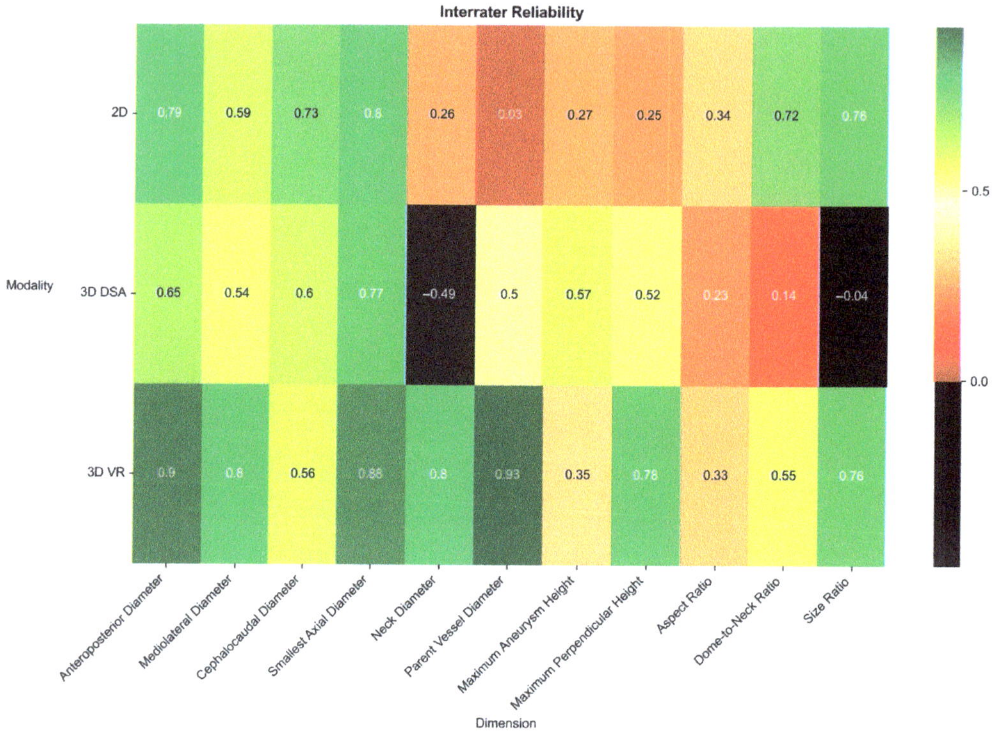

Figure 5. Heat map of ICC scores for 2D DSA, 3D DSA, and 3D VR measurements of various aneurysm dimensions. ICC values indicate reliability: below 0.5 = poor, 0.5–0.75 = moderate, 0.75–0.9 = good, and above 0.9 = excellent.

3.2.2. Interrater Reliability of Morphological Aneurysm Features Comparing 3D VR with 3D DSA and 2D DSA

Morphological classification displayed non-significantly higher interrater reliability in 3D VR (3D VR [Fleiss' $\varkappa$ (95% CI)]: 0.35 (0.13–0.57)) than 3D DSA (3D DSA [$\varkappa$ (95% CI)]: 0.16 (−0.06–0.37), p = 0.23) and significantly higher interrater reliability than 2D DSA (2D DSA [$\varkappa$ (95% CI)]: −0.045 (−0.29–0.2), p = 0.019). 3D VR (3D VR [$\varkappa$ (95% CI)]: 0.26 (−0.1–0.62) exhibited non-significant higher interrater reliability when determining the presence of an aneurysm neck than 3D DSA (3D DSA [$\varkappa$ (95% CI)]: −0.05 (−0.41–0.31), p = 0.23) and 2D DSA (2D DSA [$\varkappa$ (95% CI)]: −0.071 (−0.45–0.31), p = 0.22). Regarding aneurysm orientation, 3D VR (3D VR [$\varkappa$ (95% CI)]: 0.3 (0.17–0.43)) exhibited significantly lower interrater reliability than 2D DSA (2D DSA [$\varkappa$ (95% CI)]: 0.51 (0.38–0.63), p = 0.02) and non-significantly higher interrater reliability than 3D DSA (3D DSA [$\varkappa$ (95% CI)]: 0.17 (0.027–0.31), p = 0.18). Accurate identification of the parent vessel was achieved in 90% (n = 27) of cases using 3D VR assessment, in 70% (n = 21) using 3D DSA assessment, and in 93% (n = 28) using 2D DSA assessment.

3.3. Secondary Outcomes

3.3.1. Comparative Differences between the 3D VR Measurements and the 3D and 2D DSA Measurements

All dimensions and morphological parameters except for dome diameter, maximum height, maximum perpendicular height, and dome-to-neck ratio showed non-significant differences between 3D VR and 3D DSA (Table 3, Figure 6). Compared to 2D DSA, all dimensions and morphological parameters, except for neck diameter, parent vessel diameter, maximum height, and perpendicular height, showed non-significant differences in 3D VR (Table 3, Figure 6).

Table 3. Aneurysm dimension measurement difference comparison by modality.

	3D VR (n = 30)	3D DSA (n = 30)	2D DSA (n = 30)	3D VR vs. 3D DSA	3D VR vs. 2D DSA	3D DSA vs. 2D DSA
Aneurysm Dimension	**Mean ± Range (mm)**	**Mean ± Range (mm)**	**Mean ± Range (mm)**	***p* Value**	***p* Value**	***p* Value**
Anteroposterior Diameter	5.7 ± 5	5.8 ± 5.1	5.7 ± 5	0.84	0.84	0.68
Mediolateral Diameter	5.7 ± 5.1	5.8 ± 5.1	5.4 ± 3.7	0.62	0.69	0.46
Craniocaudal Diameter	6.3 ± 4.6	6.1 ± 5.7	5.8 ± 5	0.42	0.23	0.63
Dome Diameter	5.8 ± 4.6	6.1 ± 6.5	5.3 ± 5.8	0.004	0.14	0.85
Neck Diameter	4.4 ± 3.8	3.3 ± 4.1	3.4 ± 3.6	0.68	0.005	0.10
Parent Vessel Diameter	2.3 ± 1.8	2.3 ± 2.55	1.9 ± 2.8	0.48	0.017	0.047
Maximum Height	6.5 ± 8.5	5.8 ± 4.4	5.7 ± 3.9	0.016	0.009	0.80
Maximum Perpendicular Height	6.3 ± 4.3	5.3 ± 4.5	5.3 ± 5.3	0.016	0.004	0.95
		Morphological Parameter				
Aspect Ratio	1.6 ± 2.1	1.6 ± 1.8	1.7 ± 3.3	0.63	0.38	0.93
Dome-to-Neck Ratio	1.4 ± 2.4	1.9 ± 3.2	1.7 ± 2.6	0.0044	0.14	0.60
Size Ratio	3 ± 5.2	2.5 ± 2.4	3.3 ± 10.3	0.057	0.75	0.088

VR = virtual reality, DSA = digital subtraction angiography.

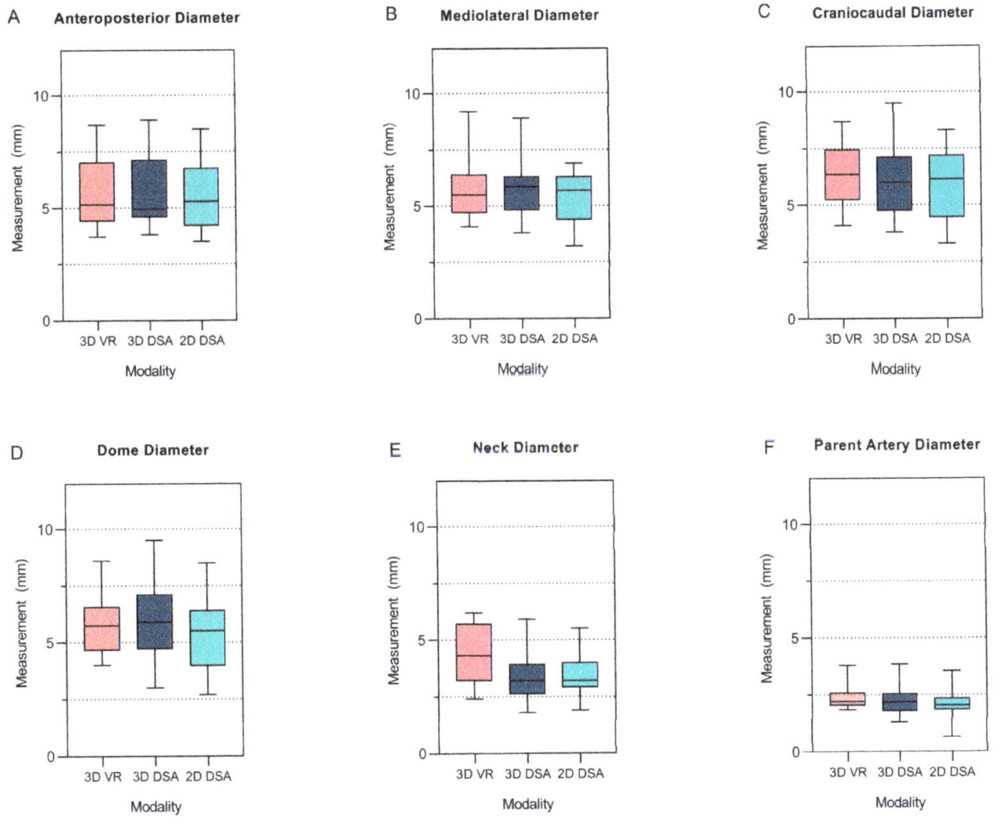

Figure 6. Box plots showing mean and range using 2D DSA, 3D DSA, and 3D VR for measurements of various aneurysm dimensions. (**A**) Anteroposterior diameter. (**B**) Mediolateral diameter. (**C**) Craniocaudal diameter. (**D**) Dome diameter. (**E**) Neck diameter. (**F**) Parent artery diameter.

A linear mixed-effects model comparing the effect of 3D VR and 3D DSA for antero-posterior, mediolateral, and craniocaudal diameter measurements found no significant difference (95% CI = −0.26–0.28, p = 0.96). Also, the model indicated no significant difference in diameter measurements between 3D VR and 2D DSA (95% CI = −0.02–0.53, p = 0.066).

3.3.2. Measurement Duration

When comparing 3D VR and 2D DSA, the 3D VR measurements were found to have a non-significantly higher mean duration (3D VR mean duration: 8.2 ± 15 min vs. 2D DSA mean duration: 7.1 ± 11 min, p = 0.15). The mean measurement duration was significantly higher for 3D VR measurements than for 3D DSA measurements (3D VR mean duration: 8.2 ± 15 min vs. 3D DSA mean duration: 4.7 ± 5 min, p = 0.000006).

The mean slope for measurement duration was higher for 3D VR than for 3D DSA and 2D DSA (3D VR: −1.14 ± 9 vs. 3D DSA: −0.66 ± 1.6 vs. 2D DSA: −0.41 ± 1.7), indicating a positive learning curve with increased usage (Figure 7). However, no statistically significant differences were noted between 3D VR and 3D DSA (p = 0.76) or between 3D VR and 2D DSA (p = 0.65).

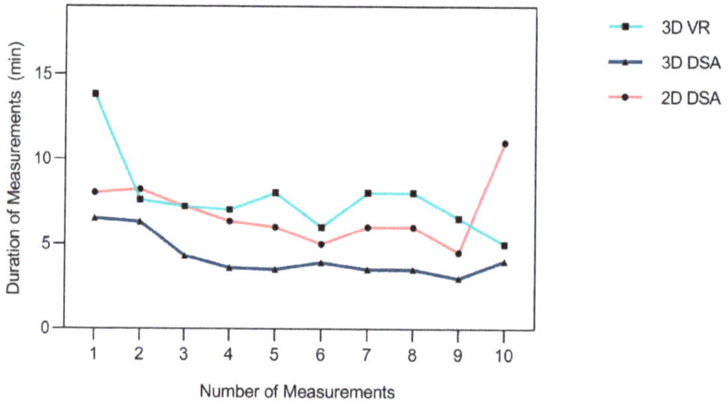

Figure 7. Line chart showing mean duration of measurement in relation to number of measurements performed.

3.3.3. Subjective Rater Experience

All raters described the 3D VR models as more intuitive to assess than the standard on-screen measurements. Furthermore, each rater expressed a desire to utilize 3D VR technology more frequently. Each rater observed phases of flow and immersion during their 3D VR measurements, with no motion sickness reported (Table 4).

Table 4. Subjective virtual reality experience.

	Rater Assessment
Which modality do you find easier to detect and describe aneurysms?	5/5 (100%) virtual reality model
	Overall agreement (1 = strongly agree, 2 = agree, 3 = neutral, 4 = disagree, 5 = strongly disagree)
	Mean (SD)
Everyday thoughts and concerns faded out during the measurement.	2.1 (0.75)
I experienced fatigue, eyestrain, difficulty focusing, headache, blurred vision, dizziness (eyes closed), or vertigo.	4.5 (0.54)

4. Discussion

Our results have shown that 3D VR measurements and the morphological characterization of aneurysms tend to exhibit higher interrater reliability than 2D DSA source images and their derived 3D reconstructions. These findings promote the potential utility of 3D VR technology as a modern tool for reproducible, precise, and reliable measurement of UIAs. Furthermore, no significant differences were found in the basic anteroposterior, mediolateral, and craniocaudal diameter measurements when comparing 3D VR to 3D DSA and 2D DSA, verifying its precision and applicability in clinical practice. Morphological parameters, including size and aspect ratio, also showed no significant difference between 3D VR, 3D DSA, and 2D DSA. To the best of our knowledge, this study is the first to compare and validate aneurysm measurements performed in a fully immersed 3D VR environment with measurements conducted on traditional 2D DSA images and 3D reconstructions. 3D DSA is widely regarded as the gold standard for assessing intracranial aneurysms, offering high-resolution 3D reconstructions that allow for precise assessment of aneurysm morphology and dimensions [31,32]. However, a comparison to 3D VR suggests that 3D VR may provide more reliable measurements than the current gold standard.

The interrater reliability of 3D VR was significantly higher than that of 3D DSA and comparable to that of 2D DSA. 3D VR measurements demonstrated higher interrater reliability in seven of eight aneurysm dimensions assessed compared to 2D DSA measurements. This may be attributed to the improved 3D visualization, which eliminates spatial superimposition, making measurements more accessible and reproducible with less investigator dependency. The comparison between 3D DSA and 2D DSA revealed no significant difference in interrater reliability. This pattern aligns with the findings of Timmins et al. [32], who also observed comparable interrater reliability when comparing 2D MRAs and their 3D reconstruction on-screen. The non-significant difference in anteroposterior, mediolateral, and craniocaudal diameters (i.e., planar dimensions of an aneurysm) between 3D VR models, 2D source images, and 3D reconstructions shows that 3D VR technology can perform planar aneurysm measurements with the same precision as on-screen measurements. This finding aligns with previous studies investigating the comparability of measurements between reconstructed 3D imaging and source imagery [33].

Regarding interrater reliability for morphological aneurysm features, we found that morphological classification exhibited non-significantly higher interrater reliability in 3D VR than in 3D DSA and significantly higher interrater reliability than in 2D DSA. The accuracy of identifying parent arteries was comparable between 3D VR and 2D DSA, whereas 3D DSA was substantially less accurate. This inaccuracy may stem from the fact that only the region of interest (ROI) surrounding the aneurysm is reconstructed in 3D, which makes it challenging to understand the full anatomy and orientation in the 3D space. Additionally, comparably low interrater reliability was observed when determining the presence of a neck in all three modalities. However, it must be noted that the ICC for 3D VR was substantially higher than that observed for 3D DSA and 2D DSA. This previously reported discrepancy in determining neck presence [34] may be explained by certain raters' tendency to infer the presence of a neck even when it may not be clearly visible. This discrepancy seemed to emerge in cases where branching vessels arise from the neck.

Interestingly, some significant differences were observed in the arguably more complex (non-planar) measurements of dome diameter, neck diameter, parent vessel diameter, maximum height, and maximum perpendicular height between 3D VR and 3D DSA and between 3D VR and 2D DSA. Upon initial assessment, this finding might lead to the conclusion that 3D VR has a diminished capability to perform such complex measurements. However, we hypothesize that the inability of 2D visualized DSAs to clearly depict aneurysm neck and parent vessel delineation substantially decreased the rater's precision in performing neck and parent vessel diameter measurements, as observed by Hochmuth et al. [21]. In contrast, the ability of 3D VR to view and measure aneurysms independently from any angle or plane and provide intraluminal visualization suggests that 3D VR can provide more precise and realistic measurements of the diameter of the neck and parent vessel. These findings indicate that 3D VR is a tool that offers comparable planar measurements while improving precision for nonplanar aneurysm dimensions with higher interrater reliability. Thus, its measurements might be closer to the ground truth.

Higher measurement durations were found for 3D VR and 2D DSA than for 3D DSA. However, it must be noted that 3D DSA measurements are performed routinely in clinical practice; therefore, raters had more experience measuring the specific dimensions in this particular sequence than for the other two modalities. More interestingly, a higher mean rate of change in measurement duration per additional measurement performed was observed in 3D VR than for both 3D DSA and 2D DSA, suggesting a positive learning curve. The observed trend of decreased duration in VR measurements aligns with the findings of the study conducted by Greuter et al. [34] that assessed the time to detect aneurysms in 3D VR. Therefore, it can be inferred that with increased training and experience, VR can likely achieve measurement durations comparable to those of 3D DSA and 2D DSA.

Raters unanimously described the 3D VR system as more intuitive than the 3D DSA and 2D DSA on-screen environments. Additionally, VR induced states of psychological flow and immersion. Notably, the raters in this study did not report any motion sickness components, possibly due to the advanced functionality of SpectoVR, which has been previously validated [29,30].

Although still emerging in cerebrovascular surgery, the ability of VR to generate accurate and interactive 3D models has proven to be a powerful tool to enhance spatial awareness and surgical precision. Studies have shown that VR significantly improves the detection of arterial anatomy in UIAs, leading to better anatomical understanding, optimized head positioning, and a more precise selection of surgical approaches [35]. Additionally, VR has been shown to reduce operating times for aneurysm clipping through more effective preoperative planning [36]. These examples are just a few of many studies highlighting the value of VR in aneurysm surgery, where it plays a crucial role in the surgical planning, execution, and teaching of complex anatomy [37–41].

However, as VR is increasingly implemented in clinical practice, verifying its validity compared to the current gold standard is fundamental. While 3D VR has demonstrated precise measurement values with higher interrater reliability in our study, there is currently a lack of data on its impact on clinical decision-making and patient outcomes. Since decision-making about treating UIAs remains strongly dependent on size and morphological characteristics, the precision and objective understanding of morphology gain importance, especially in small aneurysms, for instance [15]. Additionally, with the established practice of interdisciplinary decision-making for the treatment strategy of UIAs, increased interrater reliability supports objective discussion. Dedicated studies evaluating the particular impact of 3D VR in those situations are warranted to further validate the utility and applicability of 3D VR measurement and characterization in clinical practice.

Limitations

Several limitations should be considered when interpreting this study's findings. First, considerable variation in the number of aneurysms measured by each rater (three to ten) may have influenced correlation and reliability results. Also, no UIAs that were managed conservatively were included. Furthermore, this study had a relatively small sample size of only ten aneurysm cases, which likely does not encompass the breadth of different locations, sizes, and features of aneurysms, thus providing low power for generalizing the findings. It is essential to note that all raters were neurosurgeons rather than neuroradiologists, who more commonly perform aneurysm size measurements. Additionally, the cost of a VR system has to be considered, as it potentially limits the availability of VR in routine neurosurgical practice globally.

5. Conclusions

3D VR technology offers measurements comparable to those of 2D DSA and its 3D reconstruction while likely increasing interrater reliability. It can potentially improve the precision of measurements for non-planar aneurysm dimensions such as parent vessel, neck diameter, and height. More data regarding its utility in judging morphological changes in aneurysms are required.

Supplementary Materials: The following supporting information can be downloaded at: https://www.mdpi.com/article/10.3390/brainsci14100968/s1, Supplemental Digital Content S1: Virtual reality experience survey, Supplemental Digital Content S2: Measurement case report form, Supplemental Digital Content S3: Video demonstrating the virtual reality measurement process.

Author Contributions: Conceptualization, A.S. and R.G.; methodology, A.S. and R.G.; software, M.Ż., B.F. and P.C.C.; validation, A.S. and R.G.; formal analysis, A.S. and D.d.W.; investigation, A.S. and R.G.; resources, P.C.C., M.-N.P. and R.G.; data curation, A.S., J.R., M.R., J.S., R.G. and D.d.W.; writing—original draft preparation, A.S. and D.d.W.; writing—review and editing, all authors; visualization, A.S. and D.d.W.; supervision, J.S. and R.G.; project administration, A.S. and R.G. All authors have read and agreed to the published version of the manuscript.

Funding: This research received no external funding.

Institutional Review Board Statement: The study was conducted in accordance with the Declaration of Helsinki and approved by the Ethics Committee of Northwest and Central Switzerland (EKNZ-No. 2021-0139, 6 January 2023).

Informed Consent Statement: Informed consent was obtained from all subjects involved in the study.

Data Availability Statement: The data supporting the findings of this study are included within the article. Any additional data or materials can be made available to the corresponding author upon reasonable request.

Acknowledgments: We are grateful to the Department of Clinical Research at the University of Basel for their assistance in statistical analysis and the CNRN (Clinical Neurosurgical Research Network Basel) for administrative support.

Conflicts of Interest: The authors declare no conflicts of interest.

References

1. Vlak, M.H.M.; Algra, A.; Brandenburg, R.; Rinkel, G.J.E. Prevalence of unruptured intracranial aneurysms, with emphasis on sex, age, comorbidity, country, and time period: A systematic review and meta analysis. *Lancet Neurol.* **2011**, *10*, 626–636. [CrossRef] [PubMed]
2. Vernooij, M.W.; Ikram, M.A.; Tanghe, H.L.; Vincent, A.J.; Hofman, A.; Krestin, G.P.; Niessen, W.J.; Breteler, M.M.B.; van der Lugt, A. Incidental Findings on Brain MRI in the General Population. *N. Engl. J. Med.* **2007**, *357*, 1821–1828. [CrossRef] [PubMed]
3. Nieuwkamp, D.J.; Setz, L.E.; Algra, A.; Linn, F.H.H.; de Rooij, N.K.; Rinkel, G.J.E. Changes in case fatality of aneurysmal subarachnoid haemorrhage over time, according to age, sex, and region: A meta-analysis. *Lancet Neurol.* **2009**, *8*, 635–642. [CrossRef] [PubMed]
4. Williams, L.N.; Brown, R.D. Management of unruptured intracranial aneurysms. *Neurol. Clin. Pract.* **2013**, *3*, 99–108. [CrossRef] [PubMed]
5. Korja, M.; Lehto, H.; Juvela, S. Lifelong Rupture Risk of Intracranial Aneurysms Depends on Risk Factors. *Stroke* **2014**, *45*, 1958–1963. [CrossRef]
6. Müller, T.B.; Vik, A.; Romundstad, P.R.; Sandvei, M.S. Risk Factors for Unruptured Intracranial Aneurysms and Subarachnoid Hemorrhage in a Prospective Population-Based Study. *Stroke* **2019**, *50*, 2952–2955. [CrossRef]
7. Bijlenga, P.; Gondar, R.; Schilling, S.; Morel, S.; Hirsch, S.; Cuony, J.; Corniola, M.-V.; Perren, F.; Rüfenacht, D.; Schaller, K. PHASES Score for the Management of Intracranial Aneurysm. *Stroke* **2017**, *48*, 2105–2112. [CrossRef]
8. Greving, J.P.; Wermer, M.J.; Brown, R.D.; Morita, A.; Juvela, S.; Yonekura, M.; Ishibashi, T.; Torner, J.C.; Nakayama, T.; Rinkel, G.J.E.; et al. Development of the PHASES score for prediction of risk of rupture of intracranial aneurysms: A pooled analysis of six prospective cohort studies. *Lancet Neurol.* **2014**, *13*, 59–66. [CrossRef]
9. Etminan, N.; Brown Jr, R.D.; Beseoglu, K.; Juvela, S.; Raymond, J.; Morita, A.; Torner, J.C.; Derdeyn, C.P.; Raabe, A.; Mocco, J.; et al. The unruptured intracranial aneurysm treatment score: A multidisciplinary consensus. *Neurology* **2015**, *85*, 881–889. (In English) [CrossRef]
10. Ujiie, H.; Tamano, Y.; Sasaki, K.; Hori, T. Is the aspect ratio a reliable index for predicting the rupture of a saccular aneurysm? *Neurosurgery* **2001**, *48*, 495–502; discussion 502–503. (In English) [CrossRef]
11. Dhar, S.; Tremmel, M.; Mocco, J.; Kim, M.; Yamamoto, J.; Siddiqui, A.H.; Hopkins, L.N.; Meng, H. Morphology parameters for intracranial aneurysm rupture risk assessment. *Neurosurgery* **2008**, *63*, 185–196; discussion 196–197. (In English) [CrossRef] [PubMed]

12. Kiyosue, H.; Tanoue, S.; Okahara, M.; Hori, Y.; Nakamura, T.; Nagatomi, H.; Mori, H. Anatomic features predictive of complete aneurysm occlusion can be determined with three-dimensional digital subtraction angiography. *AJNR Am. J. Neuroradiol.* **2002**, *23*, 1206–1213. (In English) [PubMed]
13. Malhotra, A.; Wu, X.; Forman, H.P.; Grossetta Nardini, H.K.; Matouk, C.C.; Gandhi, D.; Moore, C.; Sanelli, P.G. Rupture Risk of Small Unruptured Intracranial Aneurysms: A Systematic Review. *Ann. Intern. Med.* **2017**, *167*, 26–33. (In English) [CrossRef] [PubMed]
14. Ikawa, F.; Morita, A.; Tominari, S.; Nakayama, T.; Shiokawa, Y.; Date, I.; Nozaki, K.; Miyamoto, S.; Kayama, T.; Arai, H.; et al. Rupture risk of small unruptured cerebral aneurysms. *J. Neurosurg.* **2019**, *132*, 69–78. (In English) [CrossRef]
15. Pettersson, S.D.; Salih, M.; Young, M.; Shutran, M.; Taussky, P.; Ogilvy, C.S. Predictors for Rupture of Small (<7 mm) Intracranial Aneurysms: A Systematic Review and Meta-Analysis. *World Neurosurg.* **2024**, *182*, 184–192.e14. (In English) [CrossRef]
16. Rutledge, C.; Jonzzon, S.; Winkler, E.A.; Raper, D.; Lawton, M.T.; Abla, A.A. Small Aneurysms with Low PHASES Scores Account for Most Subarachnoid Hemorrhage Cases. *World Neurosurg.* **2020**, *139*, e580–e584. (In English) [CrossRef]
17. Ujiie, H.; Tachibana, H.; Hiramatsu, O.; Hazel, A.L.; Matsumoto, T.; Ogasawara, Y.; Nakajima, H.; Hori, T.; Takakura, K.; Kajiya, F. Effects of size and shape (aspect ratio) on the hemodynamics of saccular aneurysms: A possible index for surgical treatment of intracranial aneurysms. *Neurosurgery* **1999**, *45*, 119–129; discussion 129–130. (In English) [CrossRef]
18. Beaman, C.; Patel, S.D.; Nael, K.; Colby, G.P.; Liebeskind, D.S. Imaging of Intracranial Saccular Aneurysms. *Stroke Vasc. Interv. Neurol.* **2023**, *3*, e000757. [CrossRef]
19. Backes, D.; Vergouwen, M.D.; Velthuis, B.K.; van der Schaaf, I.C.; Bor AS, E.; Algra, A.; Rinkel, G.J. Difference in Aneurysm Characteristics Between Ruptured and Unruptured Aneurysms in Patients with Multiple Intracranial Aneurysms. *Stroke* **2014**, *45*, 1299–1303. [CrossRef]
20. Kouskouras, C.; Charitanti, A.; Giavroglou, C.; Foroglou, N.; Selviaridis, P.; Kontopoulos, V.; Dimitriadis, A.S. Intracranial aneurysms: Evaluation using CTA and MRA. Correlation with DSA and intraoperative findings. *Neuroradiology* **2004**, *46*, 842–850. [CrossRef]
21. Hochmuth, A.; Spetzger, U.; Schumacher, M. Comparison of three-dimensional rotational angiography with digital subtraction angiography in the assessment of ruptured cerebral aneurysms. *AJNR Am. J. Neuroradiol.* **2002**, *23*, 1199–1205. (In English) [PubMed]
22. Zhou, Y.; Yang, P.F.; Fang, Y.B.; Xu, Y.; Hong, B.; Zhao, W.Y.; Li, Q.; Zhao, R.; Huang, Q.-H.; Liu, J.-M. Parent Artery Reconstruction for Large or Giant Cerebral Aneurysms Using the Tubridge Flow Diverter: A Multicenter, Randomized, Controlled Clinical Trial (PARAT). *Am. J. Neuroradiol.* **2018**, *39*, 807. [CrossRef] [PubMed]
23. Wong, S.C.; Nawawi, O.; Ramli, N.; Kadir, K.A.A. Benefits of 3D Rotational DSA Compared with 2D DSA in the Evaluation of Intracranial Aneurysm. *Acad. Radiol.* **2012**, *19*, 701–707. [CrossRef] [PubMed]
24. van der Kruk, S.R.; Zielinski, R.; MacDougall, H.; Hughes-Barton, D.; Gunn, K.M. Virtual reality as a patient education tool in healthcare: A scoping review. *Patient Educ. Couns.* **2022**, *105*, 1928–1942. [CrossRef]
25. Chen, S.; Zhu, J.; Cheng, C.; Pan, Z.; Liu, L.; Du, J.; Shen, X.; Shen, Z.; Zhu, H.; Liu, J.; et al. Can virtual reality improve traditional anatomy education programmes? A mixed-methods study on the use of a 3D skull model. *BMC Med. Educ.* **2020**, *20*, 395. [CrossRef]
26. Asadzadeh, A.; Samad-Soltani, T.; Salahzadeh, Z.; Rezaei-Hachesu, P. Effectiveness of virtual reality-based exercise therapy in rehabilitation: A scoping review. *Inform. Med. Unlocked* **2021**, *24*, 100562. [CrossRef]
27. Mishra, R.; Narayanan, M.D.K.; Umana, G.E.; Montemurro, N.; Chaurasia, B.; Deora, H. Virtual Reality in Neurosurgery: Beyond Neurosurgical Planning. *Int. J. Environ. Res. Public Health* **2022**, *19*, 1719. [CrossRef]
28. Saemann, A.; Schmid, S.; Licci, M.; Zelechowski, M.; Faludi, B.; Cattin, P.C.; Soleman, J.; Guzman, R. Enhancing educational experience through establishing a VR database in craniosynostosis: Report from a single institute and systematic literature review. *Front. Surg.* **2024**, *11*, 1440042. [CrossRef]
29. Maloca, P.M.; Faludi, B.; Zelechowski, M.; Jud, C.; Vollmar, T.; Hug, S. Validation of virtual reality orbitometry bridges digital and physical worlds. *Sci. Rep.* **2020**, *10*, 11815. (In English) [CrossRef]
30. Maloca, P.M.; de Carvalho JE, R.; Heeren, T.; Hasler, P.W.; Mushtaq, F.; Mon-Williams, M.; Scholl, H.P.N.; Balaskas, K.; Egan, C.; Tufail, A.; et al. High-Performance Virtual Reality Volume Rendering of Original Optical Coherence Tomography Point-Cloud Data Enhanced with Real-Time Ray Casting. *Transl. Vis. Sci. Technol.* **2018**, *7*, 2. [CrossRef]
31. Van Rooij, W.J.; Sprengers, M.E.; De Gast, A.N.; Peluso, J.P.P.; Sluzewski, M. 3D Rotational Angiography: The New Gold Standard in the Detection of Additional Intracranial Aneurysms. *Am. J. Neuroradiol.* **2008**, *29*, 976–979. [CrossRef] [PubMed]
32. Timmins, K.M.; Kuijf, H.J.; Vergouwen MD, I.; Otten, M.J.; Ruigrok, Y.M.; Velthuis, B.K.; van der Schaaf, I.C. Reliability and Agreement of 2D and 3D Measurements on MRAs for Growth Assessment of Unruptured Intracranial Aneurysms. *Am. J. Neuroradiol.* **2021**, *42*, 1598–1603. [CrossRef] [PubMed]
33. Sakamoto, S.; Kiura, Y.; Shibukawa, M.; Ohba, S.; Arita, K.; Kurisu, K. Subtracted 3D CT Angiography for Evaluation of Internal Carotid Artery Aneurysms: Comparison with Conventional Digital Subtraction Angiography. *Am. J. Neuroradiol.* **2006**, *27*, 1332. [PubMed]
34. Forbes, G.; Fox, A.J.; Huston, J., 3rd; Wiebers, D.O.; Torner, J. Interobserver variability in angiographic measurement and morphologic characterization of intracranial aneurysms: A report from the International Study of Unruptured Intracranial Aneurysms. *AJNR. Am. J. Neuroradiol.* **1996**, *17*, 1407–1415. (In English) [PubMed]

35. Zawy Alsofy, S.; Sakellaropoulou, I.; Nakamura, M.; Ewelt, C.; Salma, A.; Lewitz, M.; Welzel Saravia, H.; Sarkis, H.M.; Fortmann, T.; Stroop, R.; et al. Impact of Virtual Reality in Arterial Anatomy Detection and Surgical Planning in Patients with Unruptured Anterior Communicating Artery Aneurysms. *Brain Sci.* **2020**, *10*, 963. [CrossRef] [PubMed]
36. Steineke, T.C.; Barbery, D. Microsurgical clipping of middle cerebral artery aneurysms: Preoperative planning using virtual reality to reduce procedure time. *Neurosurg. Focus* **2021**, *51*, E12. [CrossRef]
37. Greuter, L.; De Rosa, A.; Cattin, P.; Croci, D.M.; Soleman, J.; Guzman, R. Randomized study comparing 3D virtual reality and conventional 2D on-screen teaching of cerebrovascular anatomy. *Neurosurg. Focus* **2021**, *51*, E18. [CrossRef]
38. Rychen, J.; Saemann, A.; Gehweiler, J.E.; Roethlisberger, M.; Soleman, J.; Hutter, G.; Müller-Gerbl, M.; Mariani, L.; Guzman, R. The sylvian keyhole approach for surgical clipping of middle cerebral artery aneurysms: Technical nuance to the minipterional craniotomy. *Front. Surg.* **2022**, *9*, 1078735. [CrossRef]
39. Alaraj, A.; Luciano, C.J.; Bailey, D.P.; Elsenousi, A.; Roitberg, B.Z.; Bernardo, A.; Banerjee, P.P.; Charbel, F.T. Virtual Reality Cerebral Aneurysm Clipping Simulation with Real-Time Haptic Feedback. *Oper. Neurosurg.* **2015**, *11*, 52–58. [CrossRef]
40. Kockro, R.A.; Killeen, T.; Ayyad, A.; Glaser, M.; Stadie, A.; Reisch, R.; Giese, A.; Schwandt, E. Aneurysm Surgery with Preoperative Three-Dimensional Planning in a Virtual Reality Environment: Technique and Outcome Analysis. *World Neurosurg.* **2016**, *96*, 489–499. [CrossRef]
41. Briganti, F.; Tortora, M.; Loiudice, G.; Tarantino, M.; Guida, A.; Buono, G.; Marseglia, M.; Caranci, F.; Tortora, F. Utility of virtual stenting in treatment of cerebral aneurysms by flow diverter devices. *Radiol. Med.* **2023**, *128*, 480–491. [CrossRef] [PubMed]

MDPI AG
Grosspeteranlage 5
4052 Basel
Switzerland
Tel.: +41 61 683 77 34

Brain Sciences Editorial Office
E-mail: brainsci@mdpi.com
www.mdpi.com/journal/brainsci

www.ingramcontent.com/pod-product-compliance
Lightning Source LLC
Chambersburg PA
CBHW061813210926
51850CB00006B/690
9783725874880